The Practice of Lacanian Psychoanalysis

The Practice of Lacanian Psychoanalysis lays out an Aristotelian framework to account for the different types of knowing and not-knowing operative in the theory and practice of psychoanalysis.

The book proposes a new model for diagnosis, giving preference to fewer over more diagnoses, and seeks to better organize them by distinguishing between structure and surface symptoms. It examines many principles of Lacanian clinical practice, including different types of frames and evidence, the practice of citation and listening, the resistance and desire of the analyst, transference love as a metaphor, the role of negative transference at the end of analysis, and the identification with the *sinthome* as Lacan's last formulation regarding the end of analysis. The text also suggests that there are three forms of love and hate based on the works of Lacan and Winnicott.

Underpinned by extensive practical knowledge of the clinic and case examples for clinicians, analysts, and practicing Lacanian analysts, this book should be of interest to academics, scholars, and clinicians alike.

Raul Moncayo (PhD) is a licensed psychologist in California, supervising analyst and founding member of the Lacanian School of Psychoanalysis, USA. Dr. Moncayo was previously the Training Director of a large psychiatric clinic for many years. He has been an adjunct faculty and visiting professor both locally and abroad and is the author of seven books.

"There are many, too many, introductions to Jacques Lacan; this book is not one of them. For here Raul Moncayo methodically performs a remarkable feat: he does to Lacan what Lacan did to Freud, operating a true 'return to Lacan' from a US-based clinical practice that reinvigorates psychoanalytic theory and praxis. This original book is demanding but worth the effort – a Lacan for the 21st century!"

Patricia Gherovici, PhD, psychoanalyst and author of Transgender Psychoanalysis: A Lacanian Perspective on Sexual Difference

"This original, erudite and thought-provoking book continues Raul Moncayo's unique interrogation of Lacanian theory and practice. Bringing a wide range of references, from philosophy of science to mathematics, anthropology, psychiatry and psychology, he makes Lacan's texts and seminars as fresh and surprising as they ought to be. This is a book not only for students new to the field but also for seasoned Lacanians. It is zesty, highly readable and profound."

Darian Leader, psychoanalyst and author

"Raul Moncayo offers profound and crucial linkages among clinical experience, psychoanalytic theory, and Lacanian practice. Throughout the book, matters pertaining to the clinic are inseparable from theoretical considerations that draw from the long history of Lacan's teaching. Dr. Moncayo speaks to diagnosis and desire, as well as the frame, aims, ends and structural considerations at play in various phases of a Lacanian treatment. The book is a vital resource for anyone who aspires to practice Lacanian psychoanalysis and further the promise of psychoanalysis currently in history."

Annie G. Rogers, PhD

The Practice of Lacanian Psychoanalysis

Theories and Principles

Raul Moncayo

Routledge
Taylor & Francis Group
LONDON AND NEW YORK

First published 2021
by Routledge
2 Park Square, Milton Park, Abingdon, Oxon OX14 4RN

and by Routledge
52 Vanderbilt Avenue, New York, NY 10017

Routledge is an imprint of the Taylor & Francis Group, an informa business

British Library Cataloguing-in-Publication Data
A catalogue record for this book is available from the British Library

Library of Congress Cataloging-in-Publication Data
A catalog record for this book has been requested

ISBN: 978-0-367-56286-1 (hbk)
ISBN: 978-0-367-34237-1 (pbk)
ISBN: 978-1-003-09717-4 (ebk)

Typeset in Baskerville
by Apex CoVantage, LLC

Contents

Preface

This book on the theory and practice of Lacanian psychoanalysis contains new unpublished material, as well as previously published clinical papers and chapters that have been critically updated. Prior work has been updated with Lacan's later work and new case material derived from analytical practice.

The book begins with an extensive introduction that covers the different forms of Aristotelian reason operative within psychoanalytic practice and a distinction in psychoanalysis between practical reason and technical rationality and between formal reason and Sophia or philosophical, dialectical, and historical reason. I link practical reason to the analytic act as a function of the Real and the form of knowing that Lacan calls savoir. "Must it be stated that we have to know [*connaitre*] other bodies of knowledge [*savoirs*] than that of science when it comes to dealing with the epistemological drive?" (Lacan, 2006, p. 737).

Chapter 1 outlines the usual Freudian–Lacanian diagnostic categories described in other Lacanian books but within that context argues how fewer diagnoses are better than more and how many of the DSM-5 diagnoses could be better organized by distinguishing between structure and surface symptoms, an approach that is consistent with Lacan's interest in topology. What is suggested is not oversimplification of diagnosis but in fact a way to make it more sophisticated and closer to what we observe in the clinic and in basic research. Chapter 1 proposes a new diagnostic model that differentiates between structures with and without symptoms and identifies neurosis as the norm for most subjects, as well as a 'normal' form of paranoia.

In addition, metanoia is conceived as a state beyond a neurotic form of paranoia and projection. Metanoia is linked to the analytical pass beyond castration conceptualized in the form of a topological knot of four for neurosis. So-called psychotic personalities are simply human beings that are psychotically structured but without symptoms of varying degrees of acuity. Neurotic projection in paranoid neurosis requires the prior establishment of primary repression, the Name of the Father (NoF), and a normal subjective psyche divided into a tripartite or quaternary structure. I argue that two different models emerged from Freud's study of psychosis and his understanding of projection as a defense formation in neurosis and psychosis.

Kleinian theory attributes splitting to psychoses while it presupposes a unified ego in neurosis. Lacanian theory normalizes division as necessary for the establishment of structure, while unity can also be imaginary and pathological. There are normal and pathological forms of both unity and division instead of unity being normal and division pathological. Projective identification in psychoses presupposes the foreclosure of the NoF that in the object relations school is not only taken for granted and not theorized, but projective identification, as a mode of communication resulting from foreclosure in psychosis, is then used and applied to treat all disorders as if they all represented the same structure or all disorders were psychotically structured. In psychoses, the primary repression that is needed to establish subjective and linguistic structure has failed, and therefore something new needs to be installed in its place. Projective identification, as a psychotic mode of projection, can then be seen as a foreclosing form of defense that, instead of continuing to foreclose the NoF, can be used to symbolize the NoF with the aid of the sinthome.

Chapter 2 updates the graph of desire to include Lacan's later theory, while Chapter 3 develops a psychoanalytic concept of evidence. Chapter 6 examines unavoidable forms of hate in relationship to knowledge, while Chapter 10 shows how fantasies often come in contradictory pairs and are staged in the choice of one or two simultaneous and contradictory partners of the different or same sex. While contrasting objective hate in Winnicott, and 'hateloving' in Lacan, during a talk I gave at the Center for Freudian Analysis and Research (CFAR) in London, the audience asked me about hate in the Real, or what is hate in the Real, or is there hate in the Real? This question led me to further reflections on the part played by the negative transference at the logical end of analyses. We already know that negative transference often leads analysands to end analysis in the sense of interrupting or abandoning their analyses. But can the negative transference, or so-called objective hate, play a constructive role in an analysis that has reached its destination both logically and therapeutically?

At the end of the book, I include two new appendices. The first addresses Lacan's last statements (*Radiophonie*, 1970; and *Television*, 1974) regarding the controversy within and outside psychoanalysis among energy, affect, and jouissance, and their relationships to the signifier and the signifying structure in analytic practice. The second is on the question of how Lacan considers truth, following Heidegger, as *Aléthes* and *Léthes*, truth proper and the true, truth and forgetting, and how this relates to the two 'half-truths' and to the notion that truth can only be half said as fiction.

In my work, I capitalize the Real, not out of a nostalgia for the old-time Absolute but to differentiate the Real from reality. If others write 'real,' readers may think the writer is referring to external social reality without understanding the precise differences between the two terms. Lacan links the Real to the thing and 'no-thing' and to jouissance and the drive. *Das Ding* refers to the thing-in-itself, and for Hegel and Heidegger, the thing-in itself also represents the absolute. However, this is the absolute of science or the correspondence between knowledge and truth. For Lacan, knowledge is Symbolic, while truth and the thing-in-itself are

Real. The Real is not an absolute or metaphysical spirit or knowledge. If anything, the reference to the absolute refers to the question of emptiness, space, and the holes in space. Metaphysical questions nowadays cannot avoid the insights of contemporary physics. The question of curved space and holes in space is very much part of Einstein's relativity theory and is predicted by his formulas. There is no conflict between curved space, the emptiness of space itself, and the predominance of relativity over the absolute.

Heidegger's reference to the thing-in-itself as *das Ding* is a more apt reference for psychoanalysis. The terms 'real' and 'reality' were often indistinguishable in Lacan's early work. The Real is not Freud's social or natural external environment, although at times the extra-conventional Real may be included within the ordinary sense of conventional reality. This may be obvious to some but needs to be clarified nonetheless. In addition, the concept of the Real changed from Lacan's early work to the later years, culminating in two forms of the Real that co-exist. The first Real is inconvenient and represents a threat to the Symbolic order, while the second Real is what organizes or structures the Symbolic and generates accord, consonance, and consistency between the different dimensions of the Borromean knot. What is outside structures the inside.

> Language . . . is only sustained from the function of what I called a hole in the Real . . . the proper efficacity of language . . . is supported by this function of the hole . . . the equivalence of an infinite straight line and a circle.
> (Lacan [1975–1976], Session of 12–9–75, II V)

> Far from the body there is a possibility of what I called last time a resonance, or consonance. And it is at the level of the Real that this consonance can be found. That the Real, with respect to these poles constituted by the body and on the other hand language, that the Real is here what brings about harmony. (*accord-à corps*). (Lacan [1975–1976], Session of 12–9–75 II X)

The book pays equal attention to Lacan's reformulation of Freudian principles, to original contributions to Freud's work, and to Lacan's later work with the Real and jouissance at its center. Although this is a book about Lacanian psychoanalysis, and not about psychoanalysis plain and simple, this is not a partisan book on Lacanian psychoanalysis. For the general culture, psychoanalysis is a dated and equivocal concept (an equivocation in the sense of something false, questionable, or deceptive), while Lacanian psychoanalysis is something new precisely geared to address problems within psychoanalytic theory and practice and to make psychoanalysis relevant for contemporary culture into the twenty-first century. Partisanship refers to political parties, ideology, and Machiavellian manipulations, not to correspondences and contradictions between theory, method, and truth.

In addition, partisan points of view are those of the ones who ignore other forms knowledge and practice available within the field. When the rest of the psychoanalytic world knowingly and deliberately ignores Lacanian psychoanalysis and proceeds to focus on Lacan's interests to the exclusion of Lacan (Freud, topology, mathematics, or linguistics) or uses and plagiarizes his contributions to develop its own alternative points of view, such discursive 'power moves' lead to the general delegitimization and dissembling of psychoanalysis as a discourse and a practice. Partisanship should not be confused with serious commitment or dedication to the study of Lacan. At the same time, Lacanian theory as a topological structure shares with topology the geometry of the rubber sheet. A rubber sheet can be extended, stretched, and bent so long as its structure is preserved. At many turns, the book underscores the similarities and differences between Lacanian psychoanalysis and other twenty-first–century schools of thought and practice.

In addition, I cover topics not considered in prior introductory books to the technique of Lacanian psychoanalysis (Fink, 2007; Quinet, 2018, for example). Among Lacan's contributions to the practice of psychoanalysis, the book features the notions of cure direction, the three payments of the analyst, his new practice of citation and the different levels of interpretation, the scansion of speech, the resistance of the analyst and its relationship to the analyst's desire, the transformations of the metaphor of transference love during the treatment, the part played by the negative transference in the end of analysis despite not having been interpreted during the treatment, and the identification with the sinthome as Lacan's last formulation regarding the end of analysis.

I argue that the latter concept is how Lacanian psychoanalysis can address the question of the difference between the therapeutics of symptom resolution within the treatment, versus the character analysis also required at least of an analyst in formation. The concept of the *sinthome* addresses the post-termination results of the analytic process that manifest in the self-analysis that continues after the end of the personal analysis. Finally, the book examines how Lacan's theory of the lack of rapport between the sexes changes the social and relationship outcomes expected from treatment within the contemporary landscape of human relationships.

Although born in Chile to a North American mother and a Chilean father, and having begun my studies of psychoanalysis in Buenos Aires, Argentina, with a short stop in London, the bulk of my clinical experience has been in the United States. I have worked in hospitals, therapeutic communities, and outpatient clinics and have been in private practice since obtaining a doctorate degree in psychology in California in 1985. In addition, I have been training and supervising psychotherapists and psychoanalysts for most of my professional career.

I mention this to highlight the relationship between evidence and clinical experience. The mental health system and field is set up in the United States in such a way that clinicians are not allowed to use theory (administrators censor it, driven by a passionate native belief that 'ignorance is bliss': the less theory you know, the better it is) and instead rely on the evidence of controlled studies done in universities with students as subjects and conducted by researchers without significant clinical experience. Clinical experience is not a relevant evidential factor in controlled studies, either in the sense that students used as research subjects are not representative of the general clinical population and that researchers themselves have not been exposed to clinical practice with the general clinical population. In addition, the circle of ignorance is completed when clinicians who reject theory apply the evidence from studies without theory.

For psychoanalysis, the evidence for the theory comes from the singularity of the practice itself and not from the logic of the experiment, survey, or questionnaire. In the study of human behavior, data is an artifice of the assumptions and concepts embedded in questions or instructions that match the conscious narratives of subjects that then are converted into numbers through a one-dimensional and linear Likert scale.

In case a psychoanalytic reader in Europe has never heard of it, the Likert scale, in psychological research, makes the assumption that attitudes can be measured, and it is a five-point scale used to allow a research subject to reveal how much they agree or disagree with a particular statement. A Likert scale assumes that the strength of an attitude is linear, on a continuum from strongly agree to strongly disagree, and makes the assumption that attitudes can be measured. The five-point scale and its scores are subjected to statistical analyses that yield a margin of significance. However, as I will show in the book, theory, or better, models developed with the constructs used for research scales, cannot account for the facts of mind discovered and worked with in psychoanalysis. Models developed from questionnaires, and in the absence of Western intellectual history, are not theory. However, models can successfully critique 'aspects' or 'extensions' of the theory but without claiming that models can substitute for theories. Regarding Western intellectual history, the important point is not to devalue other cultural traditions or champion the hegemony of the West, but to highlight the extensive knowledge and experience that the West has contributed to humanity and the history of science.

Before concluding this preface, I want to say something about Lacan's writing style. Lacan's writing, like poetry and the text of the unconscious, is equivocal and ambiguous. This is a positive way to describe it, since for many critics his writing is fragmentary, chaotic, incoherent, and incomplete. His texts oppose conforming to formal and unequivocal articulate systematization that in his theory is linked to ego consciousness, paranoia, and the mastery of knowledge (*connaissance*) associated with the university and master's discourse.

However, the singular form of knowing of the unconscious, or savoir, in the analytical situation, is not without connections to the logos of formal knowledge, as Freud's theory and writing widely attest. In fact, the two forms of knowledge coincide at the moment where subjects yield control and direction to the lightening of wit and the signifier (I think where I am not). To avoid confusion and misunderstanding, equivocal terms that have more than one meaning can be written in clear terms without losing sight of the import of equivocality in the analysis of the unconscious. An example of this would be the concept of jouissance, since people may forget that jouissance is a concept with antithetical meaning that Lacan often uses to represent suffering rather than satisfaction. Not knowing which way he is using the concept in any particular sentence or setting, or what type of jouissance he is addressing, can be confusing and make the text difficult to follow.

In addition, the relationship between the two forms of knowledge in Lacan (savoir and *connaissance*) can be elucidated by understanding them according to the different forms of Aristotelian reason at work within science and psychoanalytic theory. In the Introduction, I offer a detailed analysis of how the five forms of reason function within psychoanalytic theory and practice. I propose that practice and technique, often used interchangeably, actually represent two different concepts following from different forms of reason. Practice in psychoanalysis is the practice of the Real as an analytic act and not of technical rationality. Technique only involves information, while practice involves human subjectivity and psychical and mental experience.

Psychoanalysis shares with science the use of technical reason (analytic technique). At the same time, I argue that analytic practice and practical reason are more than technique and professional ethics. In addition, psychoanalysis uses formal reason (the theory explains facts observed in clinical practice and informs effective interventions) and dialectical or historical reason. The latter is necessary to understand contradictory and antithetical elements within the psyche.

The first forms of reason are unequivocal (the experimental hypothesis is either true or false), while Sophia or dialectical reason, as the word indicates, is equivocal and contradictory. In addition to the focus on the ambiguity, technique, and discipline of the signifier, psychoanalysis also requires analytic acts of practical reason without knowledge. Analytic acts are signifying points without knowledge that invoke enigmatic forms of unknown knowing (*l'insu qui sait*) and jouissance in the analysand. Savoir is also related to the Greek Nous and to an unconscious form of intuition.

I dedicate this book to my students and colleagues who over the years have worked with me, studied Lacanian psychoanalysis, and applied it to clinical practice. I want to thank Magdalena Romanowicz for her collaboration on papers previously published in journals and that I have reworked, updated, and expanded for this book. These include the chapters on diagnosis and the graph of desire. A shorter version of the first appeared in the *European Journal of Psychoanalysis*, while the second appeared in the *Irish Journal of Lacanian Psychoanalysis*.

Finally, this book will cover psychoanalytic literature both within and outside Lacanian psychoanalysis and across different schools of Lacanian psychoanalysis. Analytical discourse precisely is a discourse to get past Machiavellian politics in the discourse of the master that also, unfortunately, are not easily recognizable on the surface of topological structure. Political discourse, nowadays, no longer means the same thing, because left and right have been territorialized and deterritorialized (to use Deleuze and Guattari's [1972] terms), debased and distorted by the master's discourse. Present-day Russia would be an example of both. When any means are used for political ends, the ends end up reproducing the means. Power and violence, and Machiavellian manipulations, result in absolute forms of conservative and revolutionary corruption and the inevitable decline of civil society.

In a psychoanalytic organization, or in analytical discourse, symbolic lack (0), rather than the inexistant imaginary phallus of the master/leader, is the balancing point of symbolic exchange, or what Freud called the metaphoric foundational rock of symbolic castration and free association that every analyst has to pass through and beyond to be installed in the analytic position. Sometimes leaders and groups interpret "the rock" literally as an imaginary castration and subordination to an imaginary leader (primal father) that may be idealized or defied. This has been a problem associated with the master's discourse that has affected psychoanalytic organizations (Lacan, 1980).

References

Deleuze, G. and Guattari, F. (1972). *Anti-Oedipus*. Translated by R. Hurley, M. Seem and H. Lane. London and New York: Continuum, 2004. Volume 1 of Capitalism and Schizophrenia. 2 vols. 1972–1980.

Fink, B. (2007). *Fundamentals of Psychoanalytic Technique: A Lacanian Approach for Practitioners*. New York: Norton.

Lacan, J. (1966). Science and Truth. In: *Ecrits*. Translated by B. Fink. New York and London: Norton, 2006.

Lacan, J. (1970). *Radiophonie*. Scilicet 2/3. Translated by J. W. Stone. Paris: Seuil, pp. 55–99.

Lacan, J. (1974). *Television*. Edited by J. Copjec. New York: London, 1990.

Lacan, J. (1975–1976). *Joyce and the Sinthome: Seminar XXIII*. Translated by C. Gallagher. Unpublished. www.lacaninireland.com. Accessed December 4, 2019.

Lacan, J. (1980). *The Seminar of Jacques Lacan*. Book XXVII: Dissolution (1980). www.freud2lacan.com/docs/DISSOLUTION-July-12-1980-3col.pdf. Accessed November 26, 2019.

Quinet, A. (2018). *Lacan's Clinical Technique: Lack(a)nian Analysis*. London: Routledge.

Introduction

Although this is a book about the clinical practice of psychoanalysis, this introduction will outline the general epistemological background that underpins the theory and practice of Lacanian psychoanalysis. Psychoanalytic practice is not the easier form of applied psychoanalysis that technicians or specialists can practice in disregard of theoretical knowledge, as many in the mental health field are inclined to do. Of course, that theoretical knowledge without the experience of a personal analysis, or of being in the analytical function, does not by itself encompass the practice side of psychoanalysis.

Theoretical psychoanalysis cannot be entirely separated from the psychoanalysis associated with the requirements of analytical practice. On the other hand, academics are often more adept with the theory than practicing psychoanalysts, who are often not interested in a theory that they regard as academic. Although the separation between theory and practice may insulate the private practice of psychoanalysis, it also leads to the impoverishment of the theory and the intellectual climate within which psychoanalytic practice takes place. Eventually this state of affairs leads to the impoverishment of the technique itself.

Practical reason and techne represent two different forms of rationality. As mentioned elsewhere in my work, both practical reason and techne are two of the five forms of reason outlined by Aristotle. In the past, I have defined the types of reason within the context of my present psychoanalytic work but did not establish a closer correspondence with Aristotle's own definitions. I will use this Introduction to succinctly outline their classical and contemporary definitions with respect to science and the practice of psychoanalysis. In this book, the purpose of defining the five forms of reason in Aristotle is to differentiate practice from technique.

The forms of reason

It is interesting to note that natural science in the West uses mostly two (formal analytical reason and *technê*) of the five different types of rationality outlined by Aristotle. The humanities use the other three without much controversy except for two important facts: the social sciences are divided between those departments that restrict their investigations to the same two forms of reason used by natural science and those that use the two reasons used by science, plus the three reasons used by the humanities and the arts.

The second important fact is that the reduction of science and of social science to only two forms of reason *ipso facto* establishes a non-circular hierarchy between the different forms of reason. The two forms of reason that are linked to business, industry, and the exploitation of natural resources are privileged, prioritized, and funded over and above the funding or support that is available for the other three forms of reason that also make significant contributions to society. Social science containing the five reasons, supports the culture that must balance the biological semiotic order of nature in human beings. Industry funds scientific research because it is profitable not because it leads to the common good.

Thus, I argue that there exists a division within Western reason itself. The division is between Continental Europe or dialectical, critical, and historical reason, or rationalism, and the Anglo-American tradition that sticks to formal analytical reason and binary logic, or statistical empiricism in the social sciences. When I argue that techne in the form of statistical empiricism should not replace rational explanation (according to various levels of logic) in the social sciences, this does not mean that statistics should not be used to provide society the meaningful frequencies of various illnesses, rates of suicide, drug use, economic indicators, and so on. Even in natural science, the argument has also been made that we never know any data before interpreting it through theories (Deutsch, 2011, p. 30). All observations are theory laden. Continental Europe uses formal reason for the natural sciences and the social sciences but does not exclude dialectical and historical reason from the social sciences.

Aristotle thought of the types of reason as the 'virtues of thought,' of which there were five. The five are: *technê*, *epistémé*, *phronesis*, *Sophía*, and *Nous*. *Technê* represents applied science, instrumental reason, craft, art, and production. Although psychoanalysis includes technique and some consider it an art form, psychoanalysis is more than what can be described by this form of rationality. *Epistémé* is scientific, analytical, and theoretical; constitutes universal objective knowledge of causes, correlations, and probabilities; and in general represents the framework or the cognitive structure behind the definition of valid knowledge (whether analytical or continental, realism or transcendentalism). Analytical philosophy, or Anglo-American quantitative empiricism, is the philosophy that reduces philosophy to *Epistémé* or the epistemological foundation of natural science. The conflict with European Continental thought is that analytical philosophy wants to reduce the other forms of valid and legitimate knowledge to the *Epistémé* of natural science.

Scientific knowledge now includes experimentation and demonstration, which is something that was not the case at the time of Aristotle. *Phronêsis* is practical reason, or the principles of action that are geared towards ethical action in politics and society. Action is the result of deliberation and choice. However, for Aristotle, practical reason not only refers to ethical action in the sense of morality, but, like techne, practice is organized around the object of need and desire. Ordinarily, and in religion, the ethics of morality seek to restrain and bind the objects of desire under principles of continence and duty. However, the ethics of morality and practical reason in Aristotle (*Ethics*, p. xiv) are different. There are pleasures and convenient forms of jouissance that are suitable to our nature as rational beings. Temperance as a virtue allows the person to enjoy rational pleasures in the appropriate measure and with due reflection on the relationship between action and consequence. The temperate character takes responsibility for their desire and jouissance. The continent person struggles with self-control, while the incontinent lacks self-control without being vicious.

Finally, I link practical reason in psychoanalysis, or the psychoanalytic act, to Nous (defined subsequently) because practical reason is involved in the relationship between professional practices and the question of choice, free will, or indeterminism versus determinism. Truth as knowing opens to action or is unconcealed in a Real analytical act. For Aristotle, conclusions derived from practical reason must result in a Real act (the Lacanian scansion of speech and session). Free will refers to what we make out of what we are made of. Free will does not deny the existence of a determinate structure, especially in matter, but does refer to the fact that the elements of a structure can be combined in different ways with different results.

The unknown and unknowable (respectively indeterminate and undetermined) require both practical reason and Nous because the consequences of an act are as of yet unknown, and although we could predict such consequences based on social norms, consequences are also mediated by Nous as an undefined, undetermined, and unmixed aspect of the intellect that is immediate and surprising and not solely based on convention or formal logic. Aristotle likens Nous to the capacity of a blank tablet for all knowledge (the magical writing pad or pure awareness). For psychoanalysis, this is not a tablet that gets written with knowledge (Locke's [1632–1704] tabula rasa or white paper), because the separate active Nous must be empty, "All-alone," and unmixed. For this reason, I link Nous to Freud's Pcpt. cs. system as a form of awareness that remains unmarked despite all the marks that pass through it and are registered in the different filing systems and codes of Mind. Nous passes beyond representation and the signifier and therefore is linked to the Real of jouissance and to the first principles of science (*tà mathémata*). Finally, Nous and Psyche are the two Greek terms for Mind (not just reason) most commonly used in psychology and psychoanalysis. In psychoanalysis, Mind represents the symbolic reaches of the death drive associated with the tendency towards emptiness or the "no-thing."

Lacan says that choice is a forced choice, in the same way that a subject may choose to speak about a topic but, in the process of speech articulation, at some critical signifying point, a different logic takes over the coherence and organization of speech. At that point, it is the Other that has precedence over what the ego may think or not think, like or not like, at any particular moment. If a subject selects a particular social-symbolic environment that suits a particular advantage or capacity of the subject, let us say psychoanalysis as a discipline, for example, this also means that psychoanalysis and its historical characters also choose them.

The phenomena that we study contribute to an awareness that remains independent and undefined by the content of what is learned or who is doing the learning. Aristotle referred to it as separate and as being without attributes and unmixed. As such, it constitutes a link between the known and the unknown and even between the known and that which can never be completely known or defined. In many ways, it corresponds to what Freud called the free-floating awareness of the analyst without a specific subject or object.

This definition of Nous avoids the paradox of referring to an unconscious awareness, although Lacan does speak of unknown or enigmatic knowing or "*l'insu qui sait.*" When an analyst is in the presence of his/her analysand's speech, the quality of Nous will also be there with the analyst. And although the analyst may not be thinking of the theory, the first principles that matter (*tà mathémata*) will also be there for his/her disposition and use.

Sophia is speculative synthetic reason, or the highest form of theoretical, dialectical, or critical knowledge. Although Aristotle developed the principle of the excluded third, or the principle of non-contradiction, on which natural science depends, Aristotle also conceived of dialectical reason (principle of contradiction) as holding *Epistémé* and *Phronêsis* accountable to critical reason, or to the dialectical principle according to which things being what they are can also be something else or different. Episteme claims that things are one way, but critical reason points to all the evidence that points in a different yet unmanifest direction. "What was needed for the sustained, rapid growth of knowledge was a tradition of criticism. Before the enlightenment, that was a very rare sort of tradition: usually the whole point of a tradition was to keep things the same" (Deutsch, 2011, p. 13).

It is important to appraise the function of critical reason because it could be misunderstood for ordinary judgment or criticism. In some ways, judgment is perverted by the super ego's involvement in a personal criticism of the Other due to unresolved transference (rock of castration) and work transference (transmission of savoir from an individual to a group and from a group to a school) that often happens under conditions of "objective" hate (in institutions), although this is nothing to be proud of. To be proud of conflict, per conflict's sake, is to cast a curse on the work of Freud and Lacan. Unfortunately, institutions over time become breeding grounds for rivalry, ambition, disputation, and attacks on the leadership.

In this work, I may "critique" concepts for this or that reason, although the critique is not personal to the authors. I am addressing ideas and concepts that define the practice of psychoanalysis, and yes, along the way, I address many of the differences that many authors have had with both Freud and Lacan. However, practical reason has logical arguments and is not simply loud indignation or repudiation of a concept (the ordinary conception of an "argument").

By the same token, other forms of reason help critical reason grant other subjects the same freedom to disagree and critique critical reason despite conditions of objective hate. It was Socrates' custom, for example, to be open to criticism and persuasion while remaining free of objective hate despite being condemned to death by the Athenian state. Socrates did not aspire to attain a state of being perfectly secure in his beliefs. In this sense, Socrates stands as the glaring and transcendental exception to many things that I will say in this book about objective hate in relationship to knowledge, as seen in the words of Winnicott and Lacan. Finally, objective hate is the emotional element linked to rational arguments that will be further explored and defined in Chapter 6.

Part of the task of analytical practice is to get beyond imaginary identifications and the social imaginary. Post-analytical truth-effects include having ideals but without idealizations, having theories without complete theories that explain everything. Moreover, beliefs are held differently, more clearly, and without clinging to them. A subject can disagree with himself or herself and therefore remains open to changes in the theory and personal experience.

Finally, psychoanalytic and Lacanian institutions are not free of all the Machiavellian problems associated with politics, leadership, group psychology, and so on. Nonetheless, it is important to remember that a psychoanalytic organization is what the name indicates and what one expects from a group of psychoanalysts. A psychoanalytic organization is organized by the discourse of the analyst, not the master's discourse, or at least where the former has ascendancy over the latter.

As an analyst, one is prepared to receive forms of critique laden with hateful affect linked to the super ego, identifications, or prejudices of the particular person, although this is universal. So-called objective hate linked to knowledge is handled with the aid of the post-analytical effects of the sinthome and the self-analysis that continues after the personal analysis has reached its logical conclusion.

As a matter of fact, psychoanalysis is one of the tools available to work with critical reason and divest it of the elements of the super ego that could lead critical reason astray and misjudge key elements of the individual and of society. Criticism and ethics under the influence of the super ego is driven by imaginary aggressivity rather than by the principles of reason associated with the signifier. When history is affected by blind indignation and rage in the use of critical reason, then history produces contradictory undesired results and repetitions and identifications with the opposite. The wrath and blast of the One, or of the sword of wisdom, is a misnomer and a misunderstanding. The objects of the sword are false beliefs, ideas, and actions that need to be critically examined rather than the destruction of actual people or the goods and services that they provide. Just like equanimity in the use of reason is not indifference, a momentary ferocity that does not turn into hatred or ill-will is not opposed to kindness in its true sense.

It is interesting to observe that in cultures that were not influenced by Greek rationality (Socrates' leading example), critique manifests as angry criticism, humiliation, and shame (Asian cultures, for example, etc.). These cultures raise more objections to trying to understand nature and mind rationally than having an outburst of angry criticism. In that case, the culture simply expects that the criticized subject simply "eat the blame." "From the Greeks onward, we in the West place a high value on persuasion through rational discourse, while there was a lack of interest in China in persuasive discourse. Rather, the situation is prepared so that the listener is predisposed to follow one's advice" (Saporta, 2014, p. 78).

However, this critique could also apply to religion in general. For example, Martin Luther enjoyed preaching in an enraged state of mind, and this characteristic eventually led to virulent and violent anti-Semitism when he was naively surprised that Jews were not about to convert in droves to protestant Christianity. In the end, Luther was hatefully driven to condemn Jews to hell, just as the corrupt Catholic Church had done before him. Critical reason is a more evolved form of super ego based on rational principles rather than in the emotive argumentation where the errors/lack in the Other are hatefully blamed on the other.

In this regard, it is important to note that the Frankfurt school was well aware of the contradictions of modern enlightened reason and how formal reason and techne could pass into destructive use and abuse of others. In this respect, they did not hold back on their critique of how Marxism was used for similar purposes and, therefore, they were not favorably regarded within Marxist circles (Jeffries, 2017). The Frankfurt school arrived at their orientation through the study of Hegel, Freud, and psychoanalysis and not only Marxism and Western philosophy. In contrast to this, many Marxists, and Marxist institutions, were anti-Freudian and regarded the members of the Frankfurt school as traitors to the revolution.

This contradiction has been overcome by Hegelians and Marxists who have incorporated psychoanalytic ideas and the Frankfurt school into their analysis of contemporary culture (Zizek, for example). The developments in France associated with post-structuralism and postmodernism I address mostly through the lens of Lacanian psychoanalysis, although these movements cover a wider social field than Lacanian psychoanalysis. Lacan shared with Foucault, and his Parisian intellectual milieu, the analysis of various types of social discourses.

Hegel and the Frankfurt school, as well as Lacanian psychoanalysis, are important for human knowledge, because in their work, dialectical reason or the principle of contradiction and subjective truth (Sophia) achieves parity with formal reason or the principle of non-contradiction. This is not something out of fashion 50 years later, just like Freud is not irrelevant for our times. Moreover, since statistically based empiricism in the social sciences has not only not passed away but has become more influential in the social sciences and the governmental master's discourse, restricting knowledge to only two forms of reason, it is important to continue supporting classical and contemporary alternatives that function as a counter-balancing check on episteme and technology. This was precisely the task of critical reason envisioned by Aristotle. Europe understands this, but the United States, with its anti-intellectualism, repudiates Sophia that is often associated with a feminine characteristic: the love of Sophia, or the love of knowledge for knowledge's sake.

Beyond the eradication of old-world aristocracy, ordinary Americans also refuse to defer to those possessing, as Tocqueville put it, superior talent and intelligence and these natural elites could not enjoy much share in political power as a result. Ordinary Americans enjoyed too much power and claimed too great a voice in the public sphere to defer to intellectual superiors. This culture promoted a relatively pronounced equality, Tocqueville argued, but the same mores and opinions that ensured such equality also promoted mediocrity. Those who possessed true virtue and talent were left with limited choices.

Tocqueville said that those with the most education and intelligence were left with two choices. They could join limited intellectual circles to explore the weighty and complex problems facing society, or they could use their superior talents to amass vast fortunes in the private sector. Tocqueville blamed the omnipotence of majority rule as a chief factor in stifling thinking: "The majority has enclosed thought within a formidable fence. A writer is free inside that area, but woe to the man who goes beyond it, not that he stands in fear of an inquisition, but he must face all kinds of unpleasantness in everyday persecution" (Kaplan, 2005).

In the United States, the principle of equality led the middle class, and uneducated European Americans, rich and poor alike, to a passion or culture of ignorance that rejects abstract intellectuals and cultural elites. The individual segregation required by intellectual work is confused with individualism, and a form of reason independent from dominant ideologies. Individual talent should simply be used to make money, or to develop the formal and technical aspects of reason that translate into economic profits in the marketplace. Contemporary figures, such as Bill Gates, Steve Jobs, and Warren Buffet, immediately come to mind.

Since critical reason is also associated with love, and the passion for knowledge, or knowledge as a passion for its own sake, an anti-intellectual environment, cannot contribute to theoretical knowledge, or to theoretical knowledge in the social sciences, leaving fundamental aspects of mental and social life in the dark. Formal and technical reason are often learned in standardized environments that are experienced as a form of duty or obligation at all costs. The rejection of Sophia, as a critical type of human reason, leaves knowledge without a heart, and without the passion for knowledge required for the hard work of theory construction. A sense of obligation is required for technological, specialized, and applied reason, but theory proceeds from Sophia and the love of knowledge for its own sake.

The dispassion of formal and technical reason, and even the hate for theory and critical reason, does not allow, for example, a corporate or government technocrat to benefit from its use. This leads to a society for which the identity of humans and machines becomes self-evident as a form of natural discovery. The concept of 'objective hate' refers to either when the love of Sophia leads to hate of formal or technological knowledge, or when the dispassion linked to formal reason turns into a cold ignorance or indifference towards the ethical, philosophical, or economic implications of science. Ordinary people and natural scientists can objectively hate critical and theoretical social science, in the same way that social scientists could be critical and objectively hate the logic of the natural sciences when restrictively applied to the social sciences. In Chapter 6, I will further explore the relationship among love, hate, transference, and knowledge, and distinguish the different types of knowledge, and love and hate, across the registers of RSI that compose the Borromean knot.

Finally, Nous is intuitive knowledge or an unconscious and immediate apprehension and insight into the nature and pattern of things. Sophia knows discursively, moving from premises to conclusions. Nous instead knows non-discursively. Nous intuitively knows the unproven assumptions that in science function as starting points for the deductive reasoning that scientific knowledge requires (Aristotle, p. xvi). In science, examples of Nous are Mendeleev's dreaming the exact image of the entire periodic table, Einstein's thought experiment of riding on a beam of light, and so on.

In Lacan, we find a twofold approach to the question of intuition as reflected in two passages from Seminar X. First (Lacan [1962–1963], pp. 57 and 64), Lacan argues that there is no transparency associated with the intuition of consciousness, since consciousness is determined by linguistic, psychical, and mathematical structure. What consciousness perceives is not how it perceives. The intuitions of consciousness are of no help in knowing how we perceive. To understand how perception takes place, it is necessary to *a*pperceive the first principles governing the organization of rationality and information. However, first principles emanate not from the saturated, habitual, and learned consciousness or from established knowledge, but from an unconscious intuition (the signifier plays and wins before the subject can realize it) or from what Lacan calls unknown knowing.

Although there are five discrete forms of reason in Aristotle, these five categories have significant overlap and are not always clearly differentiated in his work. Ethical virtue is related to rationality in general, but it is also contained within one of the five forms of reason: practical reason. Practical reason imbues rationality with virtue and an equanimous enigmatic affect. Aristotle discusses *epistêmê* and *technê* in Book VI of the *Nicomachean Ethics*. The distinction between the two points to the classic division between the theoretical and the practical. However, although he does not always observe the difference between practical reason and techne, he also differentiates between them.

Practical reason is ethical more than technical, and *technê* refers to a subjective art form and craft and not only technology. For Aristotle, art was not science or episteme but was definitely rational. The romantics, of course, at the turn of the nineteenth century, would not agree with this definition. Will, purpose, emotional intensity, value, and beauty were more important than scientific rationality. From this perspective, some psychoanalysts (Fromm [1980] and Quinet [2018], for example) have defined psychoanalysis as a qualitative art form rather than a science or a technical method (qualitative or quantitative).

> In session four Lacan turns to examining the question of *savoir-faire* or 'know-how' from the point of view of the artist, the potter, and the artifice or artifact. Know-how is not techne but rather practice as a Real act or as the Real and Nous manifesting in activity. Our thinking imputes to God the artifice or artifact that we call the Universe. The Universe means that there is Oneness or something of the One (*Yadlun* or *Il y a de l'Un*). This One is the real Other within the Other so that although there is no Other **of** the Other there is an improbable and impossible real Other **in** the Other. "The real Other of the Other, namely impossible" (Lacan [1975–1976], IV 4). This real One is not only a jouissance we know nothing of and that manifests as *lalangue* within language but is also a doing that escapes us.
>
> (Moncayo, 2018, p. 55)

Lacan statement from Seminar XIX, "*Il y a de l'Un*", has a reference in Heidegger's (1947/2008, p. 238) 'Letter on Humanism' where he says "*il y a l'Etre*". Heidegger attributes the saying to Parmenides' *esti gar einai*, "for there is Being". For Lacan the One is not the same as Being, because the One includes non-being. For this reason, Lacan changes "*Il y a l'Etre*" to "*Il y a de l'Un.*" Heidegger stresses that 'there is' translates into "it gives". The Universe is an artifact or a One+1.

The doing that escapes us refers to the practice of scanning or cutting the session and the signifier. With Lacan, we have a definition of Nous (unconscious intuition) and the Real that includes the Chinese *Wu-Wei* in an act and not only in an experience, in lalangue, or mathemes. When acts have the surprising quality of the undetermined Real (*Tyche*), and not only of the conditioned social narrative or reality, although the act may be senseless or contrary to ego expectations (the ordinary Newtonian time that all clocks measure in the case of the analytical practice of the scansion of the session), there is nothing that does not get accomplished.

I compared this to the doing or activity of biological evolution. This human being that we all contribute to is completely beyond our doing. Species being is the universal activity within and beyond the doing of any particular subject. With respect to a Symbolic environment and the order of language, the larger universal activity refers to the unconscious activity that continues processing while we sleep and that far exceeds the enjoyment that we can have of it. "The fact that the signifying chain continues to unfold and continues to be organized in the Other, whether you know it or not, this is essentially Freud's discovery" (Lacan [1957–1958], p. 132). The small piece of Real enjoyment (S_1) that a subject can drain from the larger unconscious doing that escapes us is what we call an act of wit (*l'esprit*).

> What is know-how? Let us say it is art, artifice, what gives to art, a remarkable value. The real Other of the Other, namely impossible, is the idea that we have of artifice, in so far it is a doing, *faire*, do not write it *fer*, a doing that escapes us. All of this implies a notion of the Real, of course. The Real has no meaning.
>
> (Lacan [1975–1976], IV 4)

Nous and the practice of the signifier, rather than technique, are what give an action the quality of an artistic activity. Craft, the artifice or art form, and practice, are more than the techne associated with technology as a means for practical survival or the accumulation of wealth. On the other hand, the romantic perspective can be critiqued as a form of irrational and dramatic sentimentality that is, nonetheless, related to reason via irrational numbers that, although infinitesimal, for example, can still be used within the PM (Principia Mathematica) mathematical system. In fact, the so-called irrational or emotional within the psyche, Lacan conceives according to a ratio of Phi and phi, both of which are irrational numbers. But here mathematics, as episteme, is functioning in unison with craft as artifact, with Nous as the undetermined aspect of activity, and with beauty associated with the aesthetic experience.

Finally, mathematics is beyond language, at the same time that there is an uncountable dimension of jouissance in the Real that also defies any form of calculation. If anything, the uncountable, or what cannot be reached through calculation, can be reached through meditation (Heidegger, 1966). This is the same as non-thinking as a form of jouissance or thought as a singularity.

Techne, in the case of arts and crafts, shares material production with technology but is an end in itself rather than a form of instrumental rationality or a means to the accumulation of wealth and capital. Heidegger (1955) has distinguished the *technê* associated with art from the *technê* linked to technology by defining *technê* as a form of revelation and 'bringing forth' rather than manufacturing. Rather than calculation, the psychoanalytic method represents a demand to bring forth speech and the repressed psyche through free association and the trimming and scansion of speech as done by the dream work.

These distinctions among the different forms of reason have remained remarkably the same throughout the history of Western philosophy, except that under the influence of Marxism and dialectical critical reason, the Frankfurt school (Adorno and Horkheimer, 1944), but also Heidegger (1955), developed a critique of technological and instrumental rationality under capitalism (*technê*) that utilizes science and technology (computer science nowadays, for example) for purposes of domination and exploitation of nature and fellow human beings. Here dialectical reason joins forces with practical ethical rationality against non-artistic economic production or the *technê* linked to the extraction and production of the object of need and desire.

Therefore, more than a question of personal criticism what is at stake in critical reason, and perhaps so-called objective hate, is a case of reason against itself, or a battle between the different forms of reason as part and parcel of the process of civilization and the discovery and invention of what it means to be human. Practical reason and *technê* battle themselves (art and beauty against the destructive use of *technê*, and practical reason against instrumental reason). Finally, dialectical reason and Nous battle the formal reason that supports unethical or controversial technological developments or that reduce a human being to an animal or a machine (computers or robots).

Conversely, formal reason, embedded within quantitative empiricism, battles a rationalism that formal reason considers philosophical, or worse, religious forms of 'unscientific,' magical, ideological, folk, or dogmatic thinking. At other times, critical reason embedded within dialectical materialism uses the totalizing and dogmatic aspects of critical reason to deny validity to Nous as the source of unknown knowing. Nous is not a metaphysical principle: "All this abstract nonsense is the correct theory of reality." Quantum theory in physics appeared to be in conflict with objective reality from the point of view of Newtonian classical physics but in fact required Nous or an unconscious intuition to apperceive the constituents of matter that cannot be perceived or understood otherwise.

The split and conflict between Sophia, Nous, and Formal reason involves the basic staples and alphabet of investigation in both the natural and social sciences: namely the relationship among logic, numbers, concepts, and language and their reference to objects and things in the real world. Even though most people would associate math with logic and logic with language and/or symbolic representation, in fact, math is not always logical, math and logic are not always arithmetical, and metaphor cannot be reduced to logic and mathematics.

From this point of view, the equivalence that Lacan establishes early on between displacement, metonymy, combination, and succession in numbers and signifiers is replaced in Lacan's later work by the senselessness of scientific symbols in mathematics and how such emptiness of meaning is contrasted to the imaginary displacements of meaning in language unto something else or Other (S_1–S_2). Some scholars may argue that these two points of view do not exist before and after in time but rather co-existed simultaneously in Lacan's text, but this is beyond the focus of this book. The unconscious signifying chain functions more like a string or knot of mathematical symbols than a conscious narrative chain of meaning in language. Psychoanalysis does not use imaginary storytelling as theoretical building blocks or to successfully treat various disorders. The narrative or storytelling level is a necessary level of discourse but not the most fundamental speech for psychoanalysis.

Given the conflict between the different forms of reason, it is no wonder that academics within and across disciplines, as well as people in general, would find it difficult to communicate with each other. Finally, not only are there different forms of reason that speak past each other, but there are several logical levels within logic itself (either this or that, both this and that, neither this nor that), so that people ordinarily miscommunicate because they are speaking on different logical levels: they are both right in their different respective levels, and both wrong because they think they are speaking on the same logical level, pointing thereby to Real impasse and impossibility.

This is what happens when we reduce one level to another level and, for example, commit the error of analogical thinking. Because this level looks symmetrical, for example, it does not mean that the other level cannot be asymmetrical or different in some fundamental way. This applies to the difference between instinct and drive, as well as to the difference between biological sex, social gender, and psychical or symbolic sexual difference.

In physics, just because sound waves needed a medium (air) to propagate, this did not mean that light had to use a medium (the ether) to propagate. We make the same mistake when we assume that culture is a natural bedfellow with biological evolutionary systems and therefore can be reduced to the latter. Natural environment without symbols and signifiers is not the same as cultural environment, and, therefore, the latter needs different logical levels and disciplines to be understood.

When within culture, we say that the rays of the sun are like the fingers of dawn (Homer's "rosy fingered Dawn" in the Iliad) and refer to the sun with a metaphor, although a beautiful literary expression, we don't go ahead and theorize that the rays of the sun are co-bedfellows with human fingers. Metaphor uses change and movement within language to capture something Real within both fingers and the rays of the sun as visual elements of reality. But metaphor cannot be transformed into theory without risking delusion or false belief. For the theory not to be delusional, it would have to look for structural similarities between figures of language, forms of the hand, and the propagation of light, which perhaps, after all, might not be too far-fetched. Writing and the propagation of light always return to the same Real place outside signification, which does not cease from not being written.

When the question of technique is examined in the 'light' of psychoanalytic practice, technique refers to either a subjective art form, an ethical act of practical reason, or a purely technical form of rationality associated with economic productivity and involving an exchange of technical information (skills and manuals). However, the latter would be truer of psychiatry and cognitive behaviorism than psychoanalysis.

Practice in psychoanalysis is the practice or ethics of the Real and not necessarily of technical rationality. Technique only involves information (whether linguistic or mathematical data), while practice involves human subjectivity, subjective truths of desire, psychical and mental experience, and a free-floating attention rooted in the subject's own Being. Capitalized Being refers to how Freud spoke of the core of being in *The Interpretation of Dreams* (1900). There Freud construes wishing as the core of being, and Lacan adds that in the core of being, speaking beings are constituted as a lack-of-being.

Desire as lack of being, instead of wishing, seeks the lack or the emptiness of being. Wishing wants to close the gap of desire with the *objet a*, while desire leaves the lack open without an object. The subject searches for Being in the Other or in the *objet a* as a semblance of Being. However, neither the Other nor the *objet a* can make Being present for the subject. Concealment or undiscloseness, as a mystery, preserves what is most proper to truth in the Real. The half-truth that remains in the Real is the mystery of essential emptiness and jouissance. The other-half side of truth is fictional (in the sense of Bentham) existence according to the signifier as a semblance of being.

The essence of Being is ek-sistence, and so we become present to Being not through actual existence but through the 'ek-statis' or jouissance that was a prior sistence ('ex-sistence'). The object of wish fulfillment tries to fill the lack left by the structural loss of the oedipal object, which is something impossible to do. What is possible is to leave the lack open or seek for the lack instead. Such lack or emptiness, then, becomes an index of jouissance. Since there is no Being in the Other, or Being appears as empty or inexistent, Being has been defined, following Plotinus (p. 361), Hegel, Heidegger, and Lacan, as the One's own non-being, or the Being of non-being (ontology and anti-ontology, philosophy and anti-philosophy at once).

Being is not simply existence, because the essence of Being is emptiness as 'ek-stasis' or a benevolent jouissance (not a drug-induced euphoria). What Heidegger (1947) calls 'ek-sistence' (and that Lacan spells "ex-sistence") means standing on emptiness as the truth of Being. The being of non-being is the 'ek-static' aspect of 'ek-sistence' and the location of indeterminate truth among beings. It is the emptiness of Being that makes us present to our existence. The One's own non-being also refers to both the Lacanian definition of desire that remains in between metonymic objects of demand (without being confused or 'thrown' into these objects) and the definition of jouissance situated in between signifiers (jouissance as ek-stasis is both outside and inside the heart of the signifier). Since the being of desire is lack, or its own non-being, desire manifests through the different formations of the drive and its objects.

Psychoanalysis involves subjectivity in both analyst and analysand and an experience of illumination precipitated by the analytic act or a doing (the Chinese *Wu wei*: "The Way does nothing, and yet nothing remains unaccomplished") invocative of what Lacan calls the Real unconscious. The psychoanalytic act as an intervention enacts a signifying point but does not necessarily represent a form of thinking. "One is never so solid in one's being as when one does not think" (Lacan, 1967–1968, Seminar XV, Session of 10.1.68 V 5). This would be another definition of non-thinking at work in the psychoanalytic act.

The analyst has to tolerate being nothing (the One's own non-being). "I do not think, describes the method of free association as a task that implies the destitution of the subject" (Lacan idem, Session of 24 1 68. VII 6). I argue that not-knowing or non-knowing, as necessary moments in the production of subjective truth and the production of truth-effects at the level of the Real, represents *savoir* or unconscious knowing and how Nous needs to be defined within the context of psychoanalysis. In the practice of analysis, not-knowing refers to the suspension of certainty and unequivocal universal knowledge in favor of uncertainty, ambiguity, and equivocality in the use of the signifier.

There is a difference between teaching a technique and a practice of knowing how to learn that differs from the domain of education where a subject learns from a teacher or master through a process of imitation and identification. There is knowing and truth not contained in learning. In this sense, a learning theory of information acquisition is not essential to the analytic task. Instead of the acquiring of information and problem-solving skills, analysis is the invention and discovery of unconscious knowing, the subject of which is the product of the articulation of the structure.

Unconscious unknown knowing produces a new subject grounded both in the signifier and the Real of bodily jouissance that lies beyond it. The unconscious makes the subject rather than the ego being a man-made self (the self-made man). Transmission in psychoanalysis transmits something of Mind that was neither there before the invention of psychoanalysis nor is something completely new. Invention and innovation require both a tradition and an epistemological break with tradition. Unknown knowing appears as a lightening beyond the limits of what the analyst or analysand knows. Such lightening contains the logic of contradiction that constantly produces a pair of opposites that need to be set apart and brought into relation to one another.

In the saying, or the formations of the unconscious, opposites are pressed together, while in narrative statements, they are set apart. Instead of linking signifiers within narrative statements, in analysis, key signifiers are set apart and brought into relation with other unconscious signifiers. What is privileged in the practice of psychoanalysis is not the formal logic of ego narratives based on premises and conclusions, storytelling, and the rules of syntax and grammar but rather metaphoric, synchronic, homophonic, and surprising connections among ambiguous and equivocal terms. This leads not to a universal knowledge but to realizational or awakening moments of *J'ouis-Sense* or the S_1 not linked to a master knowledge or narrative but rather to the Real of the body and jouissance. Realizational or awakening moments of jouissance have a therapeutic effect and refer us back to the Greek Nous.

This singular form of knowing or savoir coincides with the universal logos based on the cognitive interests of the ego at the *moment* where the subject yields control and direction to the lightening of wit (I think where I am not). In between the logos and revelation lies Nous, or non-knowing and realization (I am where I don't think). Unknown knowing is a clarity or *claritas* that signifies without ordering. Another way of saying this is contained within the polyvocality of the word experience. Experience refers to what we already know on the basis of past history and a universal constituted knowledge, but it also refers to the experience of the Real and the new and previously unformulated.

The deciphering of speech requires not only putting an ordering symbolic code into use but also an experiential moment of illumination produced by the articulation of two chains into a Borromean structure in the here and now. The unconscious chain of enunciation, and the manifestation of the Real in the fantasy and actions of the subject, put the subject at odds with the reality of the conscious chain of the statement. Reality is where the Real is not found. The Real and reality are at odds, although the first definition of the real in Lacan shares with reality the sense of a threat and intrusion or imposition on the subject. Reality is based on symbolic information and *techné*, while the Real is an experience of jouissance outside symbolic coordinates.

With regard to the virtues of thought from the perspective of the five forms of reason, there are various forms of thought: thinking, not-thinking or the suppression/suspension of thought, and non-thinking or 'thought' that refers to thinking as a form of jouissance outside language. There are various levels of thinking and reason: action/practice (practical reason), binary and dual thinking (formal reason), self-centered and objective thinking, nondual and dialectical thinking (dialectical reason), and non-thinking that includes thinking as well as vice versa (Nous).

In psychoanalysis, we don't perform arithmetical operations to reveal the irrational within the structure but rather use the rules of substitution and metaphor to arrive at the 'what' of the underlying structure that appears not to exist within the phenomenal or manifest figures of speech and discourse. In addition, the structure can also be said not to exist, in that structure is not the same as its instantiation in the phenomenal world, and its instantiation or reiteration in a phenomenal event is not the same as the impossible and unnamable that is actually what we are seeking for in the search for truth and knowledge. The impossible and unnamable is actually the brightness or the flashing of light into the phenomenal world (that includes the brain), otherwise known as enlightenment or illumination whether analytical or synthetic, objective or subjective, within language or experiment, or within the immanence of experience and outside language and reasoning altogether.

The different forms of reason correspond to different logical levels. There is the cognitive function (understanding) associated with the measurement of forms (formal reason), and then there is the cogito (dialectical critical reason or reason proper) linked to the apperception of structure that itself requires Nous (negative dialectics and non-thinking) to apprehend its emptiness and non-existence as the impossible and unnamable at work in the emergence of structure and creation.

Practical reason or ethics in my work also has the function of preventing, collapsing, and reducing the different logical levels and dimensions of reality. Beyond nationalism, and relative and preferred cultural, linguistic, and gender identity, I argue that it is not ethical or in the best interest of humanity to define knowledge in the absence of one or more dimensions of rationality. Conflicts emerge between the different forms of reason, and their corresponding discourses, resulting in petty bickering and academic posturing and domination and the fight over economic resources that is common in the master's discourse that runs and prevails within university discourse. We have to have the courage to embrace the five forms of rationality that Aristotle and the Greeks have bequeathed us. This is truly a direct experiential transmission of a desire for knowing and realization not dependent on academic institutions and that springs forth from the human spirit itself, in which all forms of life and the universe are embedded.

Anglo American analytical philosophy, or the philosophy of science that supports technical procedures and formal reason, neglects nous or unconscious intuition, dialectical logic, and practical reason. Psychoanalysis uses the five Aristotelian categories of reason, and this is what lends it a broad, profound, and humane dimension derived from a founding genius. I say genius because many of the geniuses that the history of the university depends on were only post facto incorporated and accepted into academic discourse. I argue that they were who they were because they used more than two forms of reason, if not all five. Their ideas are controversial precisely because they are using several forms of reason that conflict with the prevailing formal reason associated with science and beliefs or prejudices held by academic and governmental institutions. Talent is generated by nature for the good life in common, and is not widely distributed, or chosen by political decision or popular vote. However, the people, or the bureaucratic order, may not accept the talent selected by nature and instead may treat natural talent as being equivalent to whatever capacity is generated by specialization within the culture.

There are many examples: Socrates, Galileo, Newton, Darwin, Einstein, Freud, and Lacan, to name only a few. We all know what the Athenian state did to Socrates. Galileo, Newton, and Darwin eventually gained wide acceptance and even controversial dominion, despite the initial rejection of the Church and the science of their time. Freud was initially rejected, then adopted, and then rejected once again. Lacan was also expelled from the psychoanalytic organization that Freud founded for his innovations in technique and for critiquing how the International Psychoanalytic Association (IPA) was abandoning Freud's teaching and practice. In this respect, Zizek (2000) has made the interesting observation that new forms of knowledge and savoir need the pathology of the *objet a* within the personal life of a hero, as a required underside that turns a person into the One as a public figure.

In the social sciences within Anglo-American academia, statistically modeled empirical science operates according to rational models based on formal analytical reason and techne (*epistêmê and technê*). The latter are shared with binary digital computers and with artificial intelligence but may lack properly human dimensions (the other forms of reason). Practical reason is so much more than technical rationality. Praxis not only includes ethics but also a practice of the Real that involves subjectivity, or an objective form of subjectivity independent from quantitative measurement or calculation.

Listening is also a Real practice (*J'ouis-sense*) facilitated by the clear state acting as a screen/filter to prevent past experience from saturating and biasing new and present experience. One listens with knowing, not-knowing or ignoring, and non-knowing that allow for the emergence of new significations. Finally, the epistémé that links theory and practice in psychoanalysis includes dialectical logic and contradiction and not simply formal logic and the principle of non-contradiction. The mind as construed by Freud includes many antithetical or contradictory phenomena, as seen in dreams, the antithetical meaning of primal words (Freud, 1910), the formations of the unconscious, symptoms, the experience of pain and pleasure, and the reversible quality of the pleasure and reality principle, of primary and secondary process thinking and feeling states (love and hate, for example). Formal reason and techne alone, although rational, cannot capture the observations of psychoanalysis and the dimensions of human subjectivity studied therein.

For Lacan (1972–1973), thought in the Real (Nous) is a form of jouissance that is also found in the gaps between ideas. Thought is jouissance, and jouissance is what grounds thought and the symbolic order with the real hands and feet of reality. The reason that science cannot define the nature of thought, and thought being a fundamental capacity and characteristic of human nature, is that thought includes the unsayable Real of jouissance.

Silence, for example, can be of various kinds, some of which are coded, and some of which are not. What is undefinable and uncoded about human thought is the same as what is undefinable about Nous as a form of human reason. Thought includes the unsayable as jouissance that goes beyond what nowadays is called emotional intelligence (like a computer asking you, "How are you today," and offering a medication or an empathic piece of advice based on information that has been uploaded into the computer), since jouissance cannot be reduced to emotions or electricity.

Finally, practical reason in psychoanalysis also means that when discussing cases, from an ethical and practical point of view, the analyst will have to continue to disguise and modify clinical material in order to say the truth about truth. It is important to remember that the challenge that we are facing is not only a question of protecting subjects' privacy but also the impossibility to describe, measure, or scale every aspect of psychoanalytic sessions. Even the best, most accurate description of it will not stand for the "real thing." This is why Aristotle's five types of reason cannot be substituted for one another nor remain unrelated. But in order not to fall into the ethical chaos of anything goes, the hierarchy and circularity of mental functions need to be preserved.

With respect to the circularity and relationship among the different categories of reason, an interesting relationship exists between practical reason and techne, method, or technique. Practice means that the singular individual has to be directly engaged in a Real practice or specific type of activity rather than simply being treated as a number or a constituent of a set, category, or experiment. The treatment method of free association, for example, constitutes ways of unchaining thoughts, feelings, truth, and signifiers from pre-determined chains of thinking, knowledge, or ideology. The theory or the first principles orient us towards the Real of a practice but do not absorb it into the closed circularity of established discourse. This way, the theory can change the practice and the practice inform the theory but without either one being reduced to the other. Both the theory and the practice have to remain open or unsaturated as well as related to one another.

It is also true that a clinician can practice psychoanalytic principles without being an expert in the theory so long as they don't split the two or favor one over the other. In general, theoretical books are written by academics, while clinical books are written by practicing psychoanalysts. I am mostly referring to Lacanian literature in English but not to important literature in French or other languages where the relationship between academia and professional experience, or analytical discourse, may be different. In Spanish, the work of Harari would be an example of analytical discourse that is both academic and practical at once, while being outside conventional academia.

There are important translations of the work of French Lacanian analysts; among them are Colette Soler and Miller's work that I have read mostly in Spanish. Finally, as I have mentioned elsewhere, the Lacanian School of Psychoanalysis (LSP) in the San Francisco Bay area was influenced by psychoanalyst Mustapha Safouan, an early colleague of Lacan and author who was a mentor to Andre Patsalides, a Belgian analyst who worked with Lacan in Paris and founded LSP.

Within the IPA and its journals, analysts write technical papers that cite prior literature on the subject to further develop the field and the practice. No longer do analysts have to write introductory books to the practice of psychoanalysis, since so many books have already been written. The same is not true of the new growing field of Lacanian psychoanalysis. Introductory books cover familiar and basic ground necessary to establish an analytical practice within a certain orientation. The IPA for years used Ralph Greenson's (1967) book as a manual to train psychoanalysts, and more recently, Horacio Etchegoyen's (1991) book came to fulfill the same task. Etchegoyen's book cites most of the relevant literature within the IPA and includes a section on Lacanian theory and the Lacanian theory of the transference.

Within Lacanian psychoanalysis, Fink's (2011) book, *Fundamentals of Psychoanalytic Technique*, is an excellent account of Lacanian practice that has the same title as Etchegoyen's book. This may not be entirely unrelated to Etchegoyen's rapprochement with Miller when Etchegoyen was the president of the IPA and to Miller's own international organization to which Fink belongs.

Although Etchegoyen's book includes a section on the Lacanian theory of the transference, it does not discuss how the transference is analyzed or used in the actual practice of Lacanian psychoanalysis. The reason for this is not mentioned either because it involves the administrative and political decision to exclude Lacan and ignore his contributions to the clinic and the practice of analysis, much to the detriment and fragmentation of psychoanalysis itself. This kind of toxic intellectual politics, together with the fragmentation of the theory into various theoretical and pragmatic clinical models, may have led to the rapid delegitimization of psychoanalysis itself.

Within the Lacanian field, both Fink (2011) and Nobus (2000), for example, are both analysts and academics practicing analysis in private practice, and this has proven very effective for the development of the field. This point about academia is interesting because Lacan's work spans both the analytical and university discourse perhaps to a greater extent than even Freud.

> But I am not a professor, since, precisely, I put in question the subject supposed to know. This is precisely what the professor never puts in question because he is essentially, qua professor, its representative.
>
> (February 28, 1968, XI 3)

Analysts do not have to be academics, but analysts and researchers-practitioners that develop psychoanalytic theory are in fact generating academic thought in the Greek sense of the term. Psychoanalytic theory is a good example of how the academia is found wherever true thought emerges rather than ordinarily being identified with the site of a prestigious academic institution. Einstein is the paradigmatic example of this, and this is why he was a man of the people and loved by people. He wrote his breakthrough papers working as a patent clerk.

Freud, like Einstein, was a 'real universal seeker after truth,' rather than a 'specialist' like his followers (Klein, for example, despite the clinical importance and contribution of Klein's work for child analysis), who tried to develop specialist theories to represent and replace the encyclopedic and historical scope of Freud's theory. Jung, Bion, and Lacan also were seekers after truth with a universalist orientation. This, of course, does not mean that they were right about everything, and thus specialists are also required to test and falsify different aspects of the theory, but the theory in its entirety can only be falsified on conceptual and mathematical grounds.

A good example of how specialists are required to falsify different aspects of the theory is how Einstein coined the term quanta to refer to light as a particle and a wave but then could not theorize the concept of entanglement between two subatomic particles and how this related to both the presence of the observer and the quality of the particle as a wave. The observations and measurements were there, but he could not think of an alternative explanation for entanglement. Niels Bohr had to do it for him.

I mentioned analytical psychology, despite the history of conflict between Freud and Jung and their respective schools, first because Jungian theory is at least partially derived from psychoanalysis, and, second, because Freud incorrectly predicted that Jungian psychology would disappear in one or two generations. Lacan stayed much closer to Freud's theory than Jung ever did, since Jung tended to trivialize Freudian thought in order to establish his own system of thought. Lacan is closer to science and rational thought than Jung, since Jung privileged images and the irrational in the psyche and tended to lump the irrational and the transrational into the same bag, something that Lacan *a*-voided by theorizing the Real in its two moments. By transrational I mean how the known and unknown interact: something beyond understanding (the unknown or jouissance, for example) is also consistent with the principles of reason.

Lacan was not interested in the occult and neither was Freud, but Freudian theory and materialism (formal and dialectical) leave the occult outside science and in the trash heap of history, while with Lacanian theory, the occult is still outside science, but not foreclosed, and therefore cannot return from foreclosure in destructive and grotesque forms (for example, the horror film genre). Bertrand Russell (1935) knew this well, since despite being an analytical philosopher, an heir to Newton in mathematics (PM system), he recognized that many great individuals have required both science and what is outside science, much to the scandal and chagrin of the specialists.

Many of the discoveries and mathematical formulae found within Newton's *Philosophiæ Naturalis* and *Principia Mathematica* can be linked to his occult studies. Newton deliberately left these writings unpublished, fearing scrutiny from the scientific community. Newton, the epitome of the new science, was the last of the magicians of past antiquity. Einstein (1956, p. 29) instead believed that he was motivated in his scientific work by a mystical form of realism for which he was criticized. This is what the truth-seekers have to do to cope with (live outside imaginary identifications – Lacan's legendary social *separation* is another example) the prejudices of their time.

A good contemporary example of a scientific form of jouissance, or of Einstein's mystical realism, is the case of Paul Murdin, an English astronomer who in 1971, motivated by the concept of a black hole, decided to investigate a cosmic sign that might reveal something unusual about a star. Murdin decided to focus on X-rays and noticed a bright X-ray source in the constellation of Cygnus. The source of the X-rays was not a supergiant star but something else that the star was orbiting that turned out to be a binary star that had become a black hole.

X-rays were caused by the black hole peeling off the outer layer from the existing sun orbiting around and being sucked down into the black hole. However, the point I want to make is orthogonal to the content of the knowledge I just described, with the latter being widely available to the general public. Once Murdin realized what he had discovered, he felt so elated and happy that he had to get up and walk about his desk to calm down. His pulse was racing; he felt such a sense of awe that he could not do any serious work for the rest of the day. This is another example of the connection between knowledge and jouissance associated with light-dawning discoveries that should not be underestimated. The Other jouissance (*J'ouis-sense*) experienced in a true scientific discovery was already there beforehand, guiding and propelling the process of discovery and realization. Scientists are simply following their passion or bliss. The word bliss is interesting, because in its homophony with the word bless, it becomes the jouissance associated with the word well said, or a work well done. The word well said (*benedicere*: bless) requires the prior acceptance of symbolic castration, or that (b)less may be more.

Lacan was not a mystic, but unlike Freud, his theory distinguishes between religious delusion based on the oceanic feeling stemming from the fusion with the mother (the jouissance of the Other or the Imaginary One) and the benevolent Third Other jouissance of the mystic (One of the Real) that requires the prior establishment of the NoF and the symbolic function of castration. The One of the Imaginary is not the One of the Real: "There is nothing more dangerous than confusion over what is involved in the One. The One is not Eros as fusion, making one from two" (Lacan [1971–1972], p. 91). Miller (Lacan, 2018) has also written that "One can't help thinking that Lacan's late teaching belonged to the same register as the esoteric teaching that found a place in the Schools of antiquity" (p. 182). However, Miller's quote does not distinguish between the archaisms of antiquity and the ancestral philosophical wisdom that is still relevant for our times. Newton's thought is both in continuity with past ancestral knowledge and wisdom and in discontinuity with the archaisms of antiquity. In addition, I have argued (Moncayo, 2012) that mystical jouissance (as one of the forms of the Third jouissance) is "ex-soteric" or quotidian rather than esoteric or otherworldly.

These considerations go beyond the question of whether empiricism is always accompanied by its pair-wise companion in philosophy: idealism (for example, the works of Hume and Berkeley), or what Zizek now is calling a new form of transcendentalism in philosophy. Both terms, idealism and transcendentalism, have pejorative connotations due to understanding the relationship between realism and idealism in dualistic ways. Hume focused on sense experience, and Berkeley focused on the ideas behind sense perception, while Lacan's later theory is organized around the Real and the question of jouissance beyond representation yet equally interacting with ideas, signifiers, and sense experience. The Real of jouissance as a Third is in fact a way of breaking out of the realism/idealism duality.

In addition, the field of psychoanalytic truth has also reduplicated and divided into a theory without practice or applied to different fields and a practice often guided by a theory that is not studied in university clinical settings and that bears no systematic relationship to the Freudian concept of the Unconscious. Lacan would not be happy with this state of affairs, given that however abstract his theory was at any given point, it was always delivered with analysts in mind or thought in relationship to analytic practice. The point being that psychoanalysis cannot be dissociated from its practice given that, among other things, Lacan, like Freud, used other fields to develop psychoanalytic theory rather than psychoanalysts using psychoanalysis to reduce other fields to psychoanalysis. This is notwithstanding the fact that psychoanalysis has been and should be taught in the university and that other fields can use psychoanalysis to develop their own fields, yet the theory itself has been developed by analytical theorists engaged in the practice of analysis working in unison with university researchers and some who are both.

Lacanian thought in the United States has been disseminated mostly in the humanities, where one supposes that people are interested in theory, as distinct from those who may be solely interested in learning the trade and practice of psychotherapy. Biological psychiatry in the United States considers Lacanian theory a form of literary analysis devoid of clinical relevance. This follows on the heels of the IPA's rejection of Lacan's innovations in the practice of analysis, as reflected in the practice of scansion of session and speech.

Psychotherapy as a purely technical procedure devoid of theory or where the theory is not linked to scientific theories or to the history of Western thought would not be applied psychoanalysis according to Lacan. Applied psychoanalysis is not the practice without the theory that otherwise is left to the "experts." Applied psychoanalysis is the practice of the theory that could in fact take place in different formats and settings and not only in private practice or the standard frame. Finally, psychoanalytic theory can be used by other fields to develop their own fields by the same token that psychoanalysis can use theory derived from other fields to develop psychoanalytic theory and practice.

References

Adorno, T. W. and Horkheimer, M. (1944). *Dialectic of Enlightenment.* London: Verso, 1997.

Aristotle. (2009). *The Nicomachean Ethics.* Oxford World Classics. Cambridge: Oxford University Press.

Deutsch, D. (2011). *The Beginning of Infinity: Explanations That Transform the World.* New York: Penguin Books.

Einstein, A. (1956). *The World as I See It.* New York: Citadel Press Books.

Etchegoyen, H. (1991). *The Fundamentals of Psychoanalytic Technique.* London: Karnac.

Fink, B. (2011). *Fundamentals of Psychoanalytic Technique: A Lacanian Approach for Practitioners.* New York: Norton.

Freud, S. (1900). The Interpretation of Dreams. *SE*, 4–5.

Freud, S. (1910). The Antithetical Meaning of Primal Words. *SE*, 11, 155–161.

Fromm, E. (1980). *The Art of Listening.* New York: Open Road.

Greenson, R. (1967). *The Technique and Practice of Psychoanalysis.* London: Karnac.

Heidegger, M. (1947). *Letter on Humanism: In Basic Writings* (Revised and Expanded Edition). Translated by D. F. Krell. London: Routledge, 1993.

Heidegger, M. (1955). *The Question Concerning Technology.* New York: Garland Publishing, 1977.

Heidegger, M. (1966). Conversation on a Country Path about Thinking. In: *Martin Heidegger, Discourse on Thinking.* Translated by J. M. Anderson and E. H. Freund. New York: Harper and Row.

Jeffries, S. (2017). *Grand Hotel Abyss: The Lives of the Frankfurt School.* London: Verso.

Kaplan, J. (2005). "Political Theory: The Classic Texts and Their Continuing Relevance". The Modern Scholar. 14 lectures; (lectures #11 & #12, – see disc 6). Recorded Books, LLC.

Lacan, J. (1957–1958). *The Formations of the Unconscious: Book V: The Seminar of Jacques Lacan.* Edited by J.-A. Miller and Translated by R. Grigg. London: Polity Press.

Lacan, J. (1962–1963). *Seminar of Jacques Lacan.* Book X on Anxiety. Translated by C. Gallagher. www.lacaninireland.com/web/published-works/seminars. Accessed November 17, 2019.

Lacan, J. (1967–1968). *The Seminar of Jacques Lacan.* Book XV: The Psychoanalytic Act. Translated by C. Gallagher. www.lacaninireland.com/web/published-works/seminars. Accessed November 17, 2019.

Lacan, J. (1971–1972). *…or Worse.* London: Polity, 2018.

Lacan, J. (1972–1973). *The Seminar of Jacques Lacan: Book XX: On Feminine Sexuality, the Limits of Love and Knowledge (Encore).* New York: Norton and Norton.

Lacan, J. (1975–1976). *The Sinthome: The Seminar of Jacques Lacan.* Book XXIII. Edited by J. A. Miller. Cambridge: Polity Press, 2018.

Lacan, J. (1977–1978). *Seminar XXV: Time to Conclude.* Translated by C. Gallagher. www.lacaninireland.com/web/published-works/seminars. Accessed March 18, 2019.

Locke, J. (1632–1704). *An Essay Concerning Human Understanding*. Cambridge: Hackett Publishing Company.

Moncayo, R. (2012). *The Signifier Pointing at the Moon: Psychoanalysis and Zen Buddhism*. London: Karnac.

Moncayo, R. (2018). *Knowing, Not-Knowing, and Jouissance: Levels, Symbols, and Codes of Experience in Psychoanalysis*. London: Palgrave McMillan.

Nobus, D. (2000). *Jacques Lacan and the Freudian Practice of Psychoanalysis*. London: Routledge.

Plotinus (CE 204–70). (1991). *The Enneads (Classics)*. Penguin Books Ltd. Kindle Edition. The Enneads. London: Penguin Books.

Quinet, A. (2018). *Lacan's Clinical Technique: Lack(a)nian Analysis*. London: Routledge.

Russell, B. (1935). *Religion and Science*. London: Oxford University Press, 1947.

Saporta, J. (2014). Psychoanalysis Meets China: Transformative Dialogue or Monologue of the Western Voice. In: *Psychoanalysis in China*. Edited by D. Scharff and S. Varvin. London: Karnac.

Zizek, S. (2000). *The Fragile Absolute*. London: Verso.

1 Lacanian theory and a multidimensional and topological approach to diagnoses

Before considering DSM-5 or the contemporary manual of psychiatric diagnoses, a few words are in order regarding the etymological roots of the word 'diagnosis.' Literally, it means to know apart, discern specific differences, or even the knowing of difference. We need to know of what and how things are made so as to know how they can fall apart, malfunction, and be repaired. When things fall apart, we can know what they are made of. Finally, the knowing of relative differences directly translates into the ability to read and interpret signs, signifiers, and symptoms. A medical doctor reads signs; a psychoanalyst reads signifiers.

DSM-5, a new updated version of DSM, has finally been published after ten years of a heated debate. DSM-5 raised a lot of controversy (American Psychiatric Association, 2013). Allen Frances, MD, who chaired the DSM-IV Task Force, expressed his concern that "DSM 5 will result in the mislabeling of potentially millions of people who are basically normal." With the new version of the manual, grief may quickly turn into major depressive disorder. In this chapter, I begin by looking at some of the DSM-5 changes mentioned previously with the help of Lacanian theory and in the light of a psychoanalytic understanding of psychopathology and diagnoses. In addition, I intend to discuss the prevalence of the diagnosis of bipolar disorder and the controversy between grief and clinical depression, examine the similarities and differences between mood swings in a personality disorder and in bipolar II disorder, and, finally, distinguish between neurotic and psychotic forms of paranoia and between paranoia and metanoia.

In contrast to Vanheule's (2014) book, this chapter will not be focused on questions surrounding the statistical validity or reliability of DSM-5 or on a detailed analysis of DSM-5 itself. Vanheule, in line with psychodynamic and social psychiatry, argues that psychiatric diagnoses are not diagnosing medical/organic conditions per se and that diagnoses are intrinsically related to social-historical and subjective conditions. Ten years earlier, Verhaegue (2004) wrote a critique of DSM from a Lacanian and psychoanalytic perspective. He criticized the DSM system as a simplistic laundry list description of symptoms that produces stigmatization, promotes conventional forms of identity and normality, is unreliable, and has no meaning for treatment.

Finally, this chapter also differs from the *Psychodynamic Psychodiagnostic Manual* (PDM) (Alliance of Psychoanalytic Organizations, 2006), meant to offer a psychodynamic manual of personality disorders, since this manual does not follow

Freud's diagnostic categories and instead relies on a laundry list of personality disorders and ego functions that also confuses symptoms/traits with personality types. Freud and Lacan's are structural diagnostic categories and, therefore, many of the traits of the various personality disorders can be subsumed under the two types of neurosis (hysteria and obsessional neurosis). For example, depression is a symptom that could appear in the two types of neurosis, as well as in psychosis, but does not warrant being classified as a personality disorder unto itself.

From a Lacanian point of view, for example, depression (Moncayo, 2008) is not only genetic and/or caused by the accidental loss of a reality object/family member but also by the lack of loss of an object in normal development. By pathologizing grief, psychiatry risks that people may not want to grieve or could feel that they should not grieve, but if they don't grieve, they may, thereby, be paradoxically predisposed to depression.

I will also discuss the popular diagnosis of bipolar disorder and explore DSM changes in the context of psychoanalytic theories. What can Lacanian theory offer to DSM? For example, is bipolar disorder a psychotic or neurotic structure? There are a number of features that point to bipolar disorder being a neurotic structure.

Introduction

The *Diagnostic and Statistical Manual of Mental Disorders, Fifth Edition,* is an interesting "encyclopedia of human madness." For centuries, human beings have wanted to categorize and find patterns in the world. It seems natural, then, that at some point we would attempt to create a taxonomy of human activity and the human mind.

The origins of DSM date back to 1840. At that time, the government wanted to collect data on mental illness. It is interesting that the census used the terms 'idiocy/insanity' without any inhibitions. In a sense, someone was either 'normal' or 'insane' – the classification was very simple. Over a 40-year period of time, 'insane' included seven categories: "mania, melancholia, monomania, paresis, dementia, dipsomania and epilepsy." But none of these classifications were yet DSM, as DSM-I was born in 1952.

DSM's main goal was to create a common language that health professionals could use to communicate across borders and collect and compare information on mental illness. Of course, the previous was supposed to lead to better treatment and better outcomes for people who happened to be outside of the 'norm.' Between 1880 and 1952, from seven categories, DSM-I featured descriptions of 106 disorders, which were referred to as 'reactions.' Sixteen years later in 1968, DSM-II further increased the number of disorders to 182. Both DSM-I and II were driven mainly by the psychodynamic view up until 1980, when DSM-III came out with a whole new perspective to focus on empirical descriptions. At that point, psychiatry had 265 diagnostic categories. With DSM-IV in 1994, the 300-category line was reached with not too many changes. DSM-5 has over 1,000 pages' worth of checklists of symptoms that psychiatrists around the world use to diagnose their patients.

There was one big change in the history of DSM that occurred between DSM-II and III. The changes reflect how mental health professionals viewed mental illness at first mostly through psychodynamic lenses and conceptualized it as the product of conflict between internal drives/wishes and defenses. DSM-III opted to follow Emil Kraepelin rather than Sigmund Freud. The idea of separate syndromes and disorders was created, and so bipolar disorder, schizophrenia, and major depressive disorder were supposed to be treated differently and had unique causes.

Certainly, many changes took place since the 1840s' 'one disorder' of insanity to the over 300 nicely described illnesses and disturbances with outlined symptoms and their duration. Unfortunately, patients don't read the textbooks. Psychiatrists and other mental health professionals are often frustrated that their clients rarely fit into neat categories. In addition, symptoms frequently change over time. It often leads to patients becoming a sort of "collectors" of different diagnoses, which can be very upsetting to them. It can also lead to polypharmacy that can be outright dangerous. We try to bring basic research to help with the clarification. Psychiatry dreams about genetic, metabolic, imaging tests that will help diagnose better and faster. Unfortunately, the biological tests only support the idea that psychiatric disorders overlap and that perhaps less is more.

> Studies with functional magnetic resonance imaging show that people with anxiety disorders and those with mood disorders share a hyperactive response of the brain's amygdala region to negative emotion and aversion. Similarly, those with schizophrenia and those with post-traumatic stress disorder both show unusual activity in the prefrontal cortex when asked to carry out tasks that require sustained attention.
>
> (Dichter, Damiano and Allen, 2012) Genetics brings similar findings (Craddock and Owen, 2010)

Publication of DSM-5 brought a lot of critique, not only from more psychodynamic providers but also biological psychiatrists and researchers. The National Institute of Mental Health (NIMH) withdrew its funding from DSM two weeks before its publication. Thomas R. Insel, M.D., director of the NIMH, criticized DSM for "its lack of validity" and suggested that, "Patients with mental disorders deserve better." He suggested that a new way for psychiatric nosology is reliance on biology and that "mapping the cognitive, neuronal circuit, and genetic aspects of mental disorders will yield new and better targets for treatment."

It is a highly promising approach, although "anatomy is not destiny" and humans are even more complicated than cognitive, neuronal circuits, and genetic aspects of their being. Somehow an individual patient/subject is lost in the classification battle. Moreover, no one is asking them how they feel about their 'disorders' or why they think they may have them. People become like broken machines spitting out symptoms at the time of diagnosis. Diagnoses can also be made by diagnostic machines capable of prescribing medication without the need for a human being. An interesting paper by Sam Kriss, "Book of Lamentations," makes such an observation:

> A person who shits on the kitchen floor because it gives them erotic pleasure and a person who shits on the kitchen floor to ward off the demons living in

> the cupboard are both shunted into the diagnostic category of encopresis. It's not just that their thought-process don't matter, it's as if they don't exist. The human being is a web of flesh spun over a void.
>
> (http://thenewinquiry.com/essays/book-of-lamentations/)

Lacanian theory and the *Diagnostic and Statistical Manual of Mental Disorders*

In his famous lectures, Lacan explored Freud's discovery of the unconscious. One of his most misrepresented statements, "the unconscious is structured like a language," allowed him to disagree with Freud's "anatomy is destiny." He also redefined the concept of drives and did not think that they are purely biologically driven. What interests us most here is that during the 1950s, he spent a lot of time trying to combine the topology of surfaces (torus, Moebius band, Klein bottles, cross caps) with mental life. He claimed that the linguistic signifier, the logic of desire, fantasy, and drives, follows the logic of topology or, in broader terms, mathematics. Lacan claimed that it is the best way we can describe the subject in his or her complexity.

When we speak of the human subject, or of the influence of language on the mind/brain, and how culture shapes our otherwise natural inclinations or how topology may describe psychical structures, we are referring to phenomena beyond the distinction between normality and pathology. Social life is a world of symbolic relationships that describe normal and abnormal facts. For every society, normal and abnormal modes of behavior are complementary.

So why is the study of psychopathology necessary and important? Why do we need psychopathology? Lévi-Strauss (1950) pointed out that in tribal cultures, "Witch doctors were recruited from the disabled, ecstatic, nervous types, outsiders" (p. 14). At the same time: "No shaman is in daily life an abnormal individual, a neurotic or paranoiac, if he were, he would be classed as a lunatic, not respected as a priest" (p. 19). "Shamans exploit psychopathology but also channel and stabilize it" (p. 20). More shamans mean less psychopathology in society.

Just as there is health and illness in the body, there is also a mental 'dis-ease' and a serenity of the mind. And nature shows that the dis-ease of the mind tends to break down in discernible patterns and structures. Psychoanalysis is distinguished from psychiatry in that for psychoanalysis, there is continuity between normality and pathology. Despite mainstream society considering psychiatrists abnormal, or needing a psychiatrist themselves, psychiatry is the field that establishes conventional and normative definitions of normality within society.

Freud was the first to call his theory of mind a topographical theory. The deep topological structures can manifest via their structures but also through what appears on the surfaces that correspond to what we call symptoms. The structure–surface relationship is even stronger in Lacan's topological theory than in Freud's topographical theory. The latter involves the spatial metaphor of adjacent rooms, or a bicameral mind composed of conscious and unconscious rooms, while Lacan's topological theory places the conscious and unconscious on a Moebius strip where the unconscious inside goes into the conscious outside and the conscious outside goes into the unconscious inside, and the two dimensions are two sides of the same band.

In Seminar V (Lacan, 1957–1958), Lacan had written that: "We are thereby introduced to a true dialectic of double meaning, where the latter already involves a third party. There are not two meanings one behind the other, with a second meaning, located beyond the first and the more authentic of the two" (p. 130). With Lacan's later theory, the Third is not the battery of signifiers (the Other), already included within the two sides of band, but the Real topological figure itself.

Neurosis as representing a divided form of subjectivity is the basic characterological condition of human beings. Human beings are caught between nature and culture, and culture demands that they shape their biological bodies and minds according to cultural forms. This is where both normality and pathology begin. Such neurosis is built into a person's characterological structure. The various types of personality traits may or may not turn into dysfunctional and incapacitating symptoms, but the possibilities lie within the traits and the corresponding brain mechanisms.

Before we go into the question of how to use topology to think about DSM diagnoses, consider first this clinical vignette. A 22-year-old female with no past psychiatric history arrives for a first consultation to your office. When asked about her goal of the assessment, she says that she "just wants to manage her highs and lows." She then goes into a detailed description of how both ends of her mood fluctuations wrecked her relationships and her entire semester in college. She says that she experienced her most intense 'high' in her senior year of high school. At that time, her boyfriend broke up with her, which almost as a chain reaction started her on a self-destruction path; she did not need to sleep and felt very energetic. She described herself as hypersexual, reckless, careless, and very impulsive. She said the episode lasted for about two weeks until her friends stopped talking to her and, completely exhausted, she 'rolled into' her 'low.'

She mentioned that her 'lows' are usually marked by extreme sadness, lack of drive, anhedonia, fatigue, and 'complete shutdown.' Interesting that she also raised the question whether she has adult ADHD – a new feature of DSM-5. She did great in elementary school, but since high school, she has been unable to focus on anything. Upon further questioning, our patient admitted to cutting as the only thing that helped her with mood swings. She said that she tends to get obsessed about people only to drop them when her interest fades away. She has a hard time tolerating being dumped by her boyfriends and lists it as the main cause of her 'highs.'

What does she have? Bipolar disorder type I, II, or maybe we could explain most of her symptoms with untreated borderline personality disorder? Does she have comorbid adult ADHD? Maybe she has all of these? Why does a seemingly 'typical' case presentation present such a challenge? Here we suggest that perhaps because DSM is not a very precise diagnostic tool, symptoms that 'create' disorders are not very specific, and they often overlap.

Lacanian topology can help us to be more precise. The main advantage of topology is that shape has no meaning there; it can even be called the "geometry of the rubber sheet." We can stretch it, bend it; it does not matter as long as its structure is preserved. If nothing else, it is a wonderful metaphor where for once we don't judge people by appearances, but we are more interested in their structure. The geometry of the rubber sheet is also a good metaphor for how to make a creative use of Freudian and Lacanian theory: concepts can be stretched like a rubber sheet while preserving the structure of the theory.

For Lacan, it would be a seemingly simple question, mainly because it is a grossly limited choice: is the person sitting in front of me in the consulting room psychotic, neurotic, or perverse? There are clearly defined differences between these three diagnostic categories that have serious implications in terms of treatment and prognosis. The differences are not only superficial, for they are also present on the level of the unconscious, Oedipal and family structure, the way the subject relates to language, and, maybe most importantly, the nature of their social link. Several excellent books already exist in English explaining the existing diagnostic groups used by Freud and Lacan (Dor, 1987; Fink, 1997; Verhaegue, 2004, etc). Instead, this chapter is a contribution to elucidating further structural differences between neurosis and psychosis, between structure and symptoms, between structures and so-called character disorders, between neurotic normality and a consistent or enlightened mind beyond normality, and, finally, the difference between normally occurring paranoia associated with the ego personality and paranoid psychoses.

I want to emphasize the fact that what I am suggesting here is not oversimplification of diagnosis but in fact a way to make it more sophisticated and closer to what we observe in the clinic and in basic research. Neuroscientific and genetic findings don't support the breakdown of many mental disorders into separate categories (Dichter, Damiano and Allen, 2012; Craddock and Owen, 2010).

Perhaps the actual state of affairs is that there are a few structural differences and diagnoses that reflect changes on the level of the unconscious but also the body (in a broad meaning of the term). Additionally, since every subject is unique, we observe different symptoms and signs 'on the surface.' For example, we may see a patient with psychotic structure and obsessive, OCD-like behaviors or hoarding on the surface. Another example would be the diagnosis of schizoaffective disorder. Here we would see it as a psychotic structure with mood symptoms on the surface.

The question posed at the beginning of the chapter still remains: How come, from one disorder of mind, there are now more than 300 illnesses, and it seems that they just keep multiplying? The reason for it is because psychiatry has tried to describe all the variations within the main categories as separate disorders. With so many of them, symptoms overlap, and this leads to diagnostic chaos and real difficulties for research.

The contribution of Lacanian theory to psychiatric and psychoanalytic diagnoses

Some psychiatrists/researchers have made attempts to modify the approach that DSM has taken. For example, Craddock and Owen (2010) proposed the model of dimensional spectrum – see Figure 1.1.

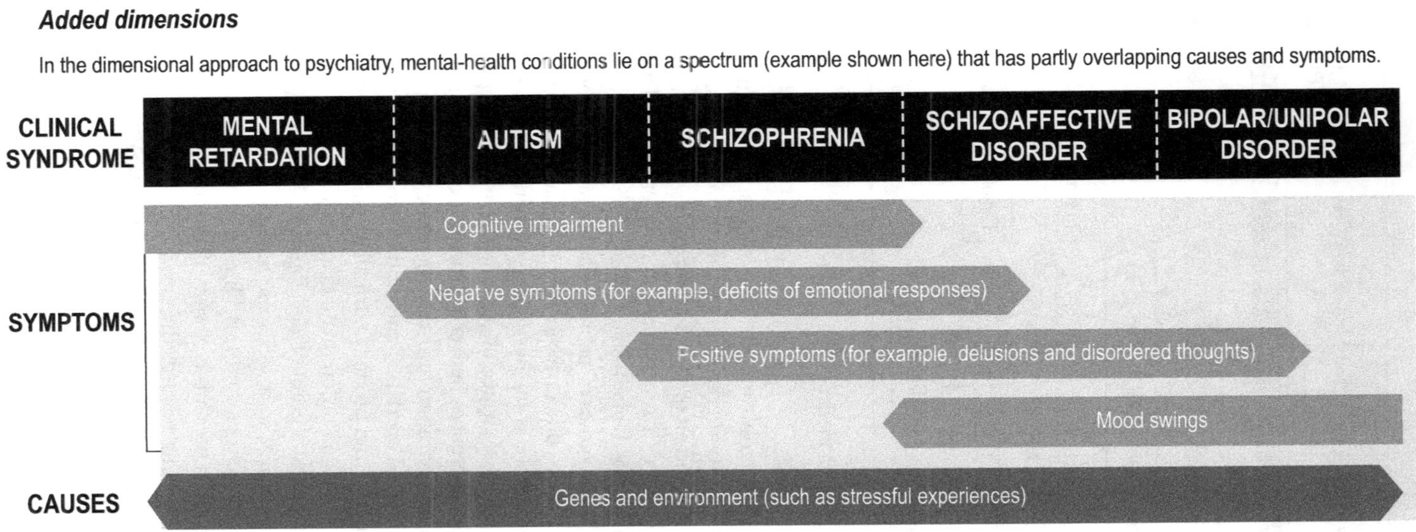

Figure 1.1 Model of dimensional spectrum

Source: From David, A., Mental health: On the spectrum, 24 April 2013; www.nature.com/news/mental-health-on-the-spectrum-1.12842

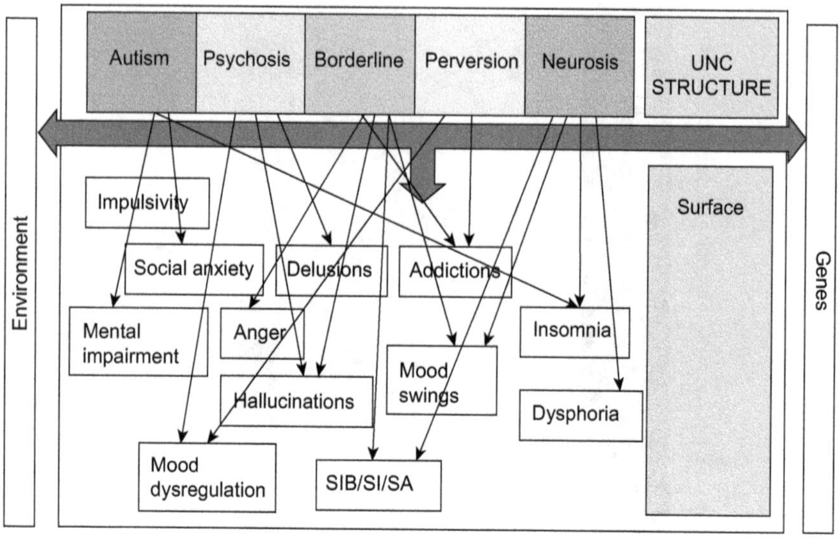

Figure 1.2 Dimensional spectrum model

Following a dimensional spectrum model, I will suggest five diagnostic structural categories: autism–psychosis–borderline–perversion–neurosis. Autism and the borderline condition are not Freudian or Lacanian diagnoses. However, autism is a pervasive developmental disorder that, according to the Centers for Disease Control, affects 1 in 59 children in the United States today. The borderline condition has many similarities with the diagnoses of neurosis but has new symptoms that need to be understood, and that has led other psychoanalysts to diagnose a separate category.

In addition, every structure is further described with specific symptoms and signs that are observed on the surface of a particular subject's topological structure. There are definite differences between structural categories; for example, a psychotic subject will be very different from a neurotic one. The symptoms and signs are on the spectrum and overlap. Genes and environment interact with each other and with the structure and produce particular symptoms accordingly.

Now, following Freud, we can differentiate diagnostic structures according to a specific defense formation and a point of developmental fixation (see Table 1.1).

The autistic pre-subject lives in a solipsistic timeless bubble that includes the individual and his mother/Other, and this One contains the entire world. The timeless bubble in this case represents a closing off or enclosure rather than what establishes a subjective opening towards the environment or what establishes any possible relationship to a natural and social environment. Autism represents the opposition between 0 and 1, either the autistic bubble or a relationship to the world, rather than the 0 that grounds any possibility of a One world (The One vs the One's own non-being). The NoF is what makes all difference between a porous symbolic enclosure (an *a*sphere) and a closed-off timeless bubble (the Imaginary rather than the Real).

Table 1.1 Diagnostic table

The Order of Unconscious Disorder	*Defense*	*Fixation*
Autism	Against being born and to live in diachronic or chronological time	Absolute primary narcissism
Psychosis	Identification with mother's imaginary phallus and foreclosure of the NoF	Relative primary narcissism
Borderline	Intersubjective splitting	On the specular image ideal ego (secondary narcissism)
Perversion	Disavowal of the law	On the lack (secondary narcissism)
Neurosis "Normal" Character Paranoia→Metanoia ↓	Identification with– avowal of the Law: repression	Ego ideal/super ego (tertiary narcissism)
The empty (*u-topia is eutopia*: no-place is a good place) subject of the Real. Benevolent Depersonalization	The Real as a structuring emptiness/openness of the subject and the signifier	(Quaternal narcissism) No fixed self or other. The word as *esprit* is a unary and slender trace of jouissance and a bodily signified of the sinthome

Freud described absolute primary narcissism as the condition of intrauterine life where the body of the mother and the baby are not differentiated. No distinction between self and other exists, yet the mother and the child are related to each other within the One bubble. The autistic pre-subject refuses to be psychically born outside the One body-bubble and may not speak or use language. The father as a function is irrelevant for the autistic pre-subject.

In psychoses, the pre-subject is identified with the breast-child as a phallic object of the jouissance of the Other (what object am I for the Other?). The psychotic is primarily a relative narcissistic object of the mother. There is no 'subject proper' or integrated specular body image. The psychotic speaks, but the order of language, by not being tied together by the paternal metaphor or NoF, results in loose associations. It is a primary form of narcissism because the subject has not been differentiated from the object and the libido rests entirely on the pre-subject as an object (of the mother's fantasy). The father is either brutal and cannot be symbolized as a function, fails, or is not allowed to mediate/symbolically castrate the mother/child fusion.

The borderline subject has attained secondary narcissism and an integrated imaginary ideal ego (body image) but remains fixated to the whole image and being the object of the mother's desire. The borderline cannot symbolize the flaws in the image or the aspect of the mother's desire that is turned towards the Other. Any flaw in the other turns the other bad and, by the same token, the borderline subject good and perfect. Conversely, if the other is seen as embodying the good and perfect specular image, then the subject becomes bad and unlovable and a failure in being the object 'cause of the other's desire.' Here the borderline is at risk of psychotic disintegration and of regression to a malevolent form of depersonalization.

To the right of the structure, or upward in development, the borderline subject can also manifest overt asocial or non-normative traits. The borderline can typically have problems with drug addiction, wear atypical clothing, have problems with impulse control, engage in sexual acting out or multiple temporary sexual 'hook-ups' that may or may not be exploitative in nature, and have many body piercings and tattoos. All these were not traditional symptoms of neurosis, although the case could be made that these are new symptoms for a contemporary form of hysterical structure.

Further study would be required to differentiate neurotic intrapsychic splitting (division) and inhibition, from intersubjective splitting, manipulating and dividing others, lack of impulse control, and the addictions and cutting associated with the borderline diagnosis. To this effect, it will be important to differentiate between a traditional grand hysteria and its social or intersubjective manifestation from the intersubjective impact of the borderline diagnosis. Grand hysterics demand the Other's love and that the other hate whom they hate. Manipulation is done out of dependence and weakness rather than a more perverse borderline desire that the other be ambivalently destroyed or degraded in some surprising way.

The pervert encountered the lack and flaw in the specular image and recognized the presence of the father, but the law, the flaw, and the name of the father are disavowed, and the subject remains fixated on the lack as a sheer negativity without a constructive function. Otherwise the pervert can appear to be perfectly normal, charming, and conventional.

The latter takes us to the neurotic structure where conventionality is structural and not only on the surface as in the pervert. The hysterical and obsessional structures avow the Law, identify with it, and inhibit and adapt themselves accordingly. The neurotic uses repression as a defense and is fixated on the narcissism of the ego ideal. The neurotic aspires to be complete and consistent by being a good boy or girl and lovable to the ego ideal and the normative values of society.

Verhaegue (2004) has described the relationship between the standards and norms by which normality is measured and the social ideals that lie behind statistical norms and the concept of normality. Normality and abnormality do not exist objectively in themselves but are relative social constructs. Wherever an ideal social norm is set up, it will automatically generate real shadows and gaps between the ideal and the real, and society will hand over the responsibility to certain individuals to constitute the abnormal statistical complement to the ideal norms of society. In addition, frequencies describe trends within society, or within social subjects, but do not reveal patterns or structures. Suicides rates have increased, while homicide rates have decreased, so this is a pattern, for example, but the question is what structural elements have caused or accompanied these changes.

The category of normal neurosis may strike the reader as having elements of things that people would consider part of normality. Normality for Lacan was a façade or a semblance of an otherwise divided subjectivity that inevitably comes with being human. This is not to say that the ego ideal or the norm could not represent an ideal that gives an orientation, yet it is often misrecognized and hardly ever realized.

The argument about a normal disorder seems ridiculous because, if this were true, one would never diagnose a condition that belongs to the general population. Thus, the assumption is that the general population does not have the symptoms of neurotic conditions and do not seek treatment. However, there is another important distinction within psychoanalytic theory that comes handy at this point: neurosis with symptoms and neurosis without symptoms (Fenichel, 1945).

In normal neurosis without symptoms, character traits occupy the place of symptoms. One could then say that a next level opens up whereby one can then classify an entire new range of personality disorders with symptoms that subjects do not believe they have. The result is that now once more diagnostic labels have proliferated with the caveat that psychiatry considers them untreatable if only because personalities are not a problem for those who have them. In this sense, we could understand character traits as the shadows that a structure sheds and sprays on the personality.

Structural paranoia and metanoia

Another outstanding related question in Lacanian theory is how to understand the structural function that Lacan's work gives to paranoia and its relationship to knowledge. Knowledge for Lacan comes in two forms. *Connaissance*, or conscious, ego-based established academic knowledge, and savoir, or unconscious knowing, or 'unknown knowing.' Lacan links paranoia to *connaissance* but not to unconscious savoir. I will have more to say about unconscious knowing in Chapter 6 when speaking about the negative transference in analysis. Lacan followed the conception of paranoic knowledge found in the work of the surrealist painter Salvador Dali (1935), where paranoia ceases to be solely a pathological category, since it also plays a constructive function in the furtherance of knowledge.

In forthcoming pages, I will link Lacan's later theory, with the Real and jouissance at its center, with how Lacan articulates paranoia in this context to continue elaborating what he had said previously in his earlier work about the relationship between knowledge (*connaissance*) and paranoia. There is no break here between the two periods, simply a relocation of the registers according to a topological knot of four.

In Seminar XXIII, Lacan redefines and relocates the function of the Real within the Borromean knot (Moncayo, 2017).

> In lesson 3 Lacan also introduces a new way of thinking of the subject, and of the subject of the Real in particular. The subject is what is supposed to the fact that the Imaginary and the Symbolic have to support and tolerate the knot of three and what ties them together.
>
> (p. 46)

> Lacan says that the Imaginary and the Symbolic are free from one another and that it is the Real that produces the impact, knot, or needlepoint that links them together (idem). "The Real is a third" (Lacan [1975–1976], Session of 9.12.75, II XIV). "The Real only has 'ex-sistence' . . . by encountering the arrest of the Symbolic and the Imaginary (idem, III 7).
>
> But the homogeneity of the Imaginary and the Real (in visual perception the perceived images appear to make the real world as we see it) in the knot of three also leads to false consistencies since we suppose an ego where the Real makes a tie, and construct a self where there is no self. (Moncayo, 2017, p. 48). "The subject is supposed to what of the Real ties the Imaginary and Symbolic together" (Lacan, Lesson of 12.16.75, III 7).

In the knot of three, the subject is socially bound by the signifier and the NoF coming from the Symbolic. "That by the fact of the said, they are arranged in a knot of three" (Lacan [1975–1976], Session of 12.16.75, III 13). The statement both reveals and constitutes the knot of three under a conventional NoF that holds it together. Instead, for the knot of four, it is the Real of jouissance that holds the knot together.

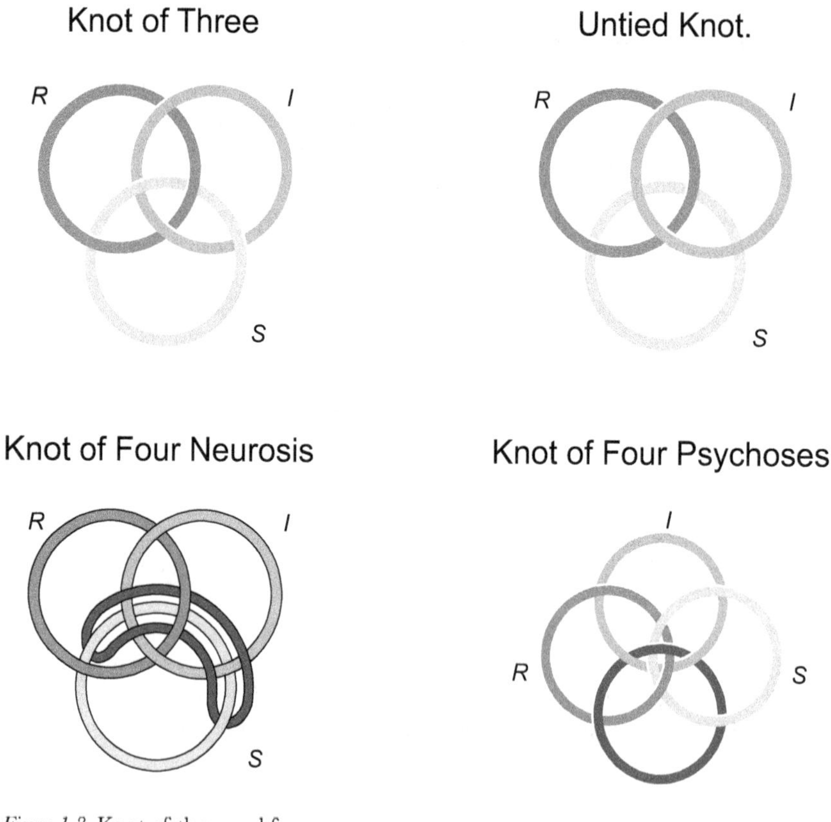

Figure 1.3 Knot of three and four

The knot of four requires that the knot of three first be untied. "I affirmed that if they have preserved themselves free among themselves, a knot of three, playing in a full application of its texture, 'ex-sists,' which is well and truly the fourth, and which is called the sinthome" (Lacan [1975–1976], Session of 12.16.75, III 13). It is interesting than in this quote, Lacan refers to the fourth as the consistency of the overall knot rather than to a fourth ring that ties a new knot of three together. "Be that as it may, the 'sistere' is already here, to be stable, to be stable on the basis of an out there" (Lacan [1971–1972], p. 122). Although the Imaginary is consistent, the second Real is the consistency of the overall knot that 'ex-sists' in the knot. "I have allowed myself to define as sinthome not what allows the knot, the knot of three, to still make a knot of three but what it preserves in such a position that it seems to be a knot of three" (Lacan [1975–1976], Session of 2/17/16, VII 5).

The second Real is duplicated as the consistency of the overall knot, which is the fourth or the sinthome. For the knot of four, the Real is duplicated (the two Reals of the early and late Lacan), and the new Real will function as the sinthome, or the NoF coming from the Real that ties the structure together. The relation between a fourth ring and the fourth as the consistency that 'ex-sists' in the overall knot remains unclear, although Lacan says that the fourth is what ties a knot of three and also what preserves the triadic structure at a level above it, or outside of it.

In addition, Lacan (1975–1976, Session of 12.16.75, II IX) said in this session that consistency is Imaginary, the Symbolic is a hole, and the Real 'ex-sists.' For the knot of four, consistency belongs to the second Real that comes to rupture the consistency that the Imaginary had initially taken from the Real that 'ex-sists.' The consistency of the knot itself is devoid of meaning or appears as senselessness or a gap that holds the signifying structure together. It is in this gap that, in analysis, the response to the message articulated by the signifiers of the subject will be how the analyst hears (*J'ouis-sens*) the Real of jouissance in both parties. When meaning appears in the saying or the subject of the enunciation, rather than in the narrative statement, the message is heard by *J'ouis-sens* rather than by listening to the distracting noise of the statement.

The ego is not only narcissistic and neurotic under the ideal ego and the ego ideal but could also be paranoid as a consequence of both. Both forms of the person, ideal ego and ego ideal, are framed and imposed by the Other of kinship, language, and culture. To have a self and a place in culture requires the acceptance of this imposition or benevolent symbolic castration. However, acceptance, or being a subject, does not come with a certain degree of frustration, coercion, and forbearance. "The manner in which each society imposes a rigorously determined use of the body upon the individual. The social structure leaves its imprint on individuals through the training of the child's bodily needs and activities" (Lévi-Strauss, 1950, p. 4). Acceptance leads to trust but also to a normal doubt or mistrust in the world.

On the surface, the idea of a normal form of paranoia could seem to be a contradiction in terms or lend some validity to the notion of a psychotic aspect within neurosis. Most people consider paranoia a form of psychoses, with paranoid schizophrenia being the paradigmatic form of psychosis. However, metanoia (from the Greek changing one's mind), and its relationship to paranoia, has been used in psychology and psychoanalysis by Jung (1960) and Laing (1968) to describe a process of fundamental change or an existential crisis in the human personality and psyche.

How are paranoia and metanoia related? In paranoia, the unconscious is projected and attributed to the Other. Since the unconscious is rejected, the Other is also treated with suspicion. Paranoid subjects are beside themselves, because their mind is outside. Metanoia is also etymologically related to the term Nous, or mind, described in the introduction. Since Nous refers to the aspect of the mind that is unknown, metanoia can be defined as trust and tolerance for the inconceivable, the unconcealed outside representation, and trust in the unknown or the unconscious. In fragment I, quoted by Heidegger (1969), Parmenides wrote that mortals lack the capacity to trust what is unknown and unconcealed.

By contrast, neurotic, or ordinary paranoia is fear of the unknown, particularly mistrust of what is unknown or unconscious about the Other. In paranoid psychoses, where the Unconscious has been foreclosed through projection, the feared unconscious returns from the outside in the form of a persecutory perception. Only neurotic paranoia can be evolved into metanoia, since paranoid psychosis forecloses the possibility of trusting the phallic function, even though at times, rudimentary forms of insight can also be observed in psychoses.

Ordinarily the body image comes from the mirror and from the Other. In the mirror phase, the ego appropriates the image from the Other, and in the process the Other is installed at the core of subjectivity, despite the apparent autonomy of the ego. The ambiguity that remains as to whether the ideal ego is the subject's own autonomous identity, or whether the ideal ego is the Other's own object, is continued in the relationship to the intersubjective other.

In structural paranoia, what is seen missing in the specular image installs a doubt in the subject with respect to the imaginary consistency and autonomy of the self-image. The Symbolic establishes a lack or something missing in the Imaginary self-image. The subject will defend against this lack by attempting to close the lack in the ego through seeking imaginary consistency in the imaginary alter ego. Unconscious knowledge about the *objet a* that has fallen off the Other to constitute the ego is projected unto the rival, fellow citizen, or alter ego. The other is seen through the cognitive veil (fantasy) of the *objet a* cause of the mother's desire that is missing in the body or specular image and that is projected unto the intersubjective other. In paranoid psychosis, the Symbolic order of language is not there to mediate the relations among the Other, the *a*, the ideal ego, and the alter ego.

Psychotic structures never attain a unified body image and a secondary form of narcissism that contains the lack within the image and instead are fixated to the relative primary narcissism of the maternal object and the mother's omnipotence. This is the source of psychotic grandiosity rather than the narcissism linked to the ideal ego. Instead of attaining the imaginary consistency of the ideal ego, the psychotic pre-subject projects the failed consistency of the ego to the consistency of the entire knot, and this is what paranoid schizophrenia consists of according to Lacan.

In "imaginary" projective intersubjectivity, every other alter ego potentially threatens to dislodge the ego from being the *objet a* cause of their mother's desire.

> Meaning is what is produced in the relationship between the Symbolic and the Imaginary. Between the Real and the Symbolic what emerges is the enjoyment of the phallus as the enjoyment of the *parletre*. In the Imaginary the enjoyment of the phallus becomes the enjoyment of the double, this is what is involved in meaning.
>
> (Lacan [1975–1976], Session of 12.16.75, III 13)

How the signifier enjoys phallic jouissance and continues processing signifiers while we sleep becomes first the enjoyment of the body image and, when this fails, the enjoyment of the imaginary double. The double refers to the alter ego (i[a']) that appears in the visual perception of reality. However, the function of the imaginary double is more than that, since it also appears in dreams wherein all the characters in a dream represent different aspects of the psyche of the dreamer. In a dream, the ideal ego (i[a]) is the alter ego (i[a']), while the subject is the dream itself. Meaning here is defined according to two axes: the displacement of images or metonymic objects in dreams and the displacement of signifiers between S_1–S_2, (S_3, S_4, . . .). Meaning is given by the dream narrative, and the intentions of the ego in the dream are often at odds with how the Other and both internal and external reality are represented in the dream. The subject and signification instead reflect the purpose of the dream itself as Other to the representation of the ego (i[a]) and its double (i[a]) in a dream. The Other appears in the dream's senseless element.

In the so-called normal paranoiac structure of the ego, the ego has a 'normal mistrust' of the impositions of the external world and the Other and enters into envious rivalry with its social counterparts. To the same extent that the ego thinks the ideal ego and ego ideal represent their autonomous agency, to that same extent, the ego may be prone to suspicion and paranoia. To the extent that the subject recognizes the Other in egoic constructions (the Other behind the mirror), or the symbolic structure of the Imaginary, this will inoculate the subject against paranoia.

During development, the subject's very core identity is defined by the Other. What is at the core of the paranoid subject is not psychosis but the proposition that "I contain multitudes," "I am an Other," and "the subject is a collectivity" (poets Whitman, Rimbaud, and Lacan, respectively). What makes this core identification normal is that the subject, wittingly or unwittingly, misrecognizes, appropriates, and takes the Other for the self.

At first, the mother and the child use the object mirror to link the mother's desire for the child to the child's specular image in the mirror, so that the Other may become the I. The child's body image is framed by the mother and the Name given to the image. That the mother as Other and mirror frames the ideal ego, or the visual representation of the body, remains an existential ambiguity for the subject. Am I me, or an Other? Who am I? If I am another, how can I be me? On the other hand, if the body image is not formed or integrated, and the protection of the mother's desire and the function of the Name is not there, then these are precisely the conditions under which the world becomes not normally but pathologically persecutory.

Once the subject realizes that the specular image has a hole or a lack built into it and that the ideal ego is not the end all or be all of the mother, because the mother's desire is turned towards the Other, the subject will turn towards the (f)Other to symbolize and articulate what is missing from the ideal ego. This leads to the formation of the ego ideal and to sexual difference. The Other and the phallic signifier will help symbolize the lack and what the social Other now demands from the subject. To be loved, it is no longer enough to be the mother's fantasy object; now the subject has to be subjected to the forms of the Law that bar or castrate the fantasy object that the child is for the mother. Under this form of primary repression, the laws of culture and signification will be established. This is what lends the ego ideal and super ego their persecutory quality.

For Lacan, the hysteric or the obsessive are both 'subjected' to the Other but in different ways. The hysteric defies subjection by finding the lack or weak points in the Other; the obsessive defies the Other according to the Law reflected in the perceived master's own standards. In either case, the subject may fear retaliation or the lack in the Other. The hysteric projects the lack unto the Other, while for the obsessive, the lack in the Other articulates the demands of the Other upon the subject. The obsessional cannot have desire because their lack of being (desire) has been taken over by the Other's desire. With respect to the lack, the obsessional fears that the Other will take from the subject the object that the subject has in fantasy taken from the Other. That the mother may have pampered, rather than frustrated the obsessive, is interpreted as the subject having taken the object mother from the Other.

In imaginary love, the imaginary Other, as imaginary *objet a*, represents the subject's own ideal ego without a lack in the image. That the imaginary other becomes a non-lacking ideal immediately places the lack on the side of the subject, therefore triggering ambivalence, if not mild forms of paranoia and apprehension. Finally, in neurosis, the subject is subjected to the imposition of the NoF and the function of symbolic castration. The words of the Other, as a result of the phallic function of symbolic castration, are experienced as a form of imaginary castration or imposition.

The other's image (object) generates a tension, as Lacan (1957–1958) calls it, whether sexual or combative, that is in the process of being reduced to nothing. The other's image (i[a']) triggers the drive and makes it seem as if the drive were outside. The image of the Other helps the subject of the drive pass through from tension to distension. In the field of photography, a visual tension is a compositional technique that creates 'dynamic' elements that activate the gaze. The dynamic elements of the visual field, its edges, regions, and textures, are the tensors that activate (tense) and satisfy (distension) the drive and also place the object at a certain distance with respect to the subject. In visual perception, it is the external object of perception that triggers the internal tensions of the drive.

Within Lacanian theory, normal (ego) paranoia begins with the mirror phase and not with the earlier ambivalence to the breast or *objet a*. The latter, which constitutes the logical basis for the Kleinian schizo-paranoid position (Klein, 1935), is stopped when the ambivalent relationship to the good and bad breast is integrated within the specular image (6 to 18 months of life). The good and bad parts, and the total image of the body, are integrated in the specular image. Now the body image in its totality can either sustain or support the subject as a stand-in for the *objet a* that caused the love of the mother for the subject, or the body image can become a new basis for a basic mistrust of a world that the subject did not make. The subject may also mistrust what the subject's ideal ego (body image) represents for the Other and what the Other wants from the subject.

In this respect, "normal" paranoia differs from the so-called schizoid personality in the same way that, for Kraepelin, schizophrenia and paranoia were two different conditions, although paranoia and paranoid delusion can also be regarded as an attempt to restore the torn cognitive links found in schizophrenia. *Schizo* in Greek refers to splitting, in the same way that hysteria represents the *spaltung* (sharp division in German) of consciousness that, far from representing pathology, represents the normal anthropological and existential condition that all human beings suffer from.

Does this apparent similarity between the two terms (*schizo/spaltung*) reflect a theoretical confusion or hide a more fundamental truth? Psychical reality is not such that the psychotic psyche is split and the neurotic psyche is unified by the ego: both are split, but neurotic division is structural or inevitable, while psychotic division could be prevented or at least silenced by the linguistic environment (NoF). With the divided subject in neurosis, the psyche is correspondingly impoverished, since the repressed is not accessible to the subject.

Spaltung and schism: neurotic projection, psychotic projective identification, and foreclosure

The distinction between neurotic and psychotic projection, in the example afforded by paranoia, is something worth considering for the purposes of this section and chapter. Neurotic projection is a formation by which repression is either achieved or reinforced. Neurotic projection presupposes a division within the subject and an expulsion into the other of the part of the self which is repressed (the subject is a crook but accuses the other of being a crook). This form of projection requires the prior establishment of primary and secondary repression. Repression, psychical or mental structure, personality or character structure, presuppose a normally divided subject.

But how is it, then, that projection is a defense of primitive origin at work in psychotic paranoia? How does projection work in psychosis where primary repression has failed?

> The most striking characteristic of symptom-formation in paranoia is the process which deserves the name of projection. An internal perception is suppressed, and, instead, its content after undergoing a certain degree of distortion, enters consciousness in the form of an external perception.
>
> (Freud, 1911, p. 169)

> The end of the world is the projection of this internal catastrophe.
>
> (idem, p. 173)

> It was incorrect for us to say that the perception which was suppressed internally was projected outwards; the truth is rather, as we now see, that what was abolished internally returns from without.
>
> (idem, p. 175)

Clearly Freud in the last quote is referring to a psychotic mechanism. The first quote could refer to the use of projection in the case of phobias as a form of neurosis. In phobia, an internal object is kept repressed, or from returning from repression, by projecting the fear unto an object in the external world. In the second step of the defensive process, the subject avoids and takes flight from the danger now represented by a phobic object. Another example of a "normal" form of neurotic projection is the case of a subject projecting unto, or blaming the Other for their own repressed desires, or accusing the Other with the very same accusations leveled by the father and the super ego against the subject.

Two different models emerged from this difference in the understanding of projection in neurosis and psychoses found in Freud. First Melanie Klein (1935) places the psychotic mechanism of projection at the origin of all normal development. In the Kleinian model, humans experience the schizo-paranoid position because she presupposes a schizoid division in the psyche as a primitive defense wherein unpleasant and satisfying experiences in relationship to the breast are split off. The experiences of rage and frustration are linked to the bad breast, while satisfaction is linked to the good breast. She theorizes that the child evacuates the bad breast and projects it unto the mother, becoming even more lethal for the subject once it is re-introjected.

Aside from the fact that projection and introjection require a distinction between inside and outside that the infant does not yet have at the time of the schizo-paranoid position, Klein's (1935) theory predicts that the primitive schism will be overcome with the integration of the good and bad breast in the depressive position. The depressive position presupposes an integration or wholeness within the subject and the object. It follows from these assumptions that, in the Kleinian model, the splitting of the psyche would be attributed to psychoses and not to neurosis. A normal ego would be unified or whole rather than divided. Since Freud's theory presupposes that primary repression establishes the structure and divisions of the normal psyche, it is unclear how splitting or division would be a characteristic solely of psychoses.

According to Freudian theory, a psychotic structure, or a stage of development, such as the schizo-paranoid position, has to represent a failure or delay in primary repression and the installation of foreclosure in lieu of primary repression, but the Kleinian model has no way of theorizing this without Freudian theory.

If primary repression has failed and foreclosure been installed in its place, then there is no way that a subject could overcome the schizo-paranoid position and move towards more advanced forms of development. To overcome a psychotic state in development, a primary repression in language is required. The treatment of psychoses requires that something else (a sinthome) be installed in lieu of both primary repression (no longer possible) and foreclosure.

This something else is what Lacan calls the sinthome or a new Name for the father and the father of the Name. In lieu of the original NoF that was foreclosed and left the subject outside the symbolic order, a new Name has to be installed. This new Name emerges from a different dimension that Lacan conceived in terms of the topological knot of four.

In the knot of three for psychosis, the links between the Symbolic and reality remain conventional, while images remain unlinked to original foreclosed signifiers. With the sinthome, images and signifiers are re-linked to one another, and isolated traumatically Real signifiers can become linked to S_2 or conventional signifieds, thanks to the Sinthome functioning in lieu of the original NoF that was foreclosed.

In the knot of three leading to psychosis, the catastrophe happens at the place and when the Imaginary is not tied to the Symbolic. When this intersection fails, the Imaginary becomes loose and is no longer tied to the rest of the knot. Psychosis alternates between loose associations and rigidified or automaton-like conventional and concrete speech devoid of symbolic signification. The sinthome is what compensates for paternal deficit and what keeps the Imaginary tied to the Symbolic. The sinthome is what compensates for the error at the place where the Symbolic ties the Imaginary to the knot of three. In neurosis, the NoF is what ties the Imaginary to the Oedipal knot. The NoF is what subsumes the imaginary relation between a–a' (the suckling infant and the mother's breast) under the signifier, and the signifier over the signified. When this fails, then a–a' remains loose and unlinked to the signifiers that define them.

The intervention of the sinthome makes a difference when it happens at the same site where the error took place. When the sinthome is set up in the same place where the slip occurred in the knot, then the primitive structure of the knot of three subsists. But why does Lacan say that the fourth ring comes out of a second Real associated with the consistency of the entire knot? The sinthome or the NoF comes out of the Real rather than from the Symbolic or the Imaginary, because the Real as the Third is self-same (empty and without differentiations as an absolute difference), while the Imaginary and the Symbolic cannot exist without each other and are not identical to themselves (I is an Other). The Real is redoubled, and this second Real is the sinthome that now links the Borromean knot of four together. Self-sameness in the Imaginary and Real are not the same. Self-sameness in the Real is always the same absolute difference. Self-sameness in the Imaginary is the projection and replication of a narcissistic structure.

The sinthome is a new metaphor for the subject that will function in lieu of the original or traditional NoF that was foreclosed in the case of the psychotic. In the treatment of psychoses, this refers not to finding any metaphors for the subject but metaphors that may make symbolic castration bearable for a particular subject. A sinthome may restore some level of functioning within the Symbolic order of social law and language. Such signifiers may be found within the symptoms of the subject that, by being symbolized within a process of nomination, become sinthomes.

As seen in the quotes previously, in Freudian theory, the primitive form of projection is best defined according to Lacan's concept of foreclosure that coincides in all essentials with the second definition given by Freud. The advantage of calling it foreclosure, instead of projection or repudiation, is that it underscores its radical nature, as well as reserving the term 'projection' for one of the ways that repression can operate within neurosis.

The difference between schism in psychoses and spaltung in neurosis translates into a split between the inside and the outside and where, by refusing primary repression and the intervention of the paternal function, the subject is not normally and neurotically divided. Instead, a wider and more intense conflict is set up between the internal world and the external social symbolic world. The internal world of the drive that has not risen to the level of symbolic desire, through the mediation of the specular image and the ideal ego, fails to be symbolized and menaces subjectivity with the chaos of unmediated sexual and aggressive drives.

In turn, the Other is perceived as threatening to annihilate the subject. The psychotic subject remains paradoxically undivided due the fusion with the mother presided over by the imaginary object that the child represents for the mother (an imaginary One, therefore). The psychotic has resisted neurotic division, only to fall into a more fundamental form of disintegration.

> According to Lacan what prevents primary repression from being established is the foreclosure (thrown out of the symbolic order) of the Name of the Father (NoF). In the defense known as foreclosure, the NoF, as the source of primary repression, is not simply repressed.
>
> (Moncayo, 2017, p. 2)

When the symbolically castrating intervention of the father does not take place and the fusion with the mother (jouissance of the Other) is not lost, the NoF and primary repression are not established. Instead, the function of castration returns in the form of a hallucination or delusion that threatens to destroy the subject. Instead of installing the NoF that normally divides the subject, the NoF is foreclosed and returns from the external world rather than from inside the subject. Instead of internalized, and after projection and foreclosure, the NoF enters consciousness in the form of a threatening external perception (the end of the world). Projection in this case is how foreclosure (rather than primary repression) is brought about. In contrast to this, projection proper can only occur after primary repression has taken place.

Freud (1930) called psychosis "a desperate attempt at rebellion" (p. 31). But according to Lacan, what returns from the outside is not the bad breast but the foreclosed NoF that comes back in persecutory form to destroy the identity of the subject. The foreclosure of the NoF, more than Klein's schizo-paranoid position or the absence of mourning, leaves the psychotic subject with concrete words but without the capacity to symbolize them.

The loss of the breast is an aspect of a larger symbolic, cultural, and mathematical operation at work in the phallic function that subtracts the imaginary phallus/*objet a* from the subject at different faces/phases of development: weaning and the breast, sphincter control and feces, sexual difference and the phallus. Grief rather than depression is the corresponding "normal" affect for all these losses. Grief only becomes depression when the object cause of the loss is repressed and hate towards the object prevails over love. The signifier is first the signifier of a lack or an absence, and this principle is more important for the theory than the empirical or lived loss of the breast during individual development, although the latter is how structure is experienced. The signifier and its laws (metaphor and metonymy, condensation and displacement) help the subject humanize the aggressiveness triggered by loss.

When self and other, subject and object, are condensed or fused into images, then this state of affairs, according to Freud, corresponds to what he calls the primary process. Condensation for Freud happens mostly in images that are the privileged mode of expression and meaning in the Unconscious (Ucs) as seen in the example of dreams. In the preconscious (Pcs), or the Unconscious in a descriptive sense (Ucs-Pcs), there is limited displacement and condensation. In this case, signifiers cannot be successfully evaded. A mnemonic link remains between signifiers in metonymy, and condensation is never complete: a trace of the opposite or of the Other remains in the subject and the signifier.

Foreclosure and psychotic projection function with images and fantasies because in psychosis, fantasy, rather than metaphor, has taken the place of perception, or the internal world has replaced the symbolically organized external world. Inside and outside, self and other, reality and fantasy are fused. It is important to notice that for Freud (1900), visual representations, in fantasies and dreams, serve as defenses against signifiers of desire. Fantasies support desire and at the same time defend against symbolic castration, as Lacan said.

> In the course of the formation of a dream these essential elements, charge as they are, with intense interest, may be treated as though they were a small value, and their place may be taken in the dream by other elements, of whose small value in the dream-thoughts there can be no question.
>
> (Freud, 1900, p. 341)

> Incidentally, reversal, or turning a thing into it opposite, is one of the means of representation most favored by the dream-work and one which is capable of employment in the most diverse direction. . . . Again, reversal is of quite special use as a help to the censorship.
>
> (idem, p. 362)

> The intensity of the elements in the one has no relation to the intensity of the elements in the other: the fact is that a complete 'transvaluation of all cyclical values' (in Nietzsche's phrase) takes place between the material of the dream-thoughts and the dream. A direct derivative of what occupies a dominating position in the dream-thoughts can often only be discovered precisely in some transitory element of the dream which is quite overshadowed by more powerful images.
>
> (idem, p. 365)

Censorship takes place by concealing dream-thoughts through two mechanisms: converting thoughts or signifiers into images and then inverting their values. What was significant in the dream-thoughts becomes insignificant in the dream-images, and what was significant in the dream images is insignificant at the level of the dream-thoughts.

Images are repressive before they are repressed, contrary to how things are usually understood. The projection and processing of images is usually understood as a primitive or archaic form of representation that escapes the laws of language and the Symbolic. Instead, visual representation in dreams and fantasy consists of adopting images that serve the purpose of drive-regulation and censorship of signifying elements. For example, Picasso's painting *Guernica* has this function for the modern world. Does the anxiety represented by the violence in the image precede its condemnation, or does the image represent a violation of a founding no with respect to violence? In either case, *Guernica* functions as a stop-sign on massacres and genocide by identifying the opposite within the image. The affirmative determination revealed in a disturbing image is its own censorship.

Of course, that visual perception, in the social construction of reality, functions differently from dreams because it is taking place at the front end rather than in the dark back cave of the mind. But since front and back are in a Moebius strip, what is received up front is interpreted at the back end, and what is a linguistic code at the back end is transformed into images at the front end. In dreams, both front (perception) and back (representation) are taking place at the back end of the mind/brain. Images in visual perception are the objective embodiment of linguistic signifiers (like algorithms behind computer images), while images in dreams and fantasies defend against and seek relief from the very same signifiers.

The symbolic process that takes place in fantasies and dreams is akin to projection and introjection, because fantasy and the other of reality are inside one another. The symbolic and discrete distance between contradictory subjects and signifiers of desire is undone by representing images containing contradictory elements. For example, an adult analysand dreamt that he was at a family gathering at the family home. When he went to the bathroom, he found a mummified corpse that transfigured into a beautiful woman.

In the associations, the corpse represented the dead father (that he killed in fantasy and had died in life) that stood in the way of him having a beautiful woman. In Oedipal structure, either a man has a father and loses the mother to the father or gains a mother that agrees with the son that the son is a better partner for the mother than the father. In this case, gaining means losing the father function along the way. In the dream, the either/or function between father and beautiful mother/woman are represented by projecting contrary elements and placing them inside the same image.

If the subject introjects the beautiful woman and now has the beautiful woman of the family home, then this satisfaction will suppress the hostility towards the father and repress the signifiers associated with the law of the father (by representing the father as a '*mummy*'). But this could also lead to the fantasy that if he has the woman of his fantasy, he himself will (through introjection) become a dead man like his father, once guilt and censorship obtain the better part of the subject. The forbidden woman becomes deadly.

In order to speak of introjection and projection, a prior distinction between inside and outside becomes necessary. Introjection and projection are symbolically structured. In this sense, defense formations are predicated on the prior existence of primary repression and the installation of the NoF as a key symbolic signifier. Once psychical structure is established through repression and consequent symbolization, then self and other, or subject and object, or any pair for that matter, could presumably be contained within a single dream image.

This differs from integrated visual images associated with waking ordinary perceptions that are symbolically structured. Integrated here means integrated by signifying elements that link up the various visual representations of objects and alter egos (i[a's] or intersubjective others) into a symbolic environmental net. But prior to that, in the perception of the unified body image in the mirror (ideal ego or specular image), for example, the subject perceives a unified body image that previously only existed as a series of uncoordinated bodily movements. What unifies the body image is both the mother's desire behind the image and the Naming of the image associated with the NoF.

Now the subject has a matheme (i[a]), or ideal ego, named and loved by the Other, with which to relate to other alter egos or i(a', a_1', a_2' . . .). The numbers in the 'a's represent the capture of the earlier a–a', then i(a)–i(a') relationship, into the battery of signifiers and net of the Symbolic order. However, since the *a* in the image of the body or ideal ego is missing, the ego will look for the alter ego to close this gap, only to discover that the *a* has also fallen off the Other as well. In an earlier book, we proposed a formula for symbolic castration,

> Mathematically Phi – phi (1,618 – 0,618) = 1. This can be seen as the formula for the phallic function of castration. Phi – phi = the "symbolic phallus" minus the "imaginary phallus" . . . -phi or the lack of the imaginary phallus generates a lack-of-being; a hole within the whole that subjects endlessly try to fill with *objets a*. It does not work because -phi is a signifier without a signified (phallic function). It is a symbolic castration that creates a gap thereby representing a point of lack in the subject.
>
> (Moncayo and Romanowicz, 2015, p. 130)

Phi – phi = 1 is the formula for symbolic castration, where only by accepting the lack (-phi) with the help of Phi can the subject arrive at One as an imaginary number or i (imaginary in the mathematical, not Lacanian, sense). Otherwise, the subject keeps looking for the fantasy object in reality and in the axis of real numbers (real in the mathematical sense and in the sense of external reality).

According to the formula Phi – phi, as the formula for symbolic castration, Phi subtracts the *a* (phi) and turns every i(a) and i(a'1,2,3,4) into a 1 that can be used as either a real or imaginary number. Phi is the quantity or power by which phi changes into 1 as either a series of real numbers or a series of imaginary numbers. In this sense, the formula for castration also qualifies as a logarithm for images.

By phi missing from Phi, Phi becomes either a real 1 or an imaginary 1. Either 1 has the *objet a* missing from it. With *a* or *-a* missing in real whole-body images, the subject tries to fill the hole with other alter egos and their missing *objet a* in a futile exercise that is played at the level of images. Instead of another whole image or number, what needs to be symbolized and made manifest in numbers is the 1 as an imaginary number that appears in the hole in the image. Otherwise the alleged whole objects and alter egos or intersubjective others go from being whole numbers to being like the song: "a little bit of Monica, and Gloria, and Veronica in my life," the partial *objet a* of the subject in its various iterations.

According to Lacan, a body image also features a blank spot or a hole that points to an absence or point of lack in the ideal ego that represents the fact that the mother's desire is also turned towards the Other (the child is not the end all and be all of the mother). The hole in the image turns the subject away from fixating to the image of the ideal ego or alter ego and indicates a turn towards the big Other that will transform the ideal ego into an ego ideal.

We don't bring together visual objects so that their prior objective resemblance is made manifest, but rather, given the existence of language and a cultural symbolic world, both difference and resemblance between visual objects are distinguished at the level of the signifier. "It would be a mistake to think that the Other (with a capital O) of discourse can be absent from any distance that the subject achieves in his relationship with the other, (with a lower-case o) of the imaginary dyad" (Lacan, 2006, p. 568).

For the psychotic, we may have to use the language of projective identification, but not for neurosis, as the object relations school more and more has been inclined to do. Eventually the Kleinian model becomes a replacement for rather than an extension of Freud's theory. In addition, the risk of using projective identification as a cognitive mode in the treatment of psychoses is that it may further loosen an Imaginary register (strengthening the disorder along the way) in the psychotic subject that is already quite detached from the symbolic order. The analyst may contain the loose Imaginary register of the psychotic, but the Imaginary may be further detached if the analyst is unable to contain the material that was projected unto the analyst. Better results might be obtained by the construction of a fourth ring that will re-link the Imaginary to the Symbolic and the Real, as Lacan recommended. The fourth ring is made with signifying material within the experience of psychosis rather than by the metaphors or elements of experience within the subjectivity of the analyst himself or herself.

I am aware that Bion and others have successfully used projective identification in the treatment of psychoses. According to this orientation, the treatment cannot proceed if the analyst is intolerant of the patient's method of communicating via projective identification. In such cases, the analyst cannot stand not using words to communicate, and the words of the analyst, under conditions of frustration or anger, will be experienced by the psychotic subject as a mutilating attack on their projective methods of communication. How can the analyst overcome this impasse? Since the psychotic cannot tolerate the Symbolic or the NoF that has been radically foreclosed, object relations theory would encourage the analyst to use projective identification, even if this is understood as a pathological formation taking place after the foreclosure of the NoF.

In psychoses, words are used concretely as objects rather than as signifiers or metaphors and are often used to describe actions without a subject or object. For example, a psychotic subject may repeatedly utter the senseless words: "arms and legs." It is a mistake for the analyst to provide the subject, object, and what of a sentence, since this aspect of language is defended against. The patient's attempts at defending from the verbal interventions of the Other, by renewing the foreclosure of the NoF, may result in psychotic decompensation. Introducing syntax or the subject, object, and verb of a sentence could lead a sentence such as "arms and legs" to mean that "the Other has cut off my arms and legs." The new sentence manifests a concrete and unsymbolized image for the symbolic castration that has been foreclosed.

An analyst can use pure signifiers or S_1 that may generate organizing metaphors for a subject but without linking them to an S_2. In the formula for the paternal metaphor or NoF (S_2/S_1), S_2 is in the place of the agent, while in the discourse of the master, S_1 is in the place of the agent. In the case of the master, S_1 is the signifier of an ideology or a delusion ($S_1 \rightarrow S_2$), while in the paternal metaphor, S_2, or the NoF, is in the place of the agent. In the treatment of psychoses, S_1 has to be used without an imposing ideology and without overtly being signifiers of a father or of the Law. S_1 is used as a signifier of jouissance in the same way that for jouissance, the signifier points to something outside the Symbolic.

In dreams and fantasies, signifiers (of lack) are replaced by the objects that represent and displace them (metonymic objects), while the link to the original signifiers is obstructed. In dreams and fantasies, signifiers and part-reality object representations, like Chinese ideograms, are embedded in the internal visual object of fantasy. However, the independence of imaginary elements is illusory. Signifiers or verbal elements are projected and introjected into images, but the images are symbolically structured. It would be a mistake, in this case, to think that projection and introjection function in a psychical process that uses only ideographs and visual representation as a medium. This is only the case in psychoses due to the foreclosure of the NoF. Psychotic statements are like dream images that treat words as objects or things, except for the fact that the underlying signifiers are not symbolically structured. In psychotic thinking, logical entailment is not possible due to a failure in the structure of language. The failure of linguistic and logical structure is clouded over by the noise generated by statements that obscure who is speaking, to whom, and about what.

The psyche cannot be neatly divided into a psychoanalysis for earlier pre-verbal stages organized by the projection and introjection of internal visual representations and a verbal psychoanalysis for later stages of development and neurotic analysands. In this formulation, transference in psychosis would be handled with the concept of projective identification, while transference in neurosis, which presupposes differentiation or difference between self and other, is understood via the concept of repression and repetition.

Things do not work this way. The psyche is a Borromean knot. Fantasy as *perception* and projection in psychosis is understood as a function of the foreclosure of the NoF. It is not the case that a defense against the NoF and the imposition of language would happen later than a prior pre-verbal commerce and communication via projected and introjected images. The latter already presupposes primary repression and the installation of the NoF.

Visual object representations are not an earlier form of fragmentary communication with the object world, since the latter is already symbolically structured. In psychoses, what happens is that a symbolically structured Imaginary does not take place due to the foreclosure of the NoF. There is no normal imaginary that is not symbolically structured.

Symbolic structure is not something that happens after a period of communication via images has taken place. Projective identification is not a normal primitive form of communication that provides a foundation for verbal communication, because in normal neurosis, the Imaginary and the Symbolic are intrinsically tied from the get-go. A neurotic subject does not start with projective identification as a medium for communication only to later graduate to primary repression and the use of language and the NoF. The latter is what happens first, and if it fails, as in foreclosure, then projective identification may become an alternative mode of communication.

Psychotic use of language gives the appearance of an imaginary language prior to language proper, but this is an illusion produced by the foreclosure of a key signifier organizer of the order of language. In psychoses, fragmentary communication via images and projective identification take place due to the foreclosure of the NoF, not because a catastrophe took place and produced a fixation to an earlier stage of development that in normal development is presided over by images of subject and object that are not symbolically structured.

Projection and introjection appear to function within a psychical process that uses only ideographs and visual representation as a medium. In normal neurosis, projection and introjection function within a symbolically structured imaginary. However, since in psychoses, the Symbolic order is compromised by the foreclosure of the NoF, images are processed differently. It is foreclosure that generates an imaginary projective plane unlinked to the Symbolic. For example, when symbolization has proceeded enough to identify Oedipal wishes in projective imaginary material, then the psychotic subject will concentrate its attacks not on a symbolic ego but on the paternal metaphor that was foreclosed. Finally, when projective identification is used in the presence of foreclosure, then imaginary fusion or the collapsing of normal self-other differentiations, results in states of confusion and malevolent depersonalization.

Projective identification as a psychotic defense functions purely in the Imaginary without symbolic structure. In the Kleinian model, symbolic structure is emotionally established by the mother (through projective identification) rather than by the intervention of the father and the Symbolic. For example, a father may say no to a child: "You are not old enough to see that horror movie without becoming disturbingly afraid" (sparing the child the malevolent jouissance), while the mother may allow the child to see the horror movie but then will listen to the recounting of the movie by the child and in the process contain and soothe the 'bad internal objects' that the horror movie triggered in the child. The mother helps the child process the horror and the no and the horror of the father's no and name (*L'e no(m) du* père). The successful use of projective identification by the mother in "normal" development is predicated on the installation of the NoF and the paternal metaphor.

Under ordinary circumstances, the combination of the no of the father and the desire of the mother to contain the fear of the child would be a good example of the paternal function. This is an alternative to solely thinking of the mother's good-enough caregiving as the necessary factor for the child's character formation. Both, in fact, are needed, but containment as a limit already is a metaphor for the father's no. In temperance, the father's no is firmly established in such a way that the subject does not even have to struggle with self-control. The continent and incontinent person struggles with self-control and is one or two steps removed from temperance and may need the Other's container. The so-called normal neurotic is able to be temperate in their self-control, while those that are continent struggle with self-control and often need the Other's help in attaining self-control. The continent and incontinent need the Other to contain the passions that they themselves cannot control.

When the subject is overwhelmed by fantasy objects, especially when presented as images generated by social reality (the film industry, for example), then the subject is functioning solely in an imaginary dream or reverie that deceives and obscures rather than revealing the fundamental structures of subjectivity. Freud himself was partly responsible for this confusion when he said something like an archaic unconscious image is made conscious with a verbal representation.

Lacan has made it clear for psychoanalysis that language cannot be reduced to consciousness or the Pcs system. The Unconscious contains signifiers and not only archaic visual pre-verbal thought, and the only reason researchers don't see this is because we are under the allure and illusions of the Imaginary. The signifier is both analytic and synthetic, and visual images, of course, are not without a synthetic element, since many would argue that this is their main characteristic. Analysis requires links that already constitute a form of synthetic element, and synthesis is synthesis of separate signifying elements brought into relation to one another.

Hysteria and psychosis

In hysteria, the basic division in the subject reflects a conflict not only between drives and defenses, defenses that are drives, as well as vice versa, but also a "cleavage" between the desire of the mother and the NoF. The desire of the mother for the child completes both in the Imaginary, while the desire of the mother for the NoF reveals the lack in the (m)Other and transfers maternal omnipotence to the father (omnipotence is curbed in the father when the imaginary father is substituted for the symbolic father). It is the lack in the Other and the subject that divides the hysteric, while it is the attributed completeness of the Other that divides the obsessional. We observe that in hysteria, and neurosis in general, the desire of the mother and the NoF (paternal/parental metaphor), as well as the specular image, have all been established.

The schizoid personality, according to Guntrip (1973, following Fairbairn), is characterized by a division between a shy, introverted, embarrassed, or a cold and aloof/detached disposition and a secret, vulnerable, needy, and fear-ridden infantile state. The schizoid individual cannot love or feel warmth towards anyone and suffers from a dreaded sense of isolation and being an automaton without a separate identity (malevolent depersonalization). The first side of the division represents repressive defenses, while the second represents the repressed. Shyness as a character trait embodies the repressive, while fear of annihilation embodies the repressed or that which is being destroyed. Therefore, the repressive and the repressed formally (homomorphically) arch over both psychosis and neurosis. In this larger framework, then, how do these two forms of split/division differ?

Theoretically, a double division should be particularly problematic for the schizoid condition. However, it is not that the psychotic subject is divided and the neurotic is unified, because the developmental upgrade involved with neurosis is another form of division. In the schizoid condition, the family environment has failed to provide the mother's desire and the containing symbolic linguistic environment presided over by the NoF. Both failures hamper the capacity of the human subject to grow within a symbolic or linguistic environment, the equivalent of what air or water would represent for a bird or a fish.

Guntrip (1973) gives a wonderful example from his practice. His analysand dreamt that she "opened a locked steel drawer and inside was a tiny naked baby with open expressionless eyes, staring at nothing" (p. 152). The breast is a nothing for the baby in this instance because "*l'petit enfant*" has not been installed as the cause of the mother's desire, and the child is either neglected, is treated solely as an impersonal object, or is treated as an object but not as a subject. These three different vicissitudes may actually result in different pathological conditions.

The repressed here constitutes not repressed desire within the subject but a repressed absence of desire in the mother that can be described as a deficit of desire (no feeling or interest in the baby) more than the lack within desire that constitutes desire. Guntrip (1973) uses the happy expression that "sensitivity has fled into the subject." The overt individual is aloof, shy, or insecure, but the hidden divided aspect is extremely sensitive and fearful. Sensitivity that is both input and output into the world is not available to a pre-subject trapped inside a steel drawer.

Winnicott calls the true self (the Lacanian S or pre-subject but with the accent placed on sensitivity) to that aspect of the child that responds to the mother's desire and to the signifiers of the (f)Other. When this fails in the family environment, the so-called true self is "put into cold storage with a secret hope of rebirth" into a bona fide mathematical/oedipal structure. The true self, in the sense of the pre-subject, does not only represent the healthy and normal growth of a child's mind or character under good-enough mothering, since it also represents the undifferentiation of self and other that will transform the pre-subject into an object of the mother's desire and fantasy. The good of development (the pleasure of the good) and the good of the fantasy (the good of pleasure) are initially bound up together. One can only artificially separate them by different theoretical models that pick and choose one or the other model, according to their psycho-social-gender predilections.

What Winnicott calls a true self is the normal sense of a divided self that, like cell mitosis, is necessary for the development of the organism and psychic structure. The division of the subject is presided over by the mother's good-enough desire for the child (that allows for fusion and for separation) and the father's good-enough intervention that helps the child separate from the mother and from the inconvenient jouissance of the Other. Separation, as a result of internal division and entry into the Symbolic order, is necessary for the replication of psychical structure.

In fact, the division (in one person) between an aloof schizoid character and a severely damaged human being is a grotesque caricature of a more structured neurotic division of subjectivity. Both the desire of the mother and the NoF are stunted in their development and remain like frozen vestiges of a future that never happened. Guntrip (1973) calls this the "loss of mental rapport with the mother at a time that the mother represents the whole object world" (p. 162).

Guntrip's (1973) model mistakes the work of division in psychoses and neuroses, due to their similarity under a structural homomorphic principle that replicates division in neurosis and psychoses, but with a difference. In the field of biological semiotics, von Uexküll (1987) proposed the concept of homomorphy to describe a fundamental principle that recurs at different levels of complexity. The normal neurotic subject is also divided rather than unified. If an observer supposes that a normal subject is unified and that only a psychotic subject is divided, then when they perceive a normal and neurotic subject's division, the initial supposition may lead them to think that this apparent hysteric or obsessional neurotic is a psychotic.

In addition, the model confuses the work of division in psychoses and neuroses with the symptoms found in the different structures. Correspondingly, the model mixes up the various forms of personality disorders: schizoid, hysterical, obsessive, depressive; even the drives become anthropomorphized into sexual and aggressive personalities, and so on (not unlike the PDM). Form and content, structure and symptom, are confused in these examples.

With Lacan, we would simply say that the schizoid character is a psychotic structure with neurotic symptoms until such a time when precipitating factors trigger a full onset of psychoses out of a pre-existing psychotic structure. In this case, there would not be a psychotic part of the personality, as Bion (1967) has argued. Instead of a difference between a schizotypal personality disorder and a psychotic disorder, there is an actual difference between manifest and unmanifest structures.

If anything, and ironically, we could say that when asymptomatic, a psychotic structure is wearing a neurotic mask. The so-called mask is composed of all the functions that were acquired in development despite the damage and deficit at the more basic core level already described. When, in some cases, the core paternal metaphor is healed and re-established with the aid of the sinthome, then a psychotically structured individual can re-inhabit their human functions now renewed and enlivened (sensitivity reestablished) thanks to the fourth ring of the sinthome and the transformation of jouissance it entails. "To the paranoid three could be knotted, under the heading of a symptom, a fourth term which would situate as such, as personality. The Borromean chain of four no longer constitutes a paranoia" (Lacan [1975–1976], Session of 12.16.75, III 10).

If the division of the subject in neurosis is taken for the division of the subject in psychosis (*spaltung for schizo*), then this would lead one to the mistaken conclusion that hysteria has roots in schizophrenia. The structural demands of a hysteric for the imaginary phallus that the mother lacks are confused for the demand to be loved by a child who has not been the object of the mother's desire. It is important to clarify here that in the Lacanian field, male hysteria is as prevalent, if not more so, than female hysteria, contrary to contemporary prejudice in the culture. The male hysteric is the one that is constantly trying to show his virility to his mother. The female hysteric is constantly trying to prove and show that she, and only she, is the ideal woman.

The first hypothesis seems objectionable to some (the demand for the imaginary phallus) from the point of phenomenological or humanistic values (that critique the objectification of other human beings), because the *objet a* is taken for a commodity and this leads to the false conclusion that if children are desired as *objet a*, then this means that they are being objectified rather than genuinely loved.

A child in the position of being an object of their mother's desire, and that this object constitutes a narcissistic form or gratification/compensation for the mother, is something inevitable, and nature would not have it any other way, since it secures adequate care-giving for the survival of the individual and the species.

At the same time, a child needs to be treated as a subject and not just an object of desire, and this is what secures the "genuine concern for the other." The concern for the child as a subject is mediated by the intervention and recognition of the father, which is something that has already been prepared by the symbolic mother and the establishment of language. Both mother and father are needed to produce a normal neurotic subject and not just good-enough mothering, as Winnicott and Bion believed.

To distinguish between *objet a* and a commodity, one must distinguish between the *objet a* proper within psychoanalysis and the surplus aspect of (phallic) jouissance that as a "*lathouse*" can be extended into the marketplace (see the second appendix for more on the subject). A "*lathouse*" is the aspect of the *objet a* that secretly (*leteia*) animates a commodity object and could also turn it into a fetish (Braunstein, 2012; Lacan, 1969–1970).

Lacan has a paradoxical way of thinking about how the object of the drive and desire, as psychical objects, interact with contemporary forms of economic and symbolic exchange. On the one hand, he is suspicious of the early phase of protestant capitalism with its focus on divine service in the world and universally spreading the service of goods on the basis of continence and the abstinence of pre-marital sex (Lacan, 1960–1961, Seminar VII, session 11/16/1960). On the other hand, he calls the *objet a* the apparel of love (Lacan Seminar XV, Session of February 28, 1969, XI 3), or what makes consumers fall in love with the objects of consumption (O' I love that car, article of clothing, housing unit, haircut, etc.).

Does this mean that Lacan favors the disclosure of the *objet a* in consumption over its quality as the dignified void at the center of productive activity? Lacan clearly rejects thinking that the *objet a* or desire can be possibly satisfied with objects of consumption and at the same time rejects the idea of an ascesis or withholding of desire. Imaginary *objets a* turn service goods or commodities into false objects (the fetishism of commodities), while the only true object is the *objet a* that, as a Real object, needs to fall off or detach from objects of consumption.

In the same way, the ethics of psychoanalysis for Lacan, or the place of psychoanalysis in civilization, includes a form of sceptic ataraxia, temperance, and equanimity necessary to sustain analytic dialogue without speaking too soon or too late, too little or too much, or at least knowing when to do one rather than the other. On the other hand, psychoanalysis does not have an ideal of dispassion, since passion also has a place in the production of subjective truth as a form of jouissance. Ataraxia or equanimity differs from ascesis, since it also includes a temperance that allows for convenient forms of jouissance and rational forms of pleasure. The middle way is not asceticism.

A psychotic has not been the *objet a* for the mother, and this is why they are objectified or treated like a bizarre or crazy creature that covers the mother's lack. They are not objectified because they are loved or desired as an object cause of desire, they are objectified because they are not in that place, and the NoF was foreclosed for them. A psychotic individual is identified with being the unbarred object of the mother's desire either because they did not occupy that place or because the referred object was not barred by the father's intervention, either because of the mother's repudiation of the NoF or because of the father being too brutal or weak to intervene and be symbolized.

Hysterical demands instead respond to structural oedipal rejections rather than environmental deficit or neglect. In addition, the psychotic subject does not demand like the hysteric. Although hysterics level many complaints against the Other, the psychotic complains of fantasized perceptions of the Other's abuse. Hysterics may or may not have been sexually abused. Psychical structure itself is sufficient reason to produce sexual trauma, even in the absence of actual abuse. Hysterical complaints are demands to receive the imaginary phallus that was barred under the paternal metaphor. Guntrip and Fairbairn could not establish these structural differentiations due to their particular and structural misreading and misunderstanding of Freudian theory.

The model associated with the study of the schizoid personality needed to be explained according to Freudian theory, or the theory adjusted, but without triggering a misleading overhaul. To a great extent, the latter is what Jung, Klein, Bion, and Winnicott actually did. Although Lacan has been critiqued for claiming a return to Freud, only to develop a new theory, Lacan was much more careful, detailed, and responsive to Freud's theory than either Bion or Winnicott. Winnicott's work, however, has added a wealth of observations regarding the part played by the mother's desire in normal development.

Freudian scholarship flowered under Lacan (i.e. Laplanche, Pontalis, and Green), and nowadays it is Lacanians that mostly pay any serious scholarly attention to Freud. The rest of psychoanalysis treats Freud as a dying dinosaur, a suppressed fossil or museum piece, despite the claim to descendancy from Freud.

Thus, Freud can no longer be studied without Lacan, since Lacan is primarily responsible for raising Freud's work to a new level of relevance for the twenty-first century and beyond. Given that the object relations school neglected and ignored, or even disavowed, the function of the father, due to confusing the paternal function with the imaginary father or mother (patriarchy and matriarchy as ideologically understood), any understanding of the function of the father in Freud will have to go through Lacanian theory.

Klein helped developed the practice of child analysis, and her work on this matter is fundamental. Along the way, Klein invented her own new theory to extend Freudian theory to earlier developmental stages than those studied by Freud. In the process, she developed an alternative *model* for psychoanalysis used to treat all conditions (fixated at different levels of development) and replacing Freud's theory (not a model).

A theory is not always right and needs to be tested (in the broad sense of the term) and improved while maintaining fundamental structural components and differentiating them from new ones. Jung did this for his part, but he trivialized Freud's theory of the formations of the unconscious, the relationship of language to the unconscious, the practice of analysis, and built an entire new theory instead of extending Freud's.

Lacan's later theory is an extension of Freud's thought, but the two theories are internally correlated and part of a single Borromean structure: from the speech equivocations of the Other of the Freudian unconscious, to the equivocations of what Lacan calls lalangue in the Real unconscious. The unconscious in the dimension of the Real uses sound (homophony more than metaphor or metonymy) to condense similar-sounding words. Condensation of sounds reverses the displacements of the metonymy of meaning in language and generates, thereby, new metaphors not previously available in the metaphors and words displaced.

The Freudian unconscious is the language of the Other, while the Real unconscious, of Lacan's later work, is the language of the One. Let me offer an example. An analysand enunciated the words experience and appearance in a way that made them sound the same. In either case, it was not clear whether experience meant appearance or vice versa. Instead, because sound is involved, rather than simply syntax, the sound points to something in common between the two words. Homophony points to a new meaning or significance for the jouissance contained in both words for a subject.

Experience and structure are what make and define a subject, and at the same time something new appears in experience, since the subject is not simply the repetition or reiteration of past experience (automaton). Experience, as automaton, only appears to represent something new. Experience is how a structure appears, not what appears. At the same time, old experience may not be relevant for new experience. Experience is structural rather than based on prior experience as a form of past contingent conditioning, and at the same time, the structure has a synchronic vanishing point instant within diachronic experience. There is an untotalized and unconditioned aspect of experience that leaves experience open for the subject to appear in an entirely new light associated with surprise or Tyche, as an event that re-articulates structure in the act of speech. Body, speech, and mind engage the interactions between language and the experience of the Real as something new outside language.

Furthermore, the Real is revealed both in *lalangue* and in mathematical structure. What does this mean? A good example is provided when the same meaning is maintained across languages. Linguists typically think these similarities in meaning or structure are just random variations. The words experience and appearance in Chinese have the same similarity in sound as in English, a difference that points to the same structural similarities and differences outlined. Chinese people and North Americans speak a different language, but both Americans and Chinese use the same mathematical language. The similarity in sound could, in fact, reflect the underlying mathematical structure involved in the transmission of sound waves.

This new significance of the signifier in the Real of speech and jouissance carries the analytical process forward by leading to a subject's illumination (in this case, Real jouissance functions as signified) by the signifier. The transformations of meaning and jouissance (from the first to the Third jouissance) associated with *lalangue* (and significance as a category within symbolic language) function as an antidote to the translocation patterns of the displacements of meaning and objects in the Imaginary that turn desire into neurotic suffering and conflicts with the Other.

Lalangue is the language of the One because *lalangue* transforms jouissance by gathering and condensing meaning under a unifying principle without repressing past meaning. Lalangue carries a metaphor forward to a new significance within jouissance that is more than feeling and emotion. The emotional truth of an analytical session (as the signified) refers to transformations of a subject's jouissance while speaking about feelings generated by the words or actions of the Other.

According to Lacanian theory, the first pre-subject (S) and the primitive psyche contain the alternating currents of love and hate towards the *objet a*. In Lacan's (1954–1955, p. 243) schema L, a vector goes from S or the pre-subject to a', or from S to the breast or a'. From the breast, or the part object of the other, the vector goes to the specular image (i[a]), the body image, and the ideal ego [when written with an i as in: i(a)].

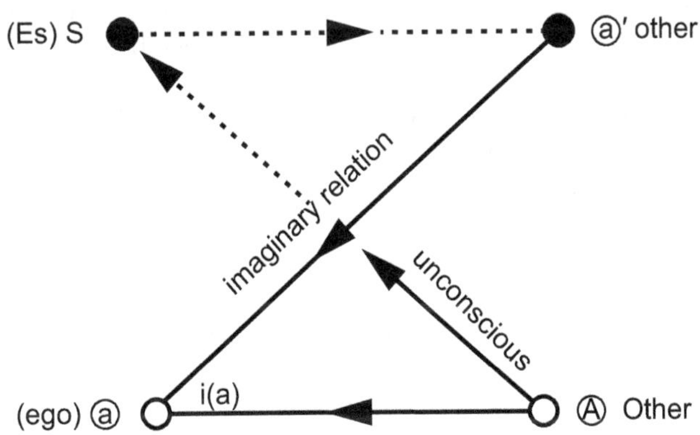

Figure 1.4 Schema L

Breast and mirror reflection, as empirical objects a' and i(a), pars and toto or 1 + a, body part and total body reflection, are mediated by the Phi function that subtracts a' from *a* (Phi – phi = 1). With the discovery of reflection, a sense of self (S) arises that is supposed to be the cause of the (m)Other's desire. This act is what finally integrates the positive and negative charges towards the same object (the good and bad breast that had been split off) as the Kleinian model predicted with respect to the breast.

The (m)Other's desire frames the subject to the same extent that the desire of the (m)Other is structured by the NoF as a law-bound signifier of desire. All normal neurotics accept this; otherwise, they would be psychotic or perverse or somewhere in between. The in between cases can be read as pointing to the borderline diagnosis or, more specifically, as the interaction between structure and symptoms in psychoses and neurosis. Just as there are psychotic structures with neurotic symptoms, the borderline diagnosis can be defined as a neurotic structure with psychotic symptoms.

But since the neurotic struggle with the NoF represents a struggle between the Imaginary and Symbolic registers and dimensions of the ego, the Real, according to Lacan, intervenes and links them inextricably to one another. The Symbolic of the earlier theory could not do this because the Symbolic was a party to the struggle (with the Imaginary), and problems cannot be resolved at the same level they were created.

Normal paranoia that feeds normal distortions and misunderstandings in communication, and normal distortions of vision, is when the ego identifies with and/or wants to supplant the binding function of the Real. For the knot of four that stabilizes a new knot of three (psychical structure), instead of the Symbolic binding the knot of three, the Real now seeks to bind the Imaginary and the Symbolic that are opposed and in conflict with one another. However, when the Real is misrecognized as the ordinary ego, then the Real, too, becomes a formidable and fear-inducing imposition that is all the more troubling given the incomprehensible aspect of the Real.

The ego instead has to become something Real or a new ego that ties RSI into a new Borromean structure of four rings. The subject of the Real or a new Real ego (Lacan, 1975–1976) has to bear the imposed or insufferable aspect of jouissance that links the body to a new metaphor of the subject. Instead of the paranoid ego supplanting the Real, the Real is what remains unconditioned in the subject beyond the conditionings of the ideal ego and ego ideal.

The deconstruction of the paranoid ego, in fact, is required to open a narrow side-path for the subject to pass beyond the precipice represented by the compulsive structure of neurosis (the automaton of repetition) and beyond the symbolic rock of castration. I have argued that this is what the knot of four entails in neurosis, as distinct from the knot of four that is needed to repair a psychotic structure (Moncayo, 2017).

The knot of four for neurosis is retied with the sinthome, or the NoF emerging from the Real, after the knot of three is untied in the analytic process. In the knot of three found in psychoses, the Imaginary is untied, while the Real and the Symbolic are still tied to each other. In this knot, the Imaginary supplants the Real, and the Symbolic fails to bind or structure the Imaginary. In the treatment of psychosis, the Imaginary is tied back to the Symbolic and the Real with the help of the sinthome.

The untying of the knot of three refers not only to deconstructing and re-signifying personal and institutional authority, the NoF, and repression, but also refers to a change in how the voice and gaze of the Other are experienced as an imposition independently from the content of the signifiers that may be at play. In psychosis, the voice is the voice of the super-ego that returns in the Real of a hallucination, while the psychotic subject is looked at from everywhere by an omnipresent gaze.

What I am calling the NoF coming from the second Real does not mean the return of the old-time Absolute, whether religious or scientific. If anything, the NoF emerging from the Real, or the sinthome, is potentially different for each singular subject and has to be found within pure signifiers of jouissance (S_1–S_0). The unconscious signifying chain contains the letters of a subject's Names, historical signifiers, and symptoms as signifiers of jouissance.

The capitalized Real as an absolute does not mean a religious Absolute, since it is a philosophical category in a pair-wise relation to relativity, which, of course, after Einstein, everyone accepts. That everything is relative is an absolute nowadays. Things being what they are can also be something else, and this something else can mean another signifier or S_2 but can also signify an experience of jouissance outside signification that I write as S_0. Everyone has to discover the particularity and singularity of the sinthome for themselves. Jouissance functions as the ultimate organizing factor for the various singularities in which a sinthome is revealed for each subject.

Jouissance represents the solidarity principle of the three Musketeers of Alexandre Dumas: Three for One and One for Three. The three jouissances are contained in the One of the Real (not the imaginary One of the first jouissance), and the Third jouissance can function in the other two, but the same is not true the other way around. As I have already explained in other works, the first jouissance is the jouissance of the Other, which becomes inconvenient if it is not replaced by phallic jouissance. The first jouissance answers the question "What object am I for the Other," or "What does the Other want from me?" The second jouissance, or phallic jouissance, is the only one of the three that passes over into the signifier (phallus = signifier of a lack).

The Third jouissance stems from the impossibility of surplus phallic jouissance and the tiresome narcissistic fact that phallic jouissance is always a question of who is or has the phallus. The symbolic phallus, or the function of symbolic castration, settles this problem by indicating the inexistence of the imaginary phallus and emphasizing that symbolic castration is an index of jouissance. These two elements transform phallic jouissance into the Third Other jouissance. The Third also comes in three forms: feminine jouissance, *J'ouis-sens* of meaning, and the jouissance of the mystic. For a more detailed examination of the three forms of jouissance (and the three forms of the Third), please refer to Chapter 3 of my book on Seminar XXIII.

The subject of the real "all-alone"

In the knot of four for neurosis, the subject drops body and mind and functions out of what Lacan (1975–1976) calls a Real ego. I call it an ego in the Real or, better, the subject of the Real. In the knot of four for neurosis, the normal and neurotic Oedipal knot of three is unknotted and then re-knotted. Instead of a paranoid and narcissistic (secondary or tertiary) ego that operates in the world in a survival and appropriative or exploitative mode, the subject of the Real is confirmed and realized by the treasury of the signifier and the 10,000 things/'no-things.'

The ego in the Real is Lacan's (1971–1972) subject 'All-alone,' or Winnicott's (1963) 'true isolate,' that, according to Lacan, appears in the place of the lack of sexual rapport between the sexes. The subject All-alone does not represent a failure in object relatedness but rather a healthy, benevolent, and satisfying form of solitude and aloneness that includes relationships and facilitates the possibility that relationships may in fact work out after all. Lacan's subject All-alone, however, is "not-All One whole Being," for also it is naught/not (Lacan, 2018, p. 218). That the Real subject is "All-alone" also means that in the Symbolic, the subject is "not-All alone." The subject (as signifier) is a collectivity within the Symbolic. But within the Real, the subject is All-alone, despite being many at the level of the signifier. From many One, and from One many, as stated in the motto of the United States (derived from Heraclitus' tenth fragment).

One cannot think of the subject All-alone, or the One that includes the many or the collectivity, as the isolated or autonomous ego of self-interest. Ego autonomy, or the fact that this is my desire, rather than the Other's desire for me, is centered around the concept of desire rather than a conflict-free sphere of the mind. The autonomy granted by the body image or the ideal ego is relative because the autonomous body image or self-image stands in as a substitute for the object of the mother's desire. The ego 'appropriates' the autonomous image of self from whom and what the ego thinks they are for the Other. As we see, the ego is not an area free of influence either from desire or language, because the ego is first an object of the Other.

Now when the ego or subject says this is my desire or this is what I want, the ego is not aware that they want something on the basis of a previously lost object. That is, ego autonomy or the ego's own desires are predicated on a subject divided between what they want and what they have lost or cannot have. In fact, the Other, or the social and public interest, represents what any human subject will come to view as their natural inclinations and capacities, along the lines established by prior human endeavor and knowledge. What establishes the public interest is the ego ideal as an identification with the (f)Other and human activities that the society expects from the subject (sleep patterns, hygiene, healthy diet, language acquisition, reading, writing, use of numbers, etc.). The ego is only autonomous on the basis of the mother's desire and an identification with the NoF and language rules. In fact, the ego often ignores the many ways in which their own interests are unconsciously determined by the Other. The ego would rather live in the illusion that their interests are self-made.

The subject of the Real, or an ego in the Real All-alone, on the one hand refers to creative activities that require solitude. Creative activities could be scientific or intellectual but could also be artistic, musical, spiritual, or physical. These are treasures of the Other found in the storehouse of the Mind and that spark a subject's desire or passion. The Other, or the heirlooms and treasury found in the storehouse of the Other, are revealed in the Other's desires for the subject that the subject acquires through identification love and an inevitable modicum of external coercion. Self-interest and the collective public interest are not opposed in the subject All-alone.

The solitude required for creative reflection and writing, for example, represents very particular types of social links. A solitary worker or researcher, for example, is alone in the sense that at the time of their research, they are not socializing or shopping or involved in family, recreational, or group activities, yet despite being alone, they are in the presence of the All-alone investigators that came before them. The subject All-alone is an integral part of the collective lineage of dead or alive minds that constitute a particular field of knowledge. In this sense, the subject is not alone but rather, in their own subjective experience of human nature and society, they are as if at One with those that came before them.

If a subject differs from others in style, content, or method, they nonetheless share the condition of being All-alone as one of the elements of the structure. This is a second characteristic of the subject in the Real: as one of the elements of a group, or a structure of interdependent elements, the subject is a '*sujet sans substance*' or without inherent nature other than that indicated by the relative relations between the signifiers or numbers that compose the structure. However, the emptiness and significance of each element, the non-being or senselessness that each element becomes when they function according to one of the names or elements designated by the structure, should not be underestimated.

Subjects become that about them, or their nature, that lies outside or is undefined or unformulated within the structure. However, this is something rather than zero and represents an experience of jouissance that lies outside the socially determined experience of desire. The letter a, as an *objet a*, is a particular letter for an alphabet of imaginary objects cause of desire (placenta, breath, breast, feces, urine, phallus, voice, gaze, and the nothing). However, the *a*, as a Real form of causality in the form of a gap, or a semblance of being, always dissipates before the Real, spreading jouissance over subject and object alike (the 'no-thing') along the way.

The subject All-alone at the place of the failure of rapport between the sexes is where self-interest and public interest meet. The failure between the sexes is presided over by the illusion of an ego individual that attempts to complete itself through the chasing after and acquisition of the object that could serve the autonomy and self-interest of the ego. When both parties to a relationship do this, and the relationship is construed on the basis of the other functioning as an object of ego-interest ($\$\lozenge a$ and I [O]), then a relationship results in irreconcilable differences or the lack of rapport between the sexes. I realize that this is not a rosy, romantic, humanistic, or 'relational' view of the relationship between the sexes. Freud's view of the love relations between the sexes is consistent with Shakespeare, who understood sexual or romantic love between the sexes as illusory, feverish (can't eat or sleep), crazy, asocial, and deadly. The impossibility is Real and, more often than not, an accurate representation of reality. However, the artifact of the sinthome can help by making a personal or sexual relationship not ideal but bearable and possible.

Every ego that is a subject lacks its object. Ego autonomy is illusory because it cannot happen without the attempt to acquire the Other as an object (i[a] or [$◊a]). The object in fact cannot be obtained because the object disappears behind the grid of numbers and signifiers that represent it. What the ego obtains instead through self-interest is a need-satisfying consumer object. The object or social good follows a collective definition of the object according to the surplus jouissance of numbers and letters that represents the object at the level of Society and its institutions. The absence of the object as an index of jouissance also meets the absence of the ego individual at the place where the subject is both a collectivity and a form of jouissance that they, and only they, are responsible for.

The subject of the Real differs both from the subject of the signifier as a collective subject and from the self-interest of the ego or the individual. The object is marked and replaced by the signifier that animates the objective existence of things and socially constructed objects, while the subject of the Real All-alone represents the non-being within the being of the signifier. Instead of the collective being of the signifier, the Real subject comes to be in non-being, or the jouissance within the being of the signifier.

Objects are socially constructed by the numbers and signifiers that represent them, while the subject comes into being at the point where the signifier ends or fails to represent the subject. We come into being at the place where the signifier represents the subject and at the same time, the signifier fails to represent the non-being of the Real subject outside the signifier. The fact that the subject, or the individual, lies outside its social representation is absolutely not the same as self-interest or the interests of an egotistical asocial individual.

The Real subject All-alone is a 'no-thing' or represents a form of infinity that is the same everywhere else and therefore is present within all subjects and objects. The subject All-alone includes signifiers without grasping them as small real or imaginary objects but only as indexes of surplus jouissance and productivity. Surplus jouissance leading to productivity beyond consumption will contribute to the overall expansion of the gross national product that benefits all subjects alike. The treasury of the signifier (empty numbers, letters, and paper) and the treasury of jouissance become One and the same thing. The subject All-alone leads to social expansion and growth, while the self-interest of the ego individual leads to contraction, deflation, and isolation and the loss of symbolic exchange and jouissance value for Society. I must remind the reader, though, that jouissance in things, as a universal activity, is not an imaginary positivity (that could be advertised and sold) and can only be negatively described as a form of *naysaying*: not this, not that, as a quiet and generative form of enjoyment.

Solitude, and the capacity to be alone, does not represent "an utterly intolerable feeling of total isolation" or a "dread of imminent annihilation" (Bion, 1967). Thus, it is important to distinguish an Imaginary autistic or psychotic fusion, or Imaginary One, from the One associated with the Real that is inextricably linked to symbolic structure. The ties of the Real function 'as if' they were a thermal wave made of tiny strings or threads of dark light (what Bion called a beam of intense darkness) in the vacuum that glue the subject to both the cultural symbolic order and the structure of matter.

Thus, to go beyond normal neurosis requires a deconstruction and restructuring of the ego that risks a border and a solidarity with psychoses (metanoia) but without ever falling into the abyss of psychoses (as antipsychiatry often did). What protects the subject from psychoses is the new NoF coming from the Real, or the sinthome, and the layer of the mind that is not saturated by the Other. This is not the usual "ego autonomy" but rather the screen of the Real, the Pcpt cs system, or the magical writing pad that remains mathematically structured and energized yet free of signifiers and representations.

When the knot of three is undone, the psyche goes back to the drawing board, or the empty screen of the Real as a form of jouissance. With the membrane of the Pcpt-Cs. system (awareness), as one of the metaphors for the NoF coming from the Real, a new knot of four can be written. With an unsayable, undetermined piece of Real, a new knot can be written that includes the white board or the page on which the knot is written. The membrane or white board, and/or screen of jouissance and pure sensitivity, cannot be separated from the knot because it is an indispensable element of the structure and its transformations.

Finally, many Lacanians argue that the borderline condition is simply the new hysteria, a hypothesis I am inclined to adopt, but would this indicate a change in the structure or only on the surface symptoms/actions? From a Lacanian perspective, a structure is in constant metonymic motion, without this indicating a change in the structure. Males or females nowadays may want to answer the question of hysteria, "Am I a man or a woman," in different ways. A female may want to adopt masculine traits and a male may adopt feminine traits. However, the regression that takes place in borderline personality disorders, or the new hysteria, from the super-ego to the ideal ego, may actually warrant the status of a different structure centered around the ideal ego and secondary narcissism.

Medical history of bipolar disorder

Another good question to pose here is whether and where to locate bipolar disorder in the maze outlined previously. The earliest written description of the illness can be traced back to 30–150 CE. Around that time, Arataeus of Cappadocia, a medical philosopher from Alexandria, wrote texts referring to a unified concept of manic-depressive illness originating in disorders of 'black bile.'

Then the illness seemed to be lost in the custom to describe all mental diseases as insanity until the middle nineteenth-century publication of Phillipe Pinel's *Treatise on Insanity* (1806) and John Haslam's *Observations on Madness and Melancholy* (1809) that reintroduced the concept of bipolar disease back into Western medicine. On January 31, 1854, Jules Baillarger described to the French Imperial Academy of Medicine a biphasic mental illness causing recurrent shifts between mania and depression that two weeks later was defined by Jean-Pierre Falret (Haustgen and

Akiskal, 2006) as *folie circulaire* ('circular insanity'). Emil Kraepelin (1921) provided a detailed clinical description for bipolar disorder, or "Manic-depressive insanity that included . . . on the one hand the whole domain of so-called periodic and circular insanity, on the other hand simple mania, [and] the greater part of the morbid states termed melancholia" (Ch. 1, p. 1).

When we think about diagnosis in terms of DSM, it was in DSM-III that the term 'bipolar disorder' replaced the term 'manic depressive disorder.' It was also DSM-III that for the first time mentioned pediatric bipolar disorder. DSM-III-R brought further classification of the disorder into subtypes such as bipolar disorder-mixed, bipolar disorder-manic, bipolar disorder-depressed, bipolar disorder-not otherwise specified, and cyclothymia. In DSM-IV and DSM-IV-TR, it was decided to divide the illness into two separate types distinguished by the type of mania: bipolar I and bipolar II. In bipolar I disorder, patients suffer from at least one manic episode and one depressive episode, while in bipolar II disorder, individuals experience at least one hypomanic episode and at least one major depressive episode. DSM-5's main change was adding the criteria of increase in energy in addition to mood changes. It is interesting, as we can look at it as an attempt to tighten the criteria.

To quickly summarize the previous, we went from simple 'manic-depressive,' one illness, to many different ones with various subgroups and additional qualifiers. The question remains: Does 'more' mean better, more accurate diagnosis or just more confusion? The question is important because diagnosis has tremendous implications in treatment, research studies, and so on.

Psychoanalytic understanding of manic depression

Early on in the psychoanalytic movement, Karl Abraham (1911) noted that in mania, complexes overcome inhibitions and the patient reverts to the care-free state of childhood.

Freud (1917) saw mania as a reversal of depression and as the psychopathological counterpart to socially sanctioned group celebration of festivals. More specifically, in some cultures, the tradition is to celebrate rather than cry and mourn during funerals. This is not unrelated to a manic reaction to loss where the subject performs euphoric ritual dances to commemorate and celebrate the loss of a loved one. What an individual does as a function of individual pathology may be equivalent to normative and normal group psychology and behavior in other cultures. This is consistent with the work of Ruth Benedict (1935) in anthropology, who observed that psychopathology is the common language between psychologists and ethnologists.

Freud (1917) distinguishes depression and mania using the relations between the ego and super ego. In depression, the super ego is the exacting and cruel (sadistic) master of the ego. In mania, the narcissistic ego has triumphed over the super-ego and performs a victory dance over the body of the dead super ego. It is the victory over the super ego that frees the narcissistic ego from the inhibitions of the super ego and allows the ego to reinstate an infantile form of omnipotence.

For Freud, mania involved the denial of the primal 'manic' and cannibalistic crime of killing and eating the primal father. However, Abraham (1911) believed that the murderous fantasies of the manic patient were primarily directed towards the mother. Manic defense was a term first used by Melanie Klein (1935) to describe a set of mental mechanisms aimed at protecting the ego from depressive and paranoid anxieties. Omnipotence, denial, and idealization are the three constituents of manic defense. Omnipotence is used to control objects but without any recognition of the object as a subject (or what object relations theory calls 'a genuine concern for the other').

The omnipotence of the subject refers back to the omnipotence of the mother-child fusion where the child functions as the imaginary phallus of the mother that completes her and closes her lack of being. In this state of affairs, the Name of the Father that symbolically castrates and humanizes the subject is not operative, at least on the surface. If the paternal function does not curve the manic omnipotence of the mother child dyad/fusion, the result will be some form of psychoses.

Once the Other intervenes, and the child is introduced into the symbolic order, then in depressive and paranoid anxieties that follow, according to Kleinian theory, there is the growing realization that the good object has been lost as a consequence of the ego's aggressivity. Beyond the self-interest in the good breast, and its survival value for the individual, once the bad breast and the good breast are realized as belonging to the same mother, the child, according to Klein, becomes worried that they may have hurt the Other to whom both the good and bad breast now belong. The manic defense constitutes the opposite wish to hurt or cannibalize the Other.

This feature of Kleinian theory, which distinguishes between the breast as a fantasized part object and the 'whole' body of the mother, is an instantiation of the logical *toto/pars pro* relation. In Lacanian psychoanalysis, the Other does not refer to the Other's whole-body image but rather to the totality of the signifying system (O or A in French). Within the totality of the signifying system, the signifier represents the lack in the Other and the subject.

The absence of the breast (i.e. bad breast due to mother's other desires/responsibilities) is symbolized in the address to the whole (m)other to whom both breasts belong, but more importantly, it is symbolized in the address to the Other as the place where signifiers reside. The object of the address is the Other, or more specifically the Other's lack/desire. A child learns how to speak by demanding to be loved as the object cause of the mother's desire.

It is a question of what *objet a* is the child for the mother more than whether the mother is represented by the breast in the child's mind. In this case, the mother's breast is an *objet a* for the child, and the child is the mother's *objet a*. The *objet a* is what the Other or the subject has lost. The mother has given off her breast for the child to appropriate and destroy (in fantasy), and therefore the question naturally arises in the child whether they had something to do with the loss of the object. The Other's desire is represented by the mother's words more than by their whole-body image as perceived by the child.

With Lacan's formula for the relationship between the *objet a* and the phallus (a/-phi = the *objet a*, as numerator, closes the gap or lack of the imaginary phallus, as denominator), the symbolic dimensions of the breast and the phallus (as golden numbers/*objet a*) can be properly understood in their structuring psychical and subjective function. Freud believed that the sadistic attacks on the frustrating bad breast phylogenetically correspond or repeat the manic oral cannibalism of the father. Through words and in time, the manic cannibalism of the infant will be curbed by the words of the symbolic mother that begin to symbolize the alternating experiences of satisfaction and frustration with the breast/*objet a*. The symbolic mother helps the child be away from the *objet a* and tolerate frustration and at the same time provides timely or good-enough satisfactions.

Once the child can accept temporary frustrations, through the words and speech of the mother, the child will develop the growing realization that the mother/breast is away because of the mother's desire for things Other than the child. More than realizing that the good and bad breast belong to the same mother, what is pivotal is the recognition of the mother's desire. It is the recognition that the mother has a desire for the Other that will shift the attention in development from the mother to the Other. At this point, the Other is no longer the total complete and whole body of the mother (phallic mother) but the Other of the address, now located in the father rather than the mother. It is the symbolic mother that paved the road for this transition to take place.

The question then becomes: What does my mother want from the (f)Other? This question brings to light the phi and the -phi, or the imaginary phallus that will function as signified for the NoF. A human subject, at this point, is a function of the intervention of the paternal metaphor and the insertion of the subject into language. The Kleinian depressive position, or the early maternal super-ego, which Klein (1935) theorized in relationship to the good and bad breast, cannot be thought of independently from the symbolic phallic function, since the latter is intrinsically linked to the *objet a* as an object that has become detached from the Other.

This quality of the *objet a* is embodied by different objects during the different phases of development, but they all follow the same overarching logical framework. The breast and the baby, as *objet a*, have equivalence in Freud's symbolic equation and Lacan's lists of *objet a*. Symbolic castration follows from a logical or mathematical structure (that subtracts an inexistent signifier and self from the subject) rather than from an oedipal myth. The myth of Oedipus is precisely that: a story that is told at the level of the Imaginary to account for a fact of the symbolic structure.

In the area shared in common between a–a' (see schema L previously), there is only a small mark of distinction that differentiates between a and a' prime, between the good breast or the mother as *objet a*, and the child occupying the place of the beloved *objet a* cause of the mother's desire; between the oral experience of satisfaction at the breast and having a biological need met. The mother's breasts and the child are both forms of the *objet a*. The child is *l'a* as '*l'petit enfant*,' and between the breast and the child as *objet a*, there is a *toto/pars pro* relationship. The mother's breast and the baby make an imaginary One that replicates the *objet a*, as a residue or leftover (1+*a*). Eventually *a–a'* will represent the relation between the child as an *objet a* for the mother and the *objet a* as both the totality of the body image and a part missing within the totality of the specular image of the child.

The breast is to the baby what the fantasy object is to the specular image and what the missing *a* or blank spot in the body image is to the totality of the image. The presence of the mother's fantasy object supports or stands invisibly behind the specular image of the child in the mirror in the same way that the absence of the mother's fantasy object in the specular image (hole or blank spot) leads the way to the recognition of the mother's desire for the Other and eventually to the NoF as the signifier of the mother's desire. Lacan theorizes that the mother's desire for a paternal object that is not the child is represented in the specular image by a blank spot or hole in the image. This is the lack within desire that everyone carries in the body image. The child is no longer a phallic object of the mother, because the part object is now missing from the ideal ego or specular image and is now linked to the Other instead.

It is symbolic loss and lack (of the *objet a*) that sensitizes the subject towards the same in the Other more than the child's supposed good nature and humanistic or altruistic moral concern for the Other that Freud considered a suspect motivation. The answer to the desire or longing for recognition from the Other goes back to the recognition of the subject's own desire. Psychoanalysis never was or can never be simplistically reduced to a moral worldview or a form of moral re-education or treatment.

When an infant is ingratiated or flattered by being his/her majesty the baby (presence of *l'a*), this may lead a child to imaginary narcissistic identifications. By the same token, *l'a* (the *a*) as the index of a luminescent non-trivial void (in the form of the agalma), and as a platform or plateau for a child's state of gratitude and satisfaction, could lead a child to act quite nobly and gallantly towards the Other (One). One can easily observe spontaneous gestures of great generosity and gratitude in a small child. Not that being a brat, or a prick, could not function as the other side of the same thing.

As stated previously, from a Lacanian point of view, lack as grief, whichis shared with the Other, is not only caused by the accidental loss of a reality object (family member) or losing the love of an important childhood figure but also by the lack of loss of an object in normal development. In either case, the losses are not grieved, in the first case because an environmental other is lost, or their love is lost, and the loss is not grieved. In the second case, the partial object is not grieved not because a loss took place that was later denied but because the necessary structural loss never happened in the first place.

According to psychoanalytic theory, a child has to lose the breast during weaning and the oral phase, feces during the anal phase and the acquisition of sphincter control, and the phallus during the genital phase and the acquisition of an ambiguous sexual identity, as a man or a woman. These are not accidental losses of a partial object but structural losses that are necessary for the development of human subjectivity.

By pathologizing grief, psychiatry risks that people may not want to grieve or could feel that they should not grieve, but if they don't grieve, they may thereby be paradoxically predisposed to depression, and this in turn could trigger manic defenses. Depression and concomitant manic defenses could be triggered not because they didn't grieve the accidental loss of a necessary and symbolic reality object but because they didn't grieve the necessary losses that take place during the course of normal development.

Pathologizing grief is consistent with the humanistic consumer society of late capitalism where everyone is expected to be happy (i.e. the "science" of happiness) and where there is no place for the positive and constructive function of lack and grief. Lack, emptiness, and grief are necessary affective components of normal and radical evolutions of psychical structure in the same way that zero is the balancing point of symbolic exchange, according to Lévi-Strauss (1950). Zero, the phallic function, or emptiness, limits the surplus of phallic jouissance and transforms the surplus into a different and convenient form of jouissance ("The road of excess leads to the palace of wisdom", Blake). However, wisdom requires the negative to transform the first, and second, into the Third jouissance. Infinity within form or the finite is a near friend that differs from the excess associated with postmodernism and neoliberal excess within the culture that leads to nihilism and chaos, for the individual, the family, and society. The Third is neither a yuppie nor a square conservative.

Regarding the psychoanalytic treatment of manic depression, the resistances to treatment have to be understood from the structure rather than from the surface of the symptoms. The manic symptom may temporarily hinder the patient's capacity for insight or the desire to know something about their symptom, take responsibility for it, and change or alter their relationship to the symptom. But once the symptom goes into remission, the question of future relapses and accessibility to treatment will be decided by the structure in which the symptom takes place.

With regard to the Lacanian understanding of manic depression proper, the following observations can be made. First of all, Lacan did not speak much about manic depression, as Freud had previously done, but from my perspective, this fact follows from a very important consideration. Lacan did not speak about manic depression because for him, the most important question was: Is this patient's bipolar disorder stemming from a neurotic, pervert, or psychotic structure? Mania is only a symptom that can be present in any structure.

If bipolar disorder stems from a neurotic structure, then the person with bipolar disorder can be stable between episodes with or without medications. This is something impossible for someone with a psychotic structure, at least without serious treatment. Moreover, in bipolar disorder with neurotic structure, psychotic features are driven by the intensity of the affect during episodes. Mood fluctuations in bipolar patients have continuity with mood fluctuations in normal neurotics (most people are neurotic) and even with the mood swings observed in the borderline character that often cannot be distinguished from the mood fluctuations in the bipolar II condition.

The question of success and failure, and of competition, is a crucial question and value, especially for contemporary capitalist societies. The intensity associated with success or failure, winning or losing, and the corresponding feelings of elation or deflation, high or low self-esteem, are part and parcel of the normal experience of a subject under contemporary capitalism. Thus, suffering is an intrinsic aspect of the human condition. It is often difficult, in fact, to separate the goals and objectives leading to success (or failure) from feelings of positive or negative self-esteem. Thinking that one is good or bad, successful or a failure, lovable or unlovable, and feeling good or bad, up or down, euphoric or dysphoric, are closely tied together and demonstrate the continuity between normal neurosis and bipolar disorder.

In addition, psychoanalytic theory prior to Lacan had a consistent way of thinking about mania in terms of what Klein called a manic defense against depression. However, in the clinic, the same mechanism or presentation is not always observed. Every bipolar patient is different, and they engage in their manic symptoms for different reasons. For some, it may be purely biological; for others, they are seriously narcissistic, and they present their grandiosity in such a way that it looks like mania, while others are psychotic, and their psychosis is presenting through grandiosity and elation (i.e. "I am god").

Case presentation

Let's use another vignette to clarify the concepts described previously. This is a 31-year-old Caucasian male with a clearly defined history of bipolar disorder. During the intake interview, he reported that his first manic episode was a week long, occurred during his teenage years, and ended in hospitalization for several months. His last major manic episode was few years prior to starting psychotherapy and apparently lasted a few months. During that time, he experienced euphoria, decreased need for sleep, racing thoughts, and some delusional thinking. He also got into some fights and spent most of his money. He stopped taking his medications and was self-medicating his racing thoughts with alcohol.

The patient started psychotherapy and continued to refuse to take any medications and instead decided to manage his mania with three hours of exercise a day. He also said that he received a lot of support from his girlfriend whom he's been seeing twice a week. Soon after beginning his treatment, he went to the psychiatric emergency room after he woke up from a beating, and it was discovered that he had skull fractures, and a plate had to be inserted in his forehead. He was temporarily bald and had ear-to-ear stitches in his skull. The only thing that he could remember was that he got drunk at a bar and had an argument with a bouncer outside the bar.

It is interesting that the patient was a very smart undergraduate philosophy student who finished all coursework but never obtained his degree. He was working at a gym and as a cook on weekends. His personal history was filled with significant mood swings, unstable relationships, and poor performance in school and work.

In significant distress, he reported odd perceptual experiences such as feeling that the walls and the floor were moving and buildings were bending over. In a closed space, he thought there was a hole in the wall and 13 floors beneath him. He also had some out-of-body experiences, where the seat of perception was removed from his body and he felt like he was one of the pieces of furniture in the room. While manic, the patient described euphoric mood, grandiosity (thinking he was god), pressured speech, and lack of sleep.

At the beginning of the treatment, the patient not only did not want to take medications but also questioned the entire therapeutic endeavor by saying that he liked suffering and his symptoms. His symptoms were not yet ego-dystonic sinthomes. He explained that the values that claim that health is better than illness were the signs of a corrupt social system that he did not want to participate in. So, then, the question arose as to why was he coming to treatment at all: What did he want, what was he looking for?

Patient could not answer any of these questions, but psychotherapist went along with his rejection of social health values and stated to the patient, "And also you don't mind when the floor moves under you or the walls undulate like water." Patient began having the symptom at that point and became very distressed. The psychotherapist responded by normalizing his experience in support of what the patient had said earlier: "Sometimes objects can stand still and sometimes they can move just like people." After psychotherapist said this, the patient's symptom disappeared just as it had appeared a minute prior. With this intervention, the therapeutic relationship was strengthened, given that it had an obvious immediate benefit to the mental state of the patient. The patient never returned again to the position of defending the suffering produced by the symptom or questioning the value of the treatment. This patient was well on his way to extracting knowledge from the symptom and becoming the symptom's disciple (sinthome).

The patient's father killed himself when he was young. Mother was about to leave the father when he shot himself. Patient saw his father as a failure in life and was never close to him. Father was illiterate. For mother, father's suicide was a relief. His mother remarried, but he never was very close with his stepfather of 20 years. He blamed his mother for oversharing details of her romantic life and of his father's death. The patient described her as a good caretaker but no more than a "gatekeeper," angry more than anything else and not very affectionate.

Original diagnosis: (DSM IV)

Axis I	Bipolar I disorder with psychotic symptoms, currently depressed, alcohol abuse, panic disorder with no agoraphobia
Axis II	Borderline personality disorder
Axis III	Multiple head injuries
Axis IV	Problems related to social environment and economic problems
Axis V	GAF: 50

DSM-5 diagnosis does not have axial representation. There is no GAF. Agoraphobia and panic disorder are now separate diagnoses. However, the part that interests us here the most is the diagnosis of bipolar disorder, which would stay the same. Perhaps this is a case where we would add anxious distress specifier. Apparently, per DSM-5 guidelines, this specifier is intended to identify patients with anxiety symptoms that are not part of the bipolar diagnostic criteria. Regardless of how we try to narrow down the diagnosis, there are still many of them to consider.

We would like to emphasize that the patient was refusing medications initially, said that they made him feel worse, that he couldn't think when he was on them, that they would take away all his motivation, and so on. Psychotherapist helped him understand that the continuum between self and no-self is normal, but in his case, what was missing was the ability to also differentiate between them. Therapist also linked this developmental achievement with the body image and the ideal ego as a product of the relationship with the mother. It is interesting that the patient showed response to the intervention. Treating his character helped his bipolar symptoms. He was also able to discuss the question of his desire.

In sessions, despite him reporting occasional psychotic-like symptoms, he did not show any language disturbances or loose associations. He was able to use metaphors well, associate to his dreams, and had some insight into his delusions. Taking all of the previous into consideration, the patient can be given the Lacanian diagnosis of a neurotic structure with psychotic symptoms, mood swings, and alcohol abuse.

With the help of treatment, the patient was able to accept that mania was a defense against depression. He recognized the difference between grief and depression and the fact that he did not have feelings when his father died when he was a teen. He then recalled becoming depressed a few years later, which was followed by his first manic episode. During the course of treatment, the patient used obsessional defiance of the law as a defense. He struggled with the idea of starting a job versus being homeless and spending his days studying in the library. His desire to be stable was first his girlfriend's desire, and he alternated between following it and defying it. So, we can observe that he had anti-social traits as symptoms without having a perverse structure.

Discussion of the case

In Frieda Fromm-Reichmann's (1953) interpersonal studies and treatment of manic-depressive patients, she observed many significant parent–child interactions that seemed to characterize the families of patients suffering from manic depression. Consistent with the findings of the histories of patients with major depression, they had sustained significant environmental losses during their childhood. It remains unclear why some patients sustain losses and do not develop major depression or why some people sustain losses and develop major depression but do not develop manic episodes/defenses.

If we follow Freud's theory of the complemental series, then the environmental traumatic factors by themselves are not sufficient to produce a symptom, or a structure for that matter. Oedipal structure is as important as, if not more important than, the family history and narrative in question. In addition, the two series may have various ways of interacting.

For example, the patient may have failed to grieve the Oedipal loss of his mother due to the family failures of the father, who was too weak to have a significant impact on the mother–son dyad. Not only did the father perform poorly as a provider and in the family, but his failure as a provider may have also affected the status and isolation of the family within the community, a finding that is consistent with the families of the patients that Fromm-Reichman studied.

Then the question is: Why the additional tendency towards mania? Well, this client may have been emboldened as the mother's 'prince' to play a 'greater' part in the family, even to the extent of replacing his father, especially upon his death. The mother may have enlisted the son to remedy the problematic situation with the father. Patient may have also experienced the suicide of his father as a personal triumph and victory in battle, similarly to how Freud described the dance of the victor over the body of the dead enemy/father. The disturbance in the patient's work ethic may also be seen as an identification with the same disturbance in the father and as an extension of the poor example and authority figure that the father represented and that the son challenged. Patient said that father's suicide made him question reality and mistrust people.

Conclusion

Lacanian topology may have a lot to offer in the process of improving our diagnostic process. Lacan's and Freud's division of people's structure into psychotic, perverted, and neurotic brings an interesting point of view in terms of nosology. There are clearly defined differences between these three diagnostic categories that are present not only on the superficial level but also in the unconscious, Oedipal, and family structure; the way the subject relates to language; and, maybe most importantly, the nature of their social link.

Such classification seems to be closer to what we observe in the clinic and in basic research. In this chapter, I suggest diagnosing patients based on their psychical structure, a description of the symptoms present on the surface, and a consideration of genetic and environmental factors that may be at play. It seems that such an approach holds a promise of being more individualized and truer to a particular subject. It could also help in tailoring therapeutic interventions in a more effective way. Most importantly, it will allow for better prognosis and plans for future treatments.

References

Abraham, K. (1911). Notes on the Psycho-Analytical Investigation and Treatment of Manic-Depressive Insanity and Allied Conditions (1911)137. In: *The International Psycho-Analytical Library*. Edited by E. Jones. London: Hogarth Press, 1927.

Alliance of Psychoanalytic Organizations (2006). *Psychodynamic Diagnostic Manual*. Maryland: Silver Springs.

American Psychiatric Association (2013). *Diagnostic and Statistical Manual of Mental Disorders* (Fifth Edition). Arlington, VA: American Psychiatric Publishing.

Benedict, R. (1935). *Patterns of Culture*. London: Routledge, 1961.

Bion, W. R. (1967). *Second Thoughts: Selected Papers on Psychoanalysis*. Northvale, NJ: Jason Aronson, 1993.

Braunstein, N. (2012). *El Inconsciente, la Tecnica y el Discurso Capitalista.* Mexico: Siglo Ventiuno.

Craddock, N. and Owen, M. J. B. (2010). *Journal of Psychiatry*, 196, 92–95.

Dali, S. (1935). The Conquest of the Irrational. https://archive.org/stream/DaliConquest Irrational/412994-Dali_ReducedPDF_djvu.txt.

Dichter, G. S., Damiano, C. A. and Allen, J. A. (2010). Reward circuitry dysfunction in psychiatric and neurodevelopmental disorders and genetic syndromes: animal models and clinical findings. *Journal of Neurodevelopmental Disorders*, 4, 19, 2012.

Dor, J. (1987). *The Clinical Lacan.* New York: Jason Aronson, 1997.

Fenichel, O. (1945). *The Psychoanalytic Theory of Neurosis.* New York: Norton.

Fink, B. (1997). *A Clinical Introduction to Lacanian Psychoanalysis.* Cambridge: Harvard University Press.

Freud, S. (1900). *The Interpretation of Dreams.* New York: Avon Books, 1965.

Freud, S. (1911). Psychoanalytic Notes Upon an Autobiographical Account of a Case of Paranoia (Dementia Paranoides). In: *Three Case Histories.* Edited by P. Rieff. New York: Collier Books.

Freud, S. (1917). Mourning and Melancholia. *SE*, 14, 239–258.

Freud, S. (1930). *Civilization and Its Discontents.* New York: Norton, 1962.

Fromm-Reichmann, F. (1953). An Intensive Study of Twelve Cases of Manic-Depressive Psychosis. *Psychiatry*, 17 (2), 103–137, 1954.

Guntrip, H. (1973). *Psychoanalytic Theory, Therapy, and the Self: A Basic Guide to the Human Personality.* Edited by E. Freud, S. Klein, H. Fairbairn and W. Jacobson. New York: Basic Books.

Haslam, J. (1809). *Observations on Madness and Melancholy.* London: J. Callow, Medical Bookseller.

Haustgen, T. and Akiskal, H. (2006). French Antecedents of 'Contemporary' Concepts in the American Psychiatric Association's Classification of Bipolar (Mood) Disorders. *Journal of Affective Disorders*, 96, 149–163.

Heidegger, M. (1969). The End of Philosophy and the Task of Thinking. In: *Basic Writings* (Revised and Expanded Edition). Translated by D. F. Krell. London: Harperperennial, 2008.

Jung, C. (1960). *The Structure and Dynamics of the Psyche.* Princeton: Princeton University Press.

Klein, M. (1935). A Contribution to the Psychogenesis of Manic-Depressive Sates. In: *The Writings of Melanie Klein.* Edited by R. Money-Kyrle (Volume 1, pp. 262–289). New York: The Free Press, 1984.

Kraepelin, E. (1921). *Manic-Depressive Insanity and Paranoia.* Edinburgh: Livingstone.

Lacan, J. (1945–1955). *The Seminar.* Book II. The Ego in Freud's Theory and in the Technique of Psychoanalysis. Translated by S. Tomaselli. New York: Cambridge University Press, 1988.

Lacan, J. (1957–1958). *Formations of the Unconscious: The Seminar of Jacques Lacan.* Book V. Edited by J. A. Miller and Translated by R. Grigg. Cambridge: Polity Press.

Lacan, J. (1961). Remarks on Daniel Lagache's Presentation: 'Psychoanalysis and Personality Structure'. In: *Écrits*, Edited by J. Lacan and J. A. Miller (pp. 543–574). New York: W. W. Norton, 2006.

Lacan, J. (1966–1967). *The Seminar of Jacques Lacan.* Book XIV. The Logic of Phantasy, . Translated by C. Gallagher from Unedited French Manuscripts. http://www.lacaninireland.com/web/translations/seminars. Accessed November 30, 2019.

Lacan, J. (1969–1970). *The Other Side of Psychoanalysis: Seminar XVII.* New York: Norton, 2007.

Lacan, J. (1971–1972). *The Seminar of Jacques Lacan.* Book XIX. Edited by J.-A. Miller. Cambridge: Polity Press, 2018.

Lacan, J. (1975–1976). *The Sinthome: The Seminar of Jacques Lacan*. Book XXIII. Edited by J. A. Miller. Cambridge: Polity Press.
Laing, R. D. (1968). *The Politics of Experience*. London: Penguin Books.
Lévi-Strauss, C. (1950). *Introduction to the Work of Marcel Mauss*. Translated by F. Baker. London: Routledge, 1987.
Moncayo, R. (2008). *Evolving Lacanian Perspectives for Clinical Psychoanalysis*. London: Karnac.
Moncayo, R. (2017). *Lalangue, Sinthome, Jouissance, and Nomination: A Reading Companion and Commentary on Lacan's Seminar XXIII*. London: Karnac.
Moncayo, R. and Romanowicz, M. (2015). *The Real Jouissance of Uncountable Numbers: The Philosophy of Science within Lacanian Psychoanalysis*. London: Karnac.
Pinel, P. (1806). *A Treatise on Insanity*. Translated from French by D. D. Davis. New York: Published under the Auspices of the Library of the New York Academy of Medicine by Hafner Publishing Co., 1962.
Vanheule, S. (2014). *Diagnosis and the DSM: A Critical Review*. London: Palgrave Pivot.
Verhaegue, P. (2004). *On Being Normal and Other Disorders*. New York: Other Press.
von Uexküll, T. (1987). The Sign Theory of Jakob von Uexküll. In: *Classics of Semiotics*. Edited by Krampen (pp. 147–179). New York: Plenum.
Winnicott, D. (1963). Communicating and Not Communicating Leading to a Study of Certain Opposites. In: *Reading Winnicott*. Edited by L. Coldwell and A. Joyce. London: Routledge, 2011.

Websites

http://thenewinquiry.com/essays/book-of-lamentations. Sam Kriss, accessed July 5, 2020
www.nature.com/news/mental-health-on-the-spectrum-1.12842. Craddock and Owen, 2010
https://archive.org/stream/DaliConquestIrrational/412994-Dali_ReducedPDF_djvu.txt

2 The signifying chain(s) in the graph of desire

Introduction

This chapter explores the various meanings attached to Lacan's famous graph of desire. Although this chapter relies heavily on the ideas presented by Lacan (1966) in his famous paper from the Ecrits, "The subversion of the subject and the dialectic of desire in the Freudian Unconscious," I believe the graph includes most of Lacan's theory, including Lacan's later concept of a Real unconscious.

This analysis of the graph will differ from other interpretations (Edelstein [2009]; Quinet [2018]) of the graph of desire that rely on Lacan's earlier work centered around the Symbolic, without the benefit of Lacan's later concepts. In the later Lacan, it is the Real and the Sinthome, rather than the Symbolic, that hold the Borromean knot together. In addition, the incompatibility of desire and speech is transferred to jouissance, while desire is understood as not without speech. Finally, jouissance is no longer only of one kind and inconvenient (jouissance of the Other), since there are three forms of jouissance and three forms of the Third jouissance no longer conceived as inconvenient.

The graph represents the relations between desire and the law, desire and the desire of the Other, and among the signifier, the subject, and the code, and among desire, jouissance, and the drive. It is proposed that the graph be constructed as an ascending and descending structure of facilitations, punctuations, and limitations, of circular repetitions and lines that escape them. Beyond the drive, the subject asks: 'What do I want from the Other and what does the Other want from me?' These questions are anything but rhetorical, as no matter what we do, we will never find complete answers to them, mainly because the answers are hidden in the questions. In other words, desire is essentially related to the loop between desire and the desire of the Other. We learn from Lacan that desire is unconscious and inseparable from the law. He also claims that despite the impossibility to describe desire – the Other lacks the signifiers to represent desire, since the signifier of desire is a missing signifier – desire can be represented with the help of mathematical graph theory.

Graph theory allows the placing of many Lacanian concepts in one picture, such as fantasy, the ideal ego, the ego ideal, the formula for the drive, the signifier of a lack in the Other, the signifying chain, and the treasury of the signifier. The most difficult part of the graph to represent is the 'beyond' castration, the non-existence of the phallus and the unthinkable Being of the subject (of the Real and the Other jouissance) that is missing within the Other and the battery of signifiers.

The graph and our questions

Graph theory is a branch of mathematics that uses mathematical structures to model pair-wise relations between objects. A 'graph' is then created from 'vertices' or 'nodes' and lines called 'edges' that connect them. In the graph of desire, the vertices or nodes are the circles that contain symbolic formulae. While I understand that the term *matheme* was not introduced by Lacan (1971–1972) until the early 1970s, the symbolic formulae of the graph introduced in 1957 will be referred to in this chapter as *mathemes:* the *matheme* for the drive ($<>D) and the *matheme* for phantasy ($<>a).

The first question that arises with regard to a graph is: How and why does Lacan formulate desire in the mathematical terms of a graph? Euler invented graph theory in mathematics to find a solution to the Konigsberg bridge problem. Graph theory allowed Euler to demonstrate that it was impossible to solve the problem and that this itself was the solution. Can the same be said about Lacan's graph of desire? Does the graph constitute a proof that the problem of desire (and by implication the problem of happiness and suffering) in human beings does not have a solution or that the solution is impossibility? If this is the case, can we still speak of a cure, a treatment, or symptom resolution in psychoanalysis, as Freud wanted and believed?

Second, why does Lacan call this graph the 'graph of desire' when desire or small 'd' has such a low profile in the graph? Many concepts apart from desire are being discussed by Lacan in his graph. He talks about fantasy, the drive, the ideal ego, the ego ideal, the formula for the drive, the signifier of a lack in the Other, the signifying chain, the treasury of signifiers, and so on. Why, then, does he name it the graph of desire?

Finally, I would like to ask the seemingly simple question as to why Lacan decides to draw several different levels or floors in his graph and a line over and above the top level. I wonder if, by drawing lines over and above the top level, he is representing the place beyond 'the rock of castration,' which in turn would indicate that there is, as Bruce Fink (1995) suggests, "a utopian moment" or a metanoia beyond neurosis, as I called it in the previous chapter. The utopian place beyond neurosis and beyond imaginary lack and the rock of castration indicates a no-place or 'u-topia.' This empty place appears as something missing within the Symbolic but 'ex-sists' in the Real as a benevolent form of jouissance holding together a knot of four beyond neurosis (sinthome).

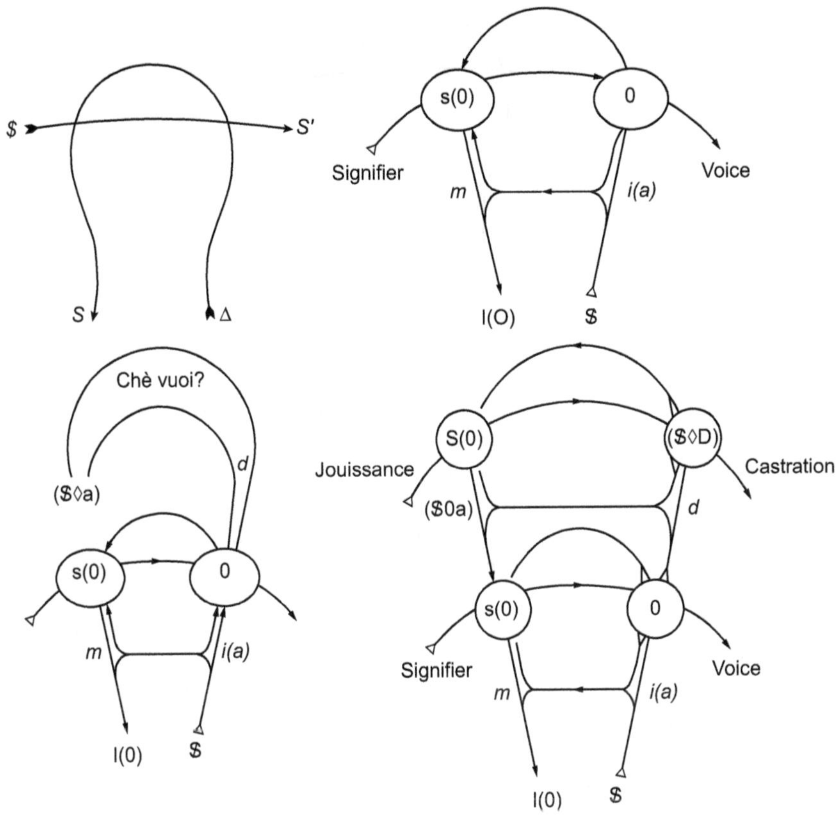

Figure 2.1 Evolution of the graph of desire

Source: Lacan, 1966. The drawings are mine. In these graphs, I have changed capital A for *Autre* in French to capital O for Other and lowercase a for *autre* to lowercase o for other

The early graph or the first level of the graph

Figure 2.4 shows the evolution of the graph of desire, which Lacan began developing in 1957 in Seminar V on the Formations of the Unconscious. It would be incorrect to consider each graph a stage of development in any genetic or biological sense. This was never Lacan's intention. I think it is better to view each version as a step in the process of constructing the graph of desire – where desire is the key word. We can also understand Lacan by reading him retroactively (from the completed graph back to the first graph), since retroactivity is part of the logic included within the graph of desire. Retroactivity can be shown in the line going in the direction S→S', which, as a result of the last word and punctuation, also goes from S'→S.

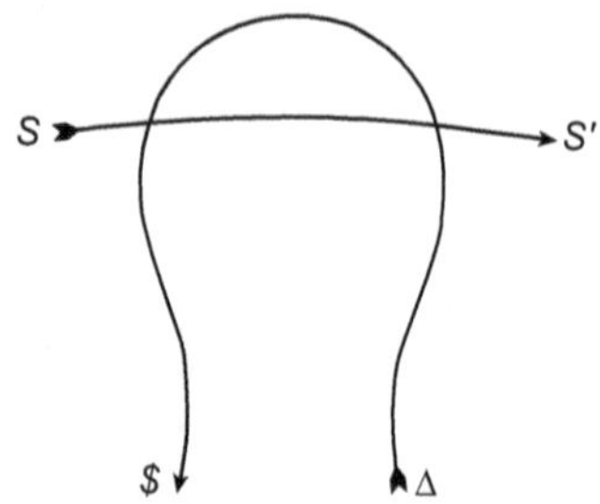

Figure 2.2 The signifying chain S→S'

For the first graph, Lacan draws two lines or edges, which, as early as 1957, he names the line of intentionality or of the subject marked by language (Δ to $) and the signifying chain (S→S'). Lacan says that the line that goes from Δ to $ is a locus or a place in space, while S→S' represents a scansion in time. From here, we could say that Δ represents the 'pre-subject' born at a particular place in space-time that then in time becomes divided thanks to the intervention of the signifier represented by S→S' [in the second graph of Figure 2.4, this comes to be written s(O)→(O)]. The loss that the bar on the subject $ produces helps generate the lack that will constitute desire. Thus, we have a first answer to our second question as to why the graph is called the graph of desire. The pathway from Δ to $ is the vector of desire, while the signifying chain S→S' in this instance is the cut produced by the law of the signifier that helps generate desire.

However, if the signifying chain bars the body of the 'pre-subject' and defines and encloses the subject within a hermeneutic circle of prohibition, how can desire aspire to any satisfaction at all? The law makes desire both possible and impossible at the same time. By forbidding the *jouissance* of the Other and the fusion with the mother, the law makes desire and phallic *jouissance* possible. At the same time, the prohibition produces a fixation on a forbidden object of desire, which then becomes impossible (i.e. the Oedipal mother/father). Let us examine the options the subject has at his/her disposal to deal with the conundrum faced by human desire both within life and within the graph of desire that represents it.

The graph of desire can be read, on the one hand, as an exchange of words and signifiers between the subject and the Other of the unconscious (the vector of unconscious desire) and, on the other hand, as an exchange between the subject and the social other in terms of speech and discourse as a form of social link [s(O)→(O)].

If we read the graph as an intrapsychic linguistic exchange between the conscious and the preconscious/unconscious, then the vector of desire (Δ to $) represents unconscious desire (of the Other) or the unconscious subject of the enunciation/saying, and the S→S' represents the subject of the statement. In the example subsequently, the vector of desire says, 'I want to have a baby,' and the statement says to the Other: 'I am going to have a baby.' In the full graph, the intrapsychic

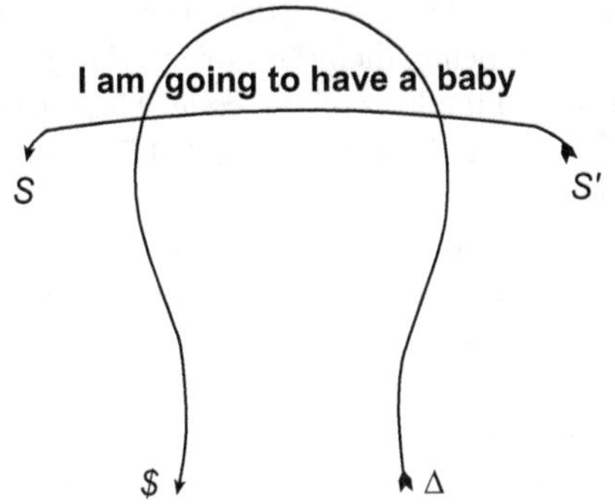

Figure 2.3 The S←S' representing the subject of the statement

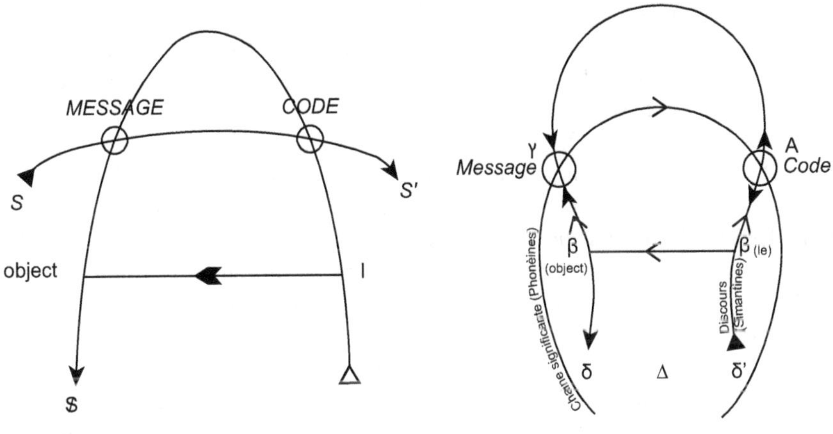

Figure 2.4 The point de capiton or anchoring/quilting point – Button tie

line of intentionality associated with desire goes all the way to the top of the graph representing Unconscious desire, the demands of the drive, and the Desire of the Other as the signifier of a lack in the Other.

S→S', the said of the statement or the *point de capiton* or anchoring/quilting point, is also known as the 'button tie,' because it ties the subject/signifier to the Other and the message to the code and provides the illusion of a fixed meaning.

The second level of the graph

The second way to read the relationship between the two vectors or lines is as intersubjective (mis)communication or interlocution, but this necessitates a second intersection.

I will use the two pictures previously to develop concepts described in the elementary graph. Both graphs show the message that goes to the code. Once the divided subject becomes a speaking being, then the subject will generate speech and messages of desire according to the laws of the code. Messages of speech reveal the subject's social intentionality and predict the probability that the subject will act in accordance with social norms.

Imagine that a girl in our example is a 16-year-old teenager who says that she is going to have a baby to her conservative parents. Or to take another example: imagine a woman in her 40s who has been dreaming about having a child for a long time and has been trying to get pregnant with her husband for the last five years. Once she learns that she is finally pregnant, she shares it with her husband. The code or the application of standards varies in the first and the second scenario, although the message is the same.

So, we have the two points of intersection: message and code. They seem symmetrical, but they are not intended to be. *The code* is a locus of the treasury of the signifiers, a place or *space* of substitution, and *the message* is a *moment* (a rhythm) for which a signification is a finished product. This simplified version of the graph helps in illustrating the relationship between subject and meaning.

The Other of the code and the Other of the unconscious respectively represent the Other of the Law and of the code, the desire of the Other, and the Other of unconscious desire. The Other of the code represents the subject's subjection to the laws of signification that articulate the relationship between signifiers. The laws of language are unconscious in a descriptive sense and at the same time are equivalent to what Freud called the function of the unconscious censor in dreams. In other words, the code and the censor can be considered aspects of an unconscious repressive force.

Then, of course, the unconscious is also associated in Freud and Lacan with the repressed force of desire. Lacan's term 'the desire of the Other' and 'desire is the desire of the Other' (1964) refer both to unconscious desire and the desires of the significant figures of childhood of the subject. Since in Lacanian theory, and implicitly in the Freudian unconscious, unconscious desire and unconscious repression have a relation of reciprocal implication – you cannot have desire without the law, and you cannot have the law without desire – the Other can represent both the code and unconscious desire.

For the sake of clarity, I would like to define the following basic terms that I am going to use in this chapter. S→S' stands here for a signifying chain and metonymy, or the relationship between the signifier and the signified. s(O) →O stands for the relationship between a message or a narrative and its meaning within the battery of the signifiers or the code.

In the *Ecrits*, Lacan (2006a) said

> For what is omitted in the platitude of modern information theory is the fact that one cannot even speak of a code without it already being the Other's code; something quite different is at stake in the message, since the subject constitutes himself on the basis of the message, such that he receives from the Other even the message he himself sends.
>
> (p. 683)

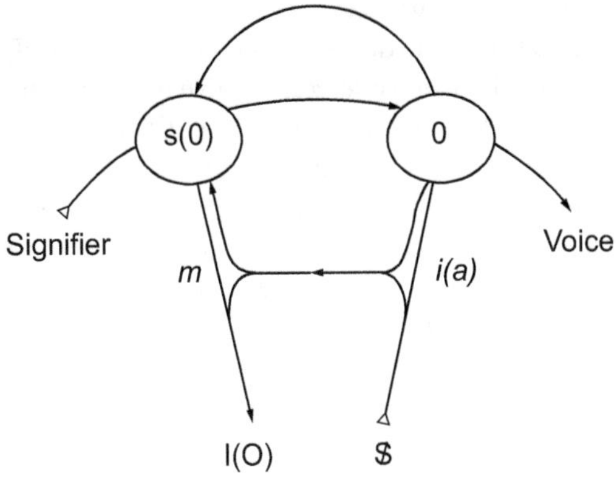

Figure 2.5 First Schema of a linguistic signifying chain with a retroactive effect.

Thus, Lacan says that the subject receives his or her message back from the other/Other in an inverted form. This means that the subject does not really know what they are saying until the meaning or their statement comes back from the Other. When a woman says, 'I am going to have a baby,' her sentence reaches punctuation through the retroaction in the point marked in the previous graph as s(O). If we could first look at the outline of it without paying attention to the lower line [i(a)-→ego or *moi*], we would take the graph as an interesting representation of identification. Let's take a look at the sentence more closely:

I (the woman who just discovered that she is pregnant) am going to have *a* baby. The message is directed to someone, and it is the 'I' of the woman who enunciates it. The person to whom she addresses the message plays a role in the process. The receiver can accept the message because of the code. If it is a husband who has been waiting for a baby, he may be very happy with the news. A matching process takes place between s(O) and O. Take a look at the place of the $. The wife, in the process of her speech, becomes the new subject who just verbalized her desire in the sentence. On the other side, we have I(O) or the ego ideal. The woman in our example may be thinking of her parents and the good things that they have transmitted to her and how it will make her a better parent, and so on. Thus, the sentence is a good example of the identification associated with the ego ideal and in general of how the subject has received its first signs from their relationship to the Other.

That is the ideal situation, but Lacan adds the lower line, one that is used quite a bit in everyday conversations. In a sense, it is an imaginary shortcut and a form of short-circuit.

Ideal ego [i(a)→e]→ego

To use our example, if the woman thinks that she practically became pregnant all by herself and tells her husband that she will be the best mother ever, this changes the picture of the sentence again. Subjectivity is lost or trapped in the Imaginary, and the exchange is closer to an object-to-object relationship (*a* to *a*', where the ego is an object rather than a signifier).

However, I have also raised the question whether the vector of desire could also be represented as the circle of normative narrative according to statements regulated by the code. The code goes back from O to s(O) and down the edge line all the way to the Ideal. The subject becomes alienated in the ego ideal. The subject is divided ($) and then re-united in the ego ideal by way of the ideal ego, the Other or code, and speech. The ego ideal, as the name indicates, represents the direction of normative speech regulated by social ideals. But the cure, treatment, or healing cannot be found at this level because the ego ideal both divides and unifies the subject. In free association, and to undo repression, social ideals and judgments need to be suspended to allow the other side of the subject and the Moebius strip to reveal itself.

For the same reasons, psychoanalysis is not a therapy based on hermeneutic or narrative discourse. Psychotherapy can be a form of narrative discourse because it supports certain social ideals and helps the individual "adapt" to society. Freud said psychoanalysis unifies the subject but does not necessarily make him/her normal from the point of view of morality or social values. Psychoanalysis temporarily suspends social values and authority to reveal the unconscious signifying chain. It will be up to the subject to take up and chose social values outside the analytic situation and post-analytically, according to a renewed understanding of their own (unconscious) subjectivity.

To use our example, the woman may think that if she has a baby, her husband will be very proud of her, he will love her more, it will make their marriage stronger, she will be a better and more complete woman, and so on. For a while, she has the impression that she has found an answer to the problem posed by the lack. The imaginary aspect of the ego ideal represents a wholeness that covers over or closes the gap in the divided subject.

Thus, to reach the heart of the question of desire arising from the paradox between desire and the law, the upper level of the graph is required. The subject now will ask the question, 'What do I want from the Other' and 'What does the Other want from me' or 'Do I know what I want or what the Other wants from me?' Desire is essentially related to the loop between desire and the desire of the Other. The subject of desire wants to receive a sign or signifier of love from the Other. To be loved by the Other, the subject has to become the object or the joy of the Other's desire.

Ultimately, the love and desire for and of the Other remain unknowingly known and/or unknowingly know about the drives linked to desire. As we notice in this step in the construction of the graph of desire, the vector of desire ($) goes up past the Other of the code and past the *d* for desire and allegedly past the upper signifying chain that will appear further on in the full graph. At the top of the graph, a ceiling even for the full graph, appears the question regarding desire. What do you or the Other want?

Although we will hear much more about the upper signifying chain, it is important to note that this particular form of the graph of desire shows how love

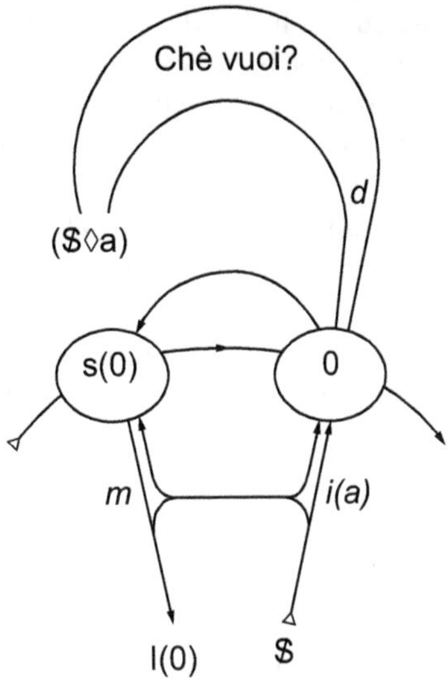

Figure 2.6 The *Che vuoi – existential questions of neurosis*

and desire remain open questions without an answer. In addition, the question of desire immediately raises the question of the law and the difference between desires that are permissible and those that are transgressive and therefore perhaps much more exciting. Permissible desires will appear in the narrative line of the statement between the enunciating ego or the ego of the statement and the Other of the code.

In the full graph, the questions of desire will appear in the form of the horizontal vector between jouissance and castration and castration as a sign of jouissance. Jouissance wants something beyond forbidden desire and phallic jouissance, the limit of which may be death itself. When jouissance meets impossibility, the result is a new form of jouissance. Death may be the final form of a series of losses and gains of jouissance of various kinds.

In this sense, the *Che vuoi*, or the question of desire in subject and Other, also refers to the existential questions of neurosis. Do you want something sexual (man or woman), or death itself (dead or alive)? These are the questions that appear in the unconscious signifying chain and the subject of the enunciation or the saying rather than in the social story and sayings regarding permissible desires.

The questions of desire are always addressed to the Other. When and where can the Law condescend to desire, and desire condescend to the drives? What the subject desires is what others have desired before them, so it is natural for the subject to look for anOther to whom address these questions.

Che vuoi? – What do you want? What *object* do you want from me or what object am I for you? – She/he asks the Other.

The pregnant woman may have figured at some point that her husband wanted her to give him a baby as a sign that he has the phallus and of the desire to inscribe the signifier into a lineage. Once the baby becomes a signifier of the NoF, and the baby is named, the baby becomes an *objet a* that represents the −1 that reveals a dignified void both within the mother and the NoF. Once named by the function of castration, the baby is no longer an imaginary phallus for either mother or father. It is enough to say at this point that the socially acceptable narrative about wanting a child acquires a different meaning in the upper signifying chain with the *objet a* of desire and the drive.

In Seminar V (1957–1958), Lacan gives an example of the two levels of the signifying chain. The formula subsequently depicts the conjunction of signifiers in two levels of the signifying chain that are pressed together, as Lacan says:

$$\frac{S\ldots\ldots\ldots}{s\ldots\ldots\ldots}$$

> In the course of their conversation, Hirsch-Hyacinth declares to Heine that he had the honors of treating the corns of the great Rothschild, Nathan the Wise. While he is trimming his corns, he says to himself that he, Hirsch-Hyacinth, is an important man. He is effectively thinking that during this procedure Nathan the Wise was mulling over the various letters that he would be sending to kings, and that if he, Hirsch-Hyacinth, should trim his corns a little too closely, this would result in an irritation in the upper regions that would in turn cause Nathan to clip the hide of kings a little more.
>
> And thus, one thing leads to another, Hirsch-Hyacinth goes on to talk about another Rothschild that he knew, Salomon Rothschild. One day, when he announces himself as Hirsch-Hyacinth, he receives a reply in nonchalant ways, "I am a lottery agent myself, for the Rothschild lottery, I do not want any colleague of mine in the kitchen." And, Hirsch-Hyacinth exclaims, "He treated me in quite a '*famillionaire*' manner."
>
> (p. 16)

The socially defined narrative or discourse refers to the fact that Hirsch-Hyacinth has the menial and low-status task of trimming the corns of the great Rothschild. To compensate for his low status, he thinks of himself as an important man, and in his resentment over his low social status, he passive-aggressively worries that he will trim the corns too closely, causing pain to the great Rothschild. In turn, he thinks this will cause Nathan the Wise to clip the hides of kings. Hirsch-Hyacinth wishes to be a millionaire, have the status of a wealthy family, and to have an influence on kings. His wish/desire comes through or breaks through the socially coded narrative or discourse. It is the neologism '*famillionaire*' that both closes the meaning of the sentence and gives it a meaning that deviates from the Code, revealing thus the intentionality of his desire within the message.

Freud (1909), for his part, in the case of the Rat man, provides another excellent example of the unconscious signifying chain. One of the Rat man's obsessions (p. 47) was that he was too fat ("Dick" in German) and that he had to make himself thinner. Freud masterfully traced this obsession to patient's jealousy of an English cousin of the lady that he loved. The cousin's name was Richard and Freud notes that in England Richards are known as Dick. In order to make himself thinner, the patient had been dashing up to a mountain top, at which point the obsessive thought occurred to him that he should jump over the precipice.

Freud observes that the suicidality or the aggressiveness towards himself revealed both the identification with Dick (get fat) and the desire not to be like him (lose the fat) and the homicidal wish or rage against the same object. In the footnote, Freud points out how names and linguistic signifiers, therefore, can be used to make connections between Ucs. thoughts (fantasies or memories) and symptoms (the thoughts about the cousin and the obsession).

Furthermore, Freud also points out that Richard comes from the French for rich man. Many French words made it into the English language through the Norman invasion of England during the 12th and 13th century CE. In England, French was the language of the wealthy aristocracy, while English remained the language of the people.

In a footnote, Freud also links this example to another case where a desire to get rid of a brother named Richard was revealed in the form of a desire of the patient to get rid of his own fortune. It is interesting to observe how Freud in these two examples, wittingly or unwittingly, is linking a desire to get rid of Richard, both in the case where Richard means fat in German, or money/wealth in French.

These examples reveal a synecdoche of the part for the whole and the self as a part/signifier of the Other stands in for the Other (fat and money as a self-object or a part object of the subject fall off the other). Fat can also be seen as the incorporation of an oral object as well as something lacking in the body image. In these two instances, the object that represents a negative, something extra in the body that adds a minus sign to the body image, or the object of the other that has been incorporated, can be both conceived as vicissitudes of the *objet a*. Finally, if we add modern North American slang to the equation, then "Dick" would also function as a signifier for the imaginary phallus. In this case, we end up with a series involving money, the *objet a*, and the phallus, an unconscious equation or signifying chain, therefore.

Before moving on to the full graph, I will pause and explain what is meant by castration within Lacanian theory in this day and age. Castration, for Freud, referred to a fantasized mutilation or dismemberment of the penis that established the psychical differences between the sexes. According to Freud, both sexes reject femininity due to the perceived fantasized castration of the mother: the mother does not have a penis because she lost it. Lacan gives more weight to the castration complex at the same time that he gives it a more structural, mathematical, and symbolic interpretation. In addition, the object of the symbolic lack, resulting from the operation of symbolic castration, is the imaginary phallus and not the penis.

The allegedly anatomical absence of the penis in the mother refers to the symbolic condition whereby the child represented an imaginary phallic and narcissistic object for the mother. The father intervenes and breaks the fantasized fusion and thus symbolically 'castrates' both mother and child. The child will no longer be an imaginary phallus for the mother, and the child becomes a subject in his/her own right. From then on, the demand for the phallus will be addressed to the father, and the omnipotence of the mother is transferred to the father.

However, at first, Lacan located the lack in the Other in the mother and considered that the father actually possessed the imaginary phallic attribution. With his later studies on the Name of the Father and the symbolic phallus/function, he comes to understand that the lack in the Other also applies to the father, however necessary the imaginary phallic attribution may be at a certain moment of the child's development. But Lacan, as far as we can tell, never went back to revise his theory of Oedipal phases/moments. Thus, I (Moncayo, 2009) have argued for a fourth moment/phase of Oedipus where the omnipotence of the father is also necessarily lost at some point.

Castration for Lacan ultimately is negotiated in relationship to the lack in the (f)Other and the realization that the phallus (and the Other) does not exist and was never there more than as a function, and this leads to the possibility of going beyond the bedrock of castration. This was Lacan's work of the early seventies, particularly in . . . *ou pire* (Seminar XIX, 1971–72) and *The Knowledge of the Psychoanalyst* (Seminar XIXa. 1971–72).

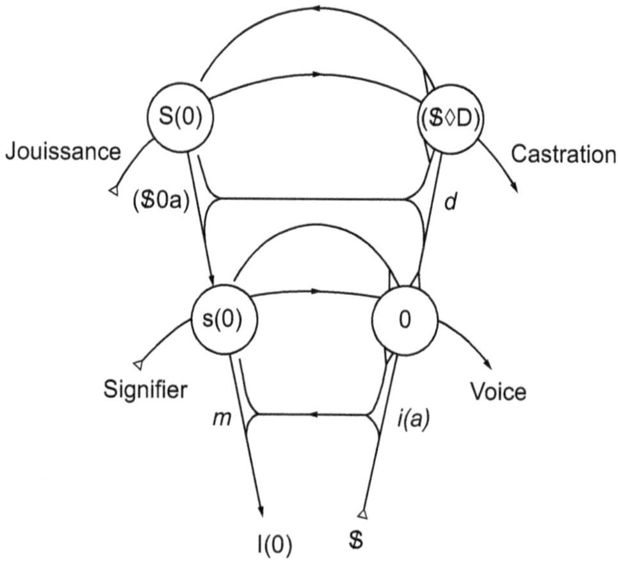

Figure 2.7 Full graph

Coming back to the full graph, there is a signifying vector that crosses from s(O) to O, and the Other (O) is not barred in that line. This would be the conscious narrative or manifest content of a patient, which expects to convey a meaning or receive a full meaning from the Other but which has the voice as a residue, since the voice says more than the narrative. Then, in the completed graph, from the O, the line goes up to desire/demand and to the *matheme* of the drive. The voice as an o-object of desire represents an aspiration of the subject to go beyond the Other of the code that generates and limits desire and divides the subject. This refers to what people often say about finding one's own voice beyond that of the super ego or beyond the prohibitive commands of the super ego.

The signifying chain can also represent the unconscious intentionality of the subject, or the subject's submission to the signifier, as Lacan puts it. The divided subject ($) at the origin of the vector of desire is rediscovered past the Other, in the matheme of the drive ($◊D).

> the strictly linguistic definition of I as signifier . . . designates the enunciating subject but does not signify him. . . . Who is speaking when the subject of the unconscious is at stake? . . . the subject constitutes a bar and a cut between signifier and signified. . . . I can come into being by disappearing from my statement. . . . Being of non-being that is how I come on the scene as a subject.
>
> (1966a, p. 678)

In the completed graph, there are not one but two signifying chains. Now these two signifying chains can be read within a single statement in the case of the lower floor, or across the two upper floors parallel to each other, with each floor representing the signifying chain differently. The lower chain (from the signifier to the voice) is the preconscious signifying chain, the level of the enunciation *énoncé* or statement. The upper chain (from *jouissance* to castration) is the signifying chain in the unconscious, the level of the enunciating, saying, or *énonciation*. The lower level represents the social link in terms of the social position of the subject in the existing social structure, while the upper chain represents both the castration and the jouissance implied in the demand/wish to be a '*famillionaire*,' for example.

The structure is thus duplicated in two ways: The sender or message is to the receiver or Code what jouissance is to castration and the demand of the drive. The lack at the point of castration or the lack in the Other is the point where the signifier passes into a jouissance without words as a response to the question of desire: 'What do I lack/want?' and 'What does the Other lack/want from me?' The unsayable about the jouissance that is desired is the place where the signifier fails or is found wanting.

Lacan emphasized this intrinsic doubling of the Other's discourse. What I mean by this doubling of the Other's discourse is that the conscious narrative or demands of the ego of the statement does not know what he/she is saying at the level of the unconscious, unconscious desire, or the enunciating subject. This double '*entendre*' or double structure of meaning, also represented in the Moebius strip, is what makes the unconscious difficult to decipher and Lacan's writing and graphs so ambiguous and difficult to understand.

Lacan used the term 'signifying chain' to describe an unconscious and automatic process of signification as embodied in his famous statement that the unconscious is structured as a language. The signifying chain is where key signifiers become linked to one another. A link of desire becomes the signified of the two signifying chains. An object of unconscious desire is represented in the upper chain of the graph. In the graph, the two chains appear the same, although they have different mathemes and different representations of the subject and the Other.

The unconscious signifier/letter is not grammatically bound by the rules of grammar and syntax. The upper chain is where desire is constituted as an unconscious signifying chain made up of senseless signifiers. Grammatical mistakes or 'slips of grammar' at times can also be formations of the unconscious. On the other hand, the passive voice in grammar indicates an impersonal activity without a subject and comes close to describing the activity of the unconscious in grammatical terms. Sexual activity is being demanded, someone is being killed, a child is being beaten, and so on. The subject makes itself do something by having the Other demand it from the subject. In phallic jouissance, the activity of the drive proceeds without speech while articulating the passive voice of the *parletre*. In sexual activity, the subject demands that the Other demand the drive from the subject as a quota of work and performance. However, the inverted form of the structure of demand is often itself unconscious or repressed.

If the subject, instead of becoming alienated in normative meaning and returning to the subject of the statement, continues along the path of desire beyond the code, then another floor or level of the graph is reached (in the completed graph). The voice, as a residue, says more than the narrative. Then, from the voice within the O, the edge or vector goes up to desire/demand and to the *matheme* of the drive.

On the left side of the graph, from the definition of the subject, starting at the lower level of the ego and passing by the fleeting symbolic moment in synchronic time (the I or Je of the signifier: s[O]), we can move up the left edge of the graph to a definition of the subject (of the Real) as a hole in the Other (S[Ø]). The Capital S represents the pure signifier but also the signifier that represents the subject. In the formula for signification shown subsequently, the S is defined as what is missing or unthinkable about the subject. Once the signifier represents/substitutes for the subject, the subject becomes something unthinkable within the Real.

> Sign, sign of What? He is precisely the sign of Nothing. If the signifier is defined as representing the subject for another signifier-indefinite referring on of meanings – and if this signifies something, it is because the signifier signifies for the other signifier this 'privileged thing' that the subject is qua nothing.
>
> (Lacan [1961–1962], XIV 8)

Subject qua nothing, or Being of non-being, are different ways that Lacan describes the '*sujet sans substance.*' Heidegger refers to Dasein as what explicates a being with regard to its Being. Since the Other represents the totality of the signifying universe for the subject, and insofar as the subject of the Real remains outside or missing within the battery of signifiers (S_2), then the subject is the subject insofar as it makes a hole in established and constituted knowledge (S_2). The subject appears where S_2 or *connaissance* is not. The S_0 remains outside group identifications, the prejudices and knowledge of the time, and represents the place from where new unconscious savoir may emerge. This is what places the subject (*nous met*) as a kind of noumenon (*noumène*) that takes us (*nous mènera*) beyond the signifier (Lacan, 1968–1969, Section V).

For the final graph, in his Seminar XVI "From Another to the other," Lacan (1968–1969) uses the symbol for the null set for the *matheme* of the signifier of the lack in the Other and says that the symbolic phallus appears in that place (Φ). The symbolic phallus is a missing signifier of jouissance, and the S is the signifier for the subject that is also missing in the Other. The Name represents something different than the signifier that represents the subject for another signifier. A Name as a unary trace (S_1) refers to the Real body of the subject rather than another signifier within language. The Name is a unary trace of jouissance that has no S_2 or another signifier that could function as its signified within the Symbolic.

In response to the lack of a signifier for the Other's lack or desire, and to the question 'What does the other want from me?' or 'Who am I?' the subject will first produce the fantasy and the *objet a* cause of the Other's desire. 'I demand of myself what you lack or desire' and 'I demand of You the ego that I am or will be.' Secondarily, and further down the graph, the ego arises as a metonymy of normative meaning that fills in or stuffs the missing place for the subject in the Other. Instead of being the S outside conventional knowledge, the normative or conventional ego searches for the social signifiers [s(O)] that could define them.

In the *matheme* for the lack in the Other in the earlier complete graph of desire (in the *Ecrits*), Lacan uses the barred A for *Autre* in French rather than the null set. The lack in the Other represents that something is missing in the Other, which could be the signifier for the o-object, capable of plugging the lack, but it could also mean that the Other is empty of signifier, letter, and representation. The barred Other appears as the signifier of a lack, or the symbolic phallus. It is the phallus as a signifier of a lack that emerges as the enjoyment of the *parletre* (speaking being). But the signifier of a lack emerges from the null set that in turn refers to the Real inexistence of the Other, the lack of a signifier, the vanishing point of the structure, and to a Third jouissance beyond the phallus.

In the Imaginary, or when the Imaginary supplants the Real, the enjoyment of the missing phallus becomes the enjoyment of the *objet a* that the fantasy of the subject generates in the place where the *objet a* is found missing in the Other. The subject's fantasy object is placed inside the hole where the object is missing in the Other. The imaginary *objet a* represents the illusory possibility of plugging the hole in the Other. In the sexual act with the imaginary Other, the subject may temporarily plug the hole and not notice what is missing, yet each repetition of the sexual act replicates the *objet a* as a missing object for the subject. The *objet a* as a residue of the sexual act shows that the sexual *partenaire* of the subject is the *objet a* rather than the other.

In this way, phallic jouissance leads to the bad infinity of surplus phallic jouissance that fails to produce a match between the *a* cause of the subject's desire and who the other is as a subject. An impossible match for a subject is not between a subject and another subject but between the *a* and the Other. *Objet a* becomes what is in the way between the desire of man and the desire of woman and directly leads to what Lacan called the lack of rapport between the sexes. With respect to the difference between the sexes, the Real manifests as the impossibility of the sexual relationship.

Lacan's first Real, as a presence disruptive of the Symbolic order, refers to the presence of the inconvenient "Thing" that appears in the place where the *a* should be missing. It is much more convenient that the *a* be missing. When the *objet a* functions as the index of a Real void (Lacan's second Real), owing to its dissolution as it approaches the Real, then this is *das Ding* in the form of the "no-thing" as a pure form of the Third jouissance beyond surplus phallic jouissance.

In neurosis, the first Real appears in the form of the impossibility of the relation between the sexes. The impasse between the sexes is traumatic given that the sexual partner is not the Other but the subject's own *objet a* that the subject will mistake for another (i[a']) subject. The first Real also appears in the *parletre* in the form of whatever is socially or conventionally said in a group about a couple, is discordant or at odds with the Real of the relationship. Whatever the ego of the statement says about a relationship, 'It's not that.'

What is traumatically Real about the sexual relation is what leads Lacan (1966–1967, Seminar XIV, Lesson 13) to consider the path of the operations of the sexual drive from the point of view of sublimation as a vicissitude of the drive. In this sense, Lacan says that the sexual act may lead to sublimation at the same time that it differs from sublimation. Phallic jouissance is the enjoyment of the sexual act where an imaginary object does not appear to be missing, and yet the sexual act perpetuates the replication of the *objet a* as a lack. Sublimation instead does not replicate the *objet a* but within sublimation, as a state or form of jouissance, the *objet a*, as an object of the sexual drive, still appears to be missing, because, after all, the subject is sublimating, and there is an end to sublimation. Sublimation does not permanently plug the hole either but stops the replication of the *objet a*.

At first Lacan linked *jouissance* to the death drive that threatens the life drive when pursuing pleasure beyond the limits of the reality principle. This follows from Freud's concept of hallucinatory wish fulfillment that can never be satisfied and always asks for more. This aspect of *jouissance* is inconvenient and needs to be brought to a stop. The drive begins with the life drive, but if unregulated, the life drive becomes the death drive. Conversely, the death drive also works within the laws and cuts of the symbolic order that refuse *jouissance* so that the law can condescend to desire, and desire can be reached in the inverted ladder of the law, as Lacan says. The law and desire put a stop to *jouissance*, and in this way, the death drive and jouissance come to work for the aims of the Life drive.

In *La Troiseme*, Lacan (1975) developed the notion of several types of *jouissance*, and the inconvenient *jouissance* became the *jouissance* of the Other that is stopped by the phallic function of symbolic castration and the symbolic order. When the jouissance of the Other is stopped, *jouissance* is attained as phallic *jouissance*. The surplus *jouissance* in the *jouissance* of the Other is transferred to phallic *jouissance* that, as we shall see subsequently, also needs to be stopped by a Third *jouissance* (defined in the previous chapter). It is the symbolic phallus, and the *Je*, S, or I, as a missing signifier of jouissance, as the form of the formless (signifier of a lack), or the no-self within the self (lack of a signifier for the I within the Other), that is an access point to the third Other jouissance.

The hole in the Other, or lack in the Other (S[Ø]), is the same as saying that there is a −1 inherent in the set of signifiers. Signifiers kill the thing, represent it, but the represented, or the signified, is missing, or outside representation. Both the dead symbolic father and the subject of the Real are 'killed' and substituted by the signifier.

Lacan says that this −1 is unpronounceable, but the operation can be pronounced whenever a proper name is pronounced in a statement. 'The operation is the calculation of signification,' as follows in the figure subsequently.

In the figure, the signifier is represented by −1, and the signified is represented as square root of −1. When the signifier represents −1 and the signified represents square root of −1, the result of their division is −1. *This means that there is a −1 or a missing signifier/subject in every statement.* However, there is a double meaning to what the missing thing is. On the one hand, there is a missing signifier as represented by −1; on the other hand, there is a signifier with no signified (the signified is not missing; it just does not exist) as represented by the square root of −1. *The −1 here represents what is missing that is unthinkable about the subject.*

"But where does this being that appears missing from the sea of proper names come from"? (Lacan p. 694). The square root of minus one represents a lot more than the phallus as an object cause of desire because it also serves as a representation of the inexistence of Being or of the One that lacks its own being. The square root of minus one, as a signifier without signified, as something more than the phallus that appears where the phallus is missing, is consistent with the Sanskrit lingam that means phallus, signifier, and the form of the formless all at once.

$$\frac{\text{S (signifier)}}{\text{s (signified)}} = \text{s (the statement)},$$

$$\text{With S} = (\text{-}1)\text{, we find: s} = \sqrt{-1}$$

$$\frac{-1}{\sqrt{-1}} = -1$$

Figure 2.8 The calculation of signification 127–128

The question of being and emptiness, present within the lack of being that constitutes desire, takes the subject/signifier beyond the confines of the signifying chain although the question of being begins at the point where the chain ends and returns to the closed circularity of language and the signifier. Being ends up gone or missing in either chain. Being is what escapes the circularity of the message and the code on the left line of the graph, while the voice is what escapes on the right side of the same graph. Being is located inside the hole of the Other [Ø] as the One's own non-being.

A question that remains outstanding is whether there is an implied relation between being and what Lacan calls the *motérialité* of lalangue, or the language of the Real unconscious. Other than association by similitude in sound, lalangue is not a metalanguage because it does not have a code (similarity in sound does not amount to a code). Further on, we will consider another aspect of Lacan's theory of the signifying chain that may contradict this last assertion. The sound of the signifier is a phonological element that refers to the Real and to the Symbolic invocation of the Real in the form of a sound wave of jouissance rather than a signifying element or particle within a system of signifiers.

Capitalized Being, that Lacan himself capitalizes (p. 694), can be thought of in terms of the Real, since, as Lacan says, the subject comes into Being and the Real when disappearing from the statement. Beyond or outside the signifier refers to a signifier that emerges from and remains linked to the Real of jouissance rather to another signifier/semblance. This is one way to read the signifier of a lack in the Other (the S_2 is missing). The capital S as a letter is a signifier of the One and of jouissance rather than the Other.

Capitalized Being in Lacan and Heidegger withdraws from the cleared ground of representation into the groundless ground of the One's own non-being. Usually Being is interpreted as the totality of subjective experience that would include many different types of beings: thoughts, words, feelings, other human or animal beings, and so on. Lacan instead refers to Being as a place of jouissance and non-thinking (I am where I do not think). In Lacanian theory, the Real is part of the Borromean knot, and although it remains mostly outside the Symbolic, the Real intersects the Symbolic and the Imaginary, nonetheless, and, therefore, is not separated from everyday imaginary and symbolic life. Heidegger sees the mystery of Being as separated from everyday ordinary life, while for Lacan, mystery or enigma, or the horizon of the Real, always bears a relationship to the spoken language.

Lalangue as the language of the One is not arranged by sinthactic conjunctions or subordinations. *Lalangue*, like wit and dreams, is impressively concise, laconic, may be structured like a riddle, and invokes a respectful Real. A house, a ship on top of it, then a letter by itself, followed by a headless subject on a beach. Logical conjunctions are missing, and instead of the 'I think,' or 'I speak' of s(O), there is a One saying that in some cases could be lacking syntaxis and grammar.

A statement states a knowledge with latent desire. Desire is the signified of those statements, yet the signified can be an unformulated desire, but as distinct from a pure desire as a form of jouissance, human desire is always in relationship to signifiers for which the statement is a substitute. Sometimes the repressed, for which the statement is a substitute, returns in the form of the saying within the statement.

In Lacan's later work, the saying refers to the subject of the enunciation and the said refers to the subject of the statement. The saying is constructed with different signifiers than the normative narrative statement and such signifiers may be "naughty" or organized in the form of a knot rather than a chain ("knots . . . are built up through developing chains of the signifying material," Lacan, 1974, p. 10).

However, Lacan will also say that these are chains of *J'ouis-sense* rather than meaning, which means that sense is not meaning, although the relations among meaning, signification, and significance are often equivocal in Lacan. With respect to the saying, in *L'etourdit*, Lacan (1972) says that the saying, despite being an enigma, follows from an enigmatic mathematical sequence. This, of course, would contradict the notion that *lalangue* is composed of the residues of language and is without a code, since a string of numbers may or may not be part of a code. A code is a differentiated part or aspect of a language that, as result of evolution, comes to regulate its meaning or function.

It may be more accurate to consider *lalangue* or the upper signifying chain not as made up of the trash, letters, or residue of language (although trashy language could certainly be the case), irrelevant to its structure, but rather of enigmatic sayings that function as senseless code that stand in at the level of language for a mathematical statement that cannot be proven within the system (linguistic or mathematical). Statements that cannot be proven according to the structure act as the foundational 'non-sense' that grounds sense in language. But how can enigmatic senseless letters of jouissance be the equivalent of mathematical or logical sequential statements that cannot be proven within the system. What would be an example of the latter?

For example, the logical statement that 0 = 1 refers to zero being the first integer of a system of whole diacritical numbers that was added to the natural numbers to increase their consistency all the way up to set theory. However, although logical, 0 = 1 is a false arithmetical statement that nonetheless grounds the arithmetical system. Zero as representing the absence of some unspecified something grounds the sequence of negative and positive integers, much the same way that non-sense grounds the sense of words within language.

Finally, the being of non-being, or the sublime outlet that Heidegger has written with an x over it, has to be brought down to earth or to '*motérialité*.' This coincides with what Joyce called an epiphany. Otherwise, a religious interpretation of Being runs the risk of solemnity or pomposity, loftiness or haughtiness, not that these traits couldn't also be found in the scientist or secular character.

The answer to the question "But where does this being, who appears in some way missing from the sea of proper names, come from?" (p. 694) comes in the form of: "I am in the place from which the universe is a flaw in the purity of Non-Being" (p. 694). Birth and death require an impurity or a loss within the pure void or emptiness. Without impurity, nothing happens, or Being does not manifest. The place of the I is the place of a flaw in the purity of Non-Being, and this place

Lacan also calls the place of *Jouissance*. The I and *jouissance* share the lack of a signifier, since the signifier is missing or is continually shifting. This is what Lacan calls the flaw in the purity of Non-being.

> the subject alternately appears and disappears in a continuous movement from signifier to signifier but can never identify with anyone – the main characteristic of the "subject of the unconscious is that of being . . . at an indeterminate place."
>
> (Lacan, 1981, p. 208 quoted by Patsalides [2001], p. 12)

In the Other, beyond a simple, particular, and self-referential name or unary trace, there is a lack of a substantial and stable referential signifier for the subject. I say self-referential in the sense that for the Name, the reference is the body rather than another signifier as is the case with metaphor and the Symbolic.

As soon as the signifier that represents a subject for another signifier names the subject, the Real subject or the subject of the Real disappears.

> the strictly linguistic definition of I as signifier . . . designates the enunciating subject but does not signify him. . . . I can come into being by disappearing from my statement. . . . Being of non-being that is how I come on the scene as a subject.
>
> (1966a, p. 678)

On the one hand, as a result of the division of the subject, the ego plugs the gap within the divided subject; on the other hand, the subject is not something substantial either that could be contraposed to the ego. The *Je* (I) of the enunciating subject for Lacan is a shifter that designates the subject but does not define it. As soon as the subject is designated by the signifier, the Real subject disappears, or goes missing. So, with Lacan's later work, the subject of the unconscious is a *'sujet sans substance.'* Does this mean then that the subject of the unconscious can only be located in the Real unconscious rather than the repressed or descriptive unconscious? The divided $ means that a subject is divided between two signifiers, but it can also refer to what about the subject is beyond the signifier and the I of the statement. The subject cannot be defined according to the signifier.

I propose that this is a different meaning of the barred subject. The subject of the Real falls in between S_1 and S_2, although it is not repressed. The subject of the unconscious appears as a discontinuity or as gap within the broken lines of the Symbolic. At this point is where Lacan defines the subject's existence as ineffable and stupid (beyond cognition). Both the ego (i[a]) and the fantasy ($\$\lozenge a$) will defensively work to plug the vacuity and lack of the subject. The subject of the Real is primarily repressed but only in the sense that there no words to describe it. In the common understanding of primary repression, what is repressed under primary repression is the pre-subject or the pre-barred imaginary phallus that the child represented for the mother. Thus, in earlier work, I have proposed that there are two types of primary repression (Moncayo, 2012; Moncayo and Romanowicz, 2015).

What falls under Freud's primary repression is the subject as the mother's imaginary phallus. Where does this subject reside, in the mind or the body? A new answer that Lacan (1966a/2006) gives is that this subject resides in the body at the level of the organ and the drive.

> So, our attention is now drawn to the subjective status of the signifying chain in the unconscious, or rather in primal repression (*Urverdrängung*). In our deduction it is easier to understand why it was necessary to question oneself regarding the function that supports the subject of the unconscious, to grasp that it is difficult to designate that subject anywhere as subject of a statement, and therefore as the articulator, when he does not even know that he is speaking. Hence the concept of drive, in which he is designated by an organic, oral, anal, etc., mapping that satisfies the requirement of being all the farther away from speaking the more he speaks.
>
> (p. 691–692)

There are two ways to understand the subject in relationship to the Real. The subject of the drive or the subject *in* the Real and the subject *of* the Real. The first refers to organ pleasure that is far away from speech, as it refers to the representation of the unbarred imaginary phallus that the child is for the mother and that is repressed under primary repression. As Edelstein (2009) states, "The organ that speaks for the subject without the subject speaking there" (p. 201). The drive rattles the subject, the subject fades before the *objet a* of the drive and desire, and in organ pleasure, the activity of the drive proceeds without speech. It is not an uncommon occurrence among human beings that the way to bypass censorship or moral judgment is simply to act out the sexual drive without discussing it first. Finally, I used to have a psychotic patient that would hear voices emanating from different internal organs. The voice of the organ would typically demand various types of perverse sexual and violent acts. The organs literally spoke to and for the subject.

The subject of the Real is something different. I pointed out previously that when the subject is named by the signifier, although the name refers to the subject, there is something Real about the subject that remains undesignated by the signifier. The Name of the subject, of course, circulates in reference to other Names/signifiers, but the reference for the Name is the subject rather another signifier. The subject as the reference for the Name is in the Real of the body. At the same time that the Name and the signifier speak for the subject, the Real subject is excluded (comes to being as the being of non-being), albeit not completely, given that the Symbolic also gives access to the Real subject that "ex-sists" outside the designation. The body as a flow of jouissance functions as signified or interpretant of the Name for the subject.

One of the fruits of a personal analysis is that the relation of the subject to the Name can change. Instead of the Name being consciously or unconsciously imposed, when the Real subject appropriates the Name in analysis, then the Name becomes imbued with the jouissance of the subject as an added value or significance.

But what is the path that goes from desire (d) to the drive? In the matheme for the drive ($◊D), D (for Demand) is in the place of the object in the formula of the phantasy ($◊*a*) whereby the object becomes a demand without a subject for the various imaginary and partial *objets* (*a*) of the drive associated with the different erogenous zones. As Edelstein (2009) has observed, in neurosis, the formula for the fantasy becomes the fantasy for the drive. In perversion, the formula for the drive becomes the formula for the fantasy.

According to Lacan, the erogenous zones have the structure of a rim with a hole inside: urinary flow and the urethra; feces and the anus; imaginary phallus and castration; breast, mouth, and weaning; voice and the void; and the absent and ubiquitous gaze of the Other as well as the opening of the eyes that never look from the place they are seen. Finally, symbolic castration is what both generates and limits the demand of the drive and the inconvenient *jouissance* of the Other.

Because of the impossibility of representing unconscious desire (the desire of the Other is an enigma) at the point of S(Ø), desire is transformed into a pure demand of the drive as represented in the top floor of the graph. To use our example again: let's say that the husband loves his wife and she loves him. They pose two questions: What do I want? And what does he/she want from me? The questions are left unanswered. The love between them is an enigma, and since they can't solve it, they reveal it through "love making," and the end result may be a baby. This is a good example of how desire is transformed into a pure demand of the drive. The One saying of desire that the subject does not know that they know is an enigma, and, as shown in the graph, the drives are partial manifestations of desire.

In the *Che Vuoi* graph, the line of desire goes up the graph, and the question of desire is posed to the Other. The *matheme* of the signifier of a lack in the Other (S[Ø]) represents the place of the enigma of the desire of the Other and the lack of a signifier in language for the enigma of desire. The vector of *jouissance* begins from this place and turns into the *matheme* and demand of the drive ($◊D).

In Seminar VI, in his commentary on Hamlet, Lacan (1958–1959) argues that Hamlet wanted to know what kind of object he was for his mother's desire/lack. Hamlet wants to know what signifier is attached to this lack. Gertrude answers Hamlet's questions by talking about her qualities as a phallic object. Lacan places some words in Gertrude's mouth that refer to the demands of the drive that follow from the signifier of a lack in the (m)Other. The words that Lacan places in Gertrude's mouth refer more to the upper signifying chain of the drive than to a normative response along the lines of how her son may or may not fulfill her social expectations as a mother. Gertrude does not have a signifier for Hamlet that he could use to define himself or tell him who he is (as an imaginary phallic object).

The enigma of the desire of the Other, however, is more than what can be framed by the formulas for the fantasy or the drive. This is the case not only because the drive wants something more than a forbidden jouissance but also because the Other lacks the signifiers to represent not only the lack of the object within desire but also the emptiness of the Other, or what the One is beyond the fantasy and the signifier.

Lacan says that desire institutes a limit on the drive but later will also say that the drive wants a satisfaction beyond the myth of a forbidden Oedipal desire (Fink, 1997, p. 208). The myth of Oedipal desire is invented to put a stop on the drive so that, in effect, the law does not constitute a true limit on desire. Thus, Lacan will say that the drive wants satisfaction rather than a forbidden pleasure or object. The drive wants something beyond unconscious Oedipal desire.

The myth and phantasy of a forbidden fruit becomes a lack in the Other or in the law or signifying system. The prohibition of incest is a structural prohibition that both limits and fuels Oedipal desire. Either the Law forbids the flaw or warns against the fall or the Law makes up the fiction of a forbidden desire. The Law implants and creates the very object that it intends to forbid. However, the Law does not end with the prohibition of incest, since the social Other places many barriers on the objects of desire and not only on Oedipal desire. The object cause of desire is the same as the object of the drive except that the object of the drive is more than a forbidden object. The lack and nostalgia for the lost object that constitute desire lead to a demand of the drive that in the end is only limited by symbolic castration as a logical structure rather than a forbidding or prohibitive tyrannical (f)Other.

What remains unclear in Lacanian theory is whether the Law stops desire and/or generates a passion for a jouissance beyond the prohibition. Such passion is also something more than the inconvenient fusion with the Other (the jouissance of Other) and more than an illusory jouissance on the other side of the wall of the Law. The drive seeks a jouissance beyond the promise of a forbidden jouissance. When desire puts a stop to jouissance so that it can be reached in the inverted ladder of the Law, an arrested jouissance does not only yield to desire but also to succeeding forms of jouissance. Inhibiting suffering or a forbidden pleasure not only facilitates desire but also the emergence of a new form of jouissance.

Lacan links jouissance and the drive to the push or impetus to act and not only to what energizes fantasy life and the life of the Imaginary, which is the realm where desire longs for a forbidden fruit. The drive and jouissance are linked to the Real, and the Real is linked to the act as a cut that brings the dimension of the Real to bear on a symbolic series or an imaginary landscape.

The subject and signifier of the social statement and narrative can escape normativity by ascending to the level of the fantasy. Here the subject represents for itself what the Other wants and what they want from the Other. But in the fantasy, the subject is blind or does not see how the fantasy has the function, yes, to support desire, but also to defend against the symbolic castration embedded in social speech. This aspect of the Code is hidden in the fantasy. The $ or divided subject in the formula ($◊a) hides the two components of the division: $\$ = S_1 - S_2$. The Other interprets/frames the fantasy, but the fantasy also contains the *objet a* in the Imaginary and the Real as a form of jouissance.

The Other of the Law generates a desire bound by the law that stops the first jouissance, but symbolic castration generates not only the demand for a phallic jouissance or act under the Law but also a jouissance consistent with the Law but beyond the Law at the same time.

Thus, the drive and *jouissance* acquire the capacity to go beyond castration and to be *not-all* under the law of castration. Once the upper floor or horizontal vector of the graph is realized, the vector of *Che Vuoi* is transformed into '*désêtre*' (unbeing or disbeing), or the emptiness of Being. Sublimation here represents both a substitutive and direct satisfaction of the drive that stops the replication of the *objet a* while at the same time not being complete or devoid of words and objects of desire. Social purposes that represent drives that are inhibited or 'castrated' in their aims constitute substitutive formations. But for Lacan, Oedipal desire, and the demands of the drives, are also substitutive forms of satisfaction. The drive also wants a direct and indeterminate satisfaction beyond oedipal desire.

The *not-all* under castration represents the possibility of a Third *jouissance* in relationship to a phallic *jouissance* made possible by the phallic function yet beyond the question of having (+phi) and not having (-phi) the phallus. Such direct satisfaction of the drive could be represented by a relationship between the symbolic function and the *objet a* in the Real as the index of a void rather than as an imaginary object.

Capital Phi, or the symbolic phallus that is missing by its very definition due to the function of castration, is the signifier of *jouissance.* It is interesting that Lacan says that the symbolic phallus is the signifier of *jouissance* and at the same time that the question of *jouissance* is 'What am I?' Both the missing I or substantial subject and the symbolic phallus can be seen as signifiers of *jouissance,* yet *jouissance* is also said not to have a signifier. Jouissance is a signless index and the outside Real that structures the internal coherence of the symbolic order. There are no signifiers of *jouissance,* or the signifiers of *jouissance* have gone missing, although jouissance can be contingently embedded in any signifier.

The signifier of a lack in the Other or as a signifier that the Other is lacking gives a different meaning to the question 'What does the other want from me?' Since ultimately the desire of the Other is a mystery or enigma without an answer, the subject produces the fantasy represented in the graph by the formula for the fantasy. The subject wishes to either complete the Other or fears that the Other wants him/her to lose something or give up the object (the Other demands the subject's castration).

Because the Other is lacking and no longer complete or whole (A or O), "The lack in the Other is called to answer (*Che Vuoi*) for the value of this treasure (the battery of signifiers or A)" (idem). The ideals of the complete Other that divided the subject will now be defined according to the signifiers of the drive/*jouissance.* The neurotic identifies the Other's lack (of ideals and signifiers) with the Other's demand, or the demands of the drive. "Indeed, the neurotic is the one who identifies the Other's lack with the Other's demand, f with D" (idem). For the neurotic, the Other's demand takes the function of the object (of the fantasy), and the fantasy is reduced to the drive ([$◊a]→[$◊D]). "In the neurotic . . . fantasy is reduced to the drive ($◊D)" (Miller, p. 26). The subject makes demands on the object of fantasy by making a demand to be demanded. In the drive, the object makes demands on the subject as a result of the subject's demand to be demanded (by the o-objects, the function of the Other's demand).

When the vector of desire goes up from the place of the Code and towards the *matheme* of the drive, the subject seems to get past the closed repetitive circle of the law and desire but only to fall into the circle of demand. The circle of demand is represented by the retroactive line that goes from the *matheme* of the drive to the signifier of the lack in the Other and back to the *matheme* of the drive.

In his interesting paper, "The Drive is Speech," Jacques-Alan Miller (1997) mentions that Lacan describes at least three types of demand. "There is the demand of need by which the quest for the object of need must pass through the apparatus of language. It is developed in Seminar IV, for example, and one sees there the vector of desire as a derived effect" (p. 27).

Miller then writes about the demand for love that as a function introduces the Other as such. "Not simply the object it can give, but nothing other than the love sign. And in Lacan's *Écrits* he inscribes desire between those two forms of demand. As he says, "desire overextends itself on this side and beyond. You see the desire between the demand for need and the demand for love" (p. 26). The most interesting, for the purpose of this chapter, is a third demand for *jouissance*, which, as Miller says, is drive.

The unconscious demand to be demanded from the place of the lack in the Other is articulated both in phallic *jouissance* and the *jouissance* of the Other. Symbolic castration is what limits the demand of the drive for the inconvenient *jouissance* of the Other, as well as the inconvenience of surplus phallic jouissance. The *jouissance* of the Other stands for the disappearance of the subject when the subject becomes an object of the Other's fantasy.

Forbidden Oedipal desire is a myth created to substitute and conceal the true limits imposed by symbolic castration. "But what is not a myth, although Freud formulated it just as early on as he formulated the Oedipus myth, is the castration complex" (p. 695). In addition, Lacan also says that "Castration means that *jouissance* has to be refused in order to be attained on the inverse scale of the law of desire" (p. 700). Right before making this statement, Lacan had said, "Desire is a defense against going beyond a certain limit in *jouissance*" (p. 699). Desire is caused by the apparent symbolic castration of the object. In an ascending and descending movement, desire is replaced and represented by the signifiers of the drive, and the signifiers of desire (Capital Phi) replace the drive.

Obviously, the acceptance of the lack, or symbolic castration, would be one of the ways we can get past the demands of the drive. But how can castration be overcome? For Freud, a personal analysis was shipwrecked on the rock of castration. The analysis of masculinity does not go beyond the point the passing through of which would indicate a giving in, a submission into passivity before the father. Correspondingly, the analysis of femininity collides with the demand for the phallus, the impossibility of which makes for varied dissatisfactions and complaints, if not for plain depressions.

To go beyond castration requires the benevolent depersonalization of the analyst and the subjective destitution of the analysand. The analyst has to forego being in the position of the Ideal, and the analysand has to find their being in non-being or emptiness beyond their narcissistic ego anxieties and beyond the preoccupation with being or not being, having and not having, the imaginary phallus.

I propose that for Freud, castration meant the symbolic loss of the penis, while for Lacan, castration represents the realization that the imaginary phallus does not exist.

Mark Danielewski (2000) once said, "Youth always tries to fill the void, an old man learns to live with it." Lacan says that in the case of the signifier of a lack in the Other (S[Ø]), what we are dealing with is the signifier of the lack of the zero symbol. Lacan has also said that the symbolic phallus appears in the place of the lack in the Other, but because it is missing or non-existent, what is not there cannot be negated.

The inexistence of the phallus is the balancing point of symbolic exchange. According to this definition of the zero symbol, following Lévi-Strauss (1950), if the symbol is missing, then no symbolic exchange is possible. The zero symbol is a missing place that represents the balancing point of symbolic exchange. By itself, the zero symbol does not exist, because it represents the absence of something. Thus, the phallus, as a unit of analysis, functions as a zero point of symbolic exchange and at the same time does not exist. That it does not exist is another way of saying that the zero symbol is missing.

The phallus functions but does not exist. The zero symbol is lacking because we are not dealing with a state of affairs where the penis existed and then was lost or cut off. The zero symbol in that case would represent the absence of the previously present penis, like an apple that was there and then eaten. When the zero symbol itself is missing, then this is equivalent to the Lacanian realization that the missing phallus does not exist or "ex-sists" in 'ex-stasis' in a Platonic mathematical realm.

Conclusion

In conclusion, Lacan's graph of desire is a mathematical/topological representation of the relations between desire and the law, the signifier/subject and the code. It also helps to describe concepts such as desire and the desire of the Other, *jouissance*, and the drive. Desire cannot exist without the law and vice versa. Also, desire can only be represented with the help of mathematical graph theory, since it lacks signifiers that could describe it. The most difficult part at the top of the graph I formulated in terms of the going beyond castration. It is a question posed throughout the chapter. Following Lacan and his graph, I argue that the place (which is a no-place) beyond castration is realized through the non-existence of the imaginary phallus and the unthinkable Being of the subject that is missing within the Other and the battery of signifiers.

References

Danielewski, M. (2000). *House of Leaves*. New York: Pantheon.
Edelstein, A. (2009). *The Graph of Desire*. London: Karnac.

Fink, B. (1995). *The Lacanian Subject: Between Language and Jouissance*. Princeton, NJ: Princeton University Press.

Fink, B. (1997). *A Clinical Introduction to Lacanian Psychoanalysis*. Cambridge: Harvard University Press.

Freud, S. (1909). Notes upon a Case of Obsessional Neurosis. In: *Three Case Histories*, New York: Collier Books, 1973.

Lacan, J. (1957–1958). *The Formations of the Unconscious: Book V: The Seminar of Jacques Lacan*. Edited by J.-A. Miller and Translated by R. Grigg. London: Polity Press.

Lacan, J. (1958–1959). *Desire and Its Interpretation: The Seminar of Jacques Lacan*. Book VI. Edited by J.-A. Miller and Translated by B. Fink. Cambridge: Polity Press, 2019.

Lacan, J. (1960–1961a). *Transference: Book VIII*. Unpublished translation by C. Gallagher, c.f. www.lacaninireland.com.

Lacan, J. (1960–1961b). *Transference: The Seminar of Jacques Lacan*. Book VIII. London: Polity Press, 2017.

Lacan, J. (1961–1962). *The Seminar of Jacques Lacan IX: On Identification*. Translated by C. Gallagher. London: Karnac.

Lacan, J. (1964). *The Four Fundamental Concepts of Psychoanalysis*. New York: Norton, 1981.

Lacan, J. (1966a). *Ecrits, the First Complete Edition in English*. Translated by B. Fink. New York and London: Norton, 2006.

Lacan, J. (1966b). The Subversion of the Subject and the Dialectic of Desire in the Freudian Unconscious. In: *Ecrits*. Translated by B. Fink. New York and London: Norton, 2006.

Lacan, J. (1966–1967). *The Seminar of Jacques Lacan: Book XIV: The Logic of Phantasy*. Unofficial translation by C. Gallagher from unedited French manuscripts.

Lacan, J. (1968–69). *From Another to the Other*. Book XVI. Unpublished translation by C. Gallagher, www.lacaninireland.com.

Lacan, J. (1971–72) . . . *ou pire* (or worse). Book XIX. Unpublished translation by C. Gallagher. www.lacaninireland.com.

Lacan, J. (1971–72). *The Knowledge of the Psychoanalyst*. Book XIXa. Unpublished translation by C. Gallagher. www.lacaninireland.com.

Lacan, J. (1972). L'etourdit. *The Letter*, 41, 31–80, 2009.

Lacan, J. (1974). *Television*. Edited by J. Copjec. New York: London, 1990.

Lacan, J. (1975). *La Troiseme*. *Lettres de l'école freudienne*, (16), 178–203.

Lévi-Strauss, C. (1950). *Introduction to the Work of Marcel Mauss*. Translated by F. Baker. London: Routledge, 1987.

Miller, J. A. (1997). The Drive Is Speech: Umbr(a): On the Drive. *Journal of the Center for Psychoanalysis and Culture*, 1, 1997.

Moncayo, R. (2009). *Evolving Lacanian Perspectives for Clinical Psychoanalysis*. London: Karnac.

Moncayo, R. and Romanowicz, M. (2015). *The Real Jouissance of Uncountable Numbers: The Philosophy of Science within Lacanian Psychoanalysis*. London: Karnac.

Quinet, A. (2018). *Lacan's Clinical Technique: Lack(a)nian Analysis*. London: Routledge.

3 The clinical evidence for psychoanalysis, standard and non-standard frames, and the question of pure and applied psychoanalysis

Before going into the content, process, and details of the actual practice of Lacanian analysis later on, this chapter will examine the evidence and epistemology behind the form, frame, and symbolic effectiveness of analytic treatment.

Although I will largely focus on psychoanalysis in private practice as the exemplary site for the practice, in Chapter 12, I also address the application of psychoanalysis to psychotherapy in the public and private clinic. When speaking of private practice, I do not refer to services solely available to the upper classes, which is how psychoanalysis was first understood in the United States. This was primarily due to the long past association between psychoanalysis and the business-based medical establishment. Private here refers to Freud's belief that psychoanalysis can only thrive in democratic rather than totalitarian societies. It is in the private sector where psychoanalysis can give the subject some relief from the family, society, and the state. Not sure the same can be said of other forms of psychotherapeutic treatment.

Both applied and non-standard analysis take different shapes in both private and public or institutional settings. When describing non-standard analyses, this chapter is primarily referring to psychoanalysis in a private-practice setting. However, it is also possible to apply Lacanian psychoanalysis to a public or institutional setting, but this would be a related but different topic. In an analytical school, both the personal and control analysis of an analyst in formation take place in private practice.

I will first introduce and define some of the basic terms I will be using in this chapter. Let's start with defining pure and applied psychoanalysis. Pure psychoanalysis refers to psychical or mental phenomena and interventions or practices associated with and only with psychoanalysis in a strict sense. The speech or mental phenomena addressed by pure psychoanalysis refers to unconscious material and true speech regarding desire rather than to conscious narratives or stories about everyday things, although desire can also be embedded in the latter. Psychoanalysis successfully finds its object as a science in the upper floor of the signifying chain within the graph of desire, as explained in the previous chapter.

In addition, pure can also refer to interventions that are justified by theoretical criteria and not solely by practical rules. However, pure psychoanalysis should not be construed as only theoretical or academic, since it also refers to the derivation of the theory from the formations of the unconscious as manifested in the clinic and in the graph of desire. Applied psychoanalysis refers to the application of psychoanalysis to clinical practice and treatment in general, but more specifically, it refers to the alleviation of symptoms and mental or emotional suffering (Miller, 2015).

Psychoanalysis as a treatment cannot be reduced to the alleviation of symptoms, since the personal analysis of an analyst in formation also requires the analysis of character, which is something that lay persons may not bring to an analysis. Personality traits are typically ego-syntonic. Finally, applied psychoanalysis can also refer to the application of psychoanalytic ideas to the treatment of conditions that fall outside the neuroses for which psychoanalysis was traditionally considered the recommended treatment.

These two categories are also intimately related to the next set of basic categories: the standard and the non-standard analysis or treatment. Typically people think of the standard or classical treatment and pure psychoanalysis as being the same, but this is not necessarily the case. Pure psychoanalysis is defined by the material or mental and emotional phenomena disclosed and worked on during the treatment. The standard analysis refers to the setting, the furniture and tools or technology used, and the frequency and length of both sessions and treatments. The non-standard treatment may vary with respect to the frame (variable length and frequency of sessions and treatment) but works on pure analytical material and thus may achieve the same or better results than a classical or standard analysis and applied psychoanalysis (a focus on symptom improvement or resolution). Conversely, a standard analysis may work on material that may not be consistent with pure psychoanalysis and achieve or not the results expected from applied psychoanalysis.

The third set of categories refers to the distinction between psychoanalysis and psychotherapy. On the one hand, psychotherapy refers to the definition of applied psychoanalysis and to the conception of psychoanalysis as a method of clinical treatment. Psychoanalysis is a form of psychotherapeutic treatment. On the other hand, psychotherapy can be differentiated from psychoanalysis as a sub-category of psychoanalysis in the case of psychoanalytic psychotherapy or as an alternative to psychoanalysis in the case of treatments that have been developed after psychoanalysis and against psychoanalysis. I will have more to say about this further in the chapter.

The concept of evidence in psychoanalysis

The concept of evidence is both similar and different across disciplines. In medicine, the concept of evidence-based practices is very simple and straightforward. A medicine either helps the symptom or it does not, and the difference matters because the professional oath of medical doctors is to help others and make sure that treatments do no harm. In addition, regardless of what the research says, a medication, for example, has to be able to help particular patients in their natural environment without producing too many adverse side effects. In law, and court proceedings leading to conviction or acquittal, the consequences are just as serious, and yet the evidence is often not quantitative because qualitative and non-computational logical analyses may also be used to arrive at legal decisions.

In a similar way to the legal concept of evidence, psychological science uses both quantitative and qualitative research methods. In fact, evidence-based practice in psychology adheres to a broad definition of what constitutes an empirical science. There exist multiple sources of scientific evidence. So long as actual therapeutic treatment involves assessment, diagnosis, and treatment procedures, any contemporary form of psychotherapy could be considered to be utilizing empirically supported principles so long as there is consensus among recognized experts within a particular psychotherapeutic orientation.

However, many professionals nowadays, especially psychoanalysts and those analytically trained, believe that evidence-based practice exclusively refers to treatments that have been proven successful in randomized trials using experimental and control groups. However, as stated previously, the American Psychological Association (APA, 2006) recognizes that best practices in psychotherapy refers to a much wider definition of clinical evidence and observation. The APA endorses multiple types of research evidence, including outcome research, clinical observation, qualitative research, and in-depth case studies.

In social science research, the term 'logic' is used loosely and refers to the stock of background beliefs used by investigators. Despite the various levels of reason and logic presented in the introduction to this book, logic in research generally refers to the likelihood of evidence given a hypothesis or its negation. Hypotheses in this case could refer to lose or prejudicial beliefs or to theories constructed according to historical precedent and various levels of logic and demonstration.

So, although social scientists in North American academia are of two kinds: those who believe in atheoretical science ('brainiatry' or brain research, for example) and those who only believe in scientific concepts built on Likert scales and the like, the end result ends up being almost the same. So-called scientific theories end up being trivial and completely divorced from intellectual history and the stream of knowledge that has been transmitted and corrected throughout the generations. In fact, and paradoxically, this is only the fate of the social sciences, including psychology, within Anglo American Academia.

The hard sciences, especially in Europe, have no problem proceeding from theoretical or mathematical premises that only later become confirmed by experiment. As Einstein (1944) said,

> A knowledge of the historic and philosophical background gives that kind of independence from prejudices of his generation from which most scientists are suffering. This independence created by philosophical insight is – in my opinion – the mark of distinction between a mere artisan or specialist and a real seeker after truth.
>
> (EA 61–573)

Einstein's understanding points to the conflict between the different forms of reason, between the specialist/technician, telescope designer/builder and observer, and the seeker after truth, between formal and technological reason and the historical and philosophical forms of reason that Einstein mentions. Although typically it is the specialist and the institution who suppress the seeker-theoritician, the two can also cooperate, since theorists are never right about everything. However, established theory cannot be entirely rejected without adequate argumentation or legitimate evidence at the correct logical or rational level.

An experiment, for example, never proves the entirety of a theory that can still contain both false and true untested presuppositions. Einstein also said that there is no direct correspondence between the individual parts of a theory and the empirical phenomena in question. *Only parts of the theory and parts of the totality of empirical facts correspond to one another, and yet it is the internal coherence of the theory that stands the best chance of explaining the structure of empirical facts, even though theory and facts don't entirely correspond with one another.* In fact, Einstein believed that the internal coherence of the theory was more important than its verification by external evidence or data. For Einstein, theory is undetermined by evidence. As a scientist once put it: "All this abstract non-sense is the correct theory of reality." Einstein used dreams, thought experiments, visualizations, and abstract mathematics to investigate what cannot be seen through the senses.

A theory cannot be falsified or invalidated by facts, for facts can only contradict certain aspects of the theory, not its structure. The structure itself can only be falsified on theoretical and/or mathematical grounds and at the correct logical level. Therefore, specialists cannot falsify the theory; they can only confirm it, develop some aspect of it, or critique it by focusing on those facts that contradict certain elements of the theory. Einstein corrected or contributed to Newton's theory of gravity on conceptual and mathematical grounds, and then the new theory could explain facts that the previous theory could not.

Specialists in the mental health field trying out new treatment methods that could work better for certain populations, particularly those who are not good candidates for intensive talk therapy, personal disclosure, and free association several times a week, are not in a position to falsify the theory, not only because some of the new techniques may have been derived from psychoanalytic ideas but because of the fact that if some elements of the theory prove to be erroneous, this does not invalidate the structure of the theory itself. The structure of the theory has to be replaced by a new structure that gives a better explanation of the majority of the facts and events of the field. How things appear are not the structure of what appears. If the structure of the theory is rejected because of some false or misunderstood elements in it, and a new reduced or simplified structure is put in its place, the new structure will not withstand the test of time.

Let us use a clinical example within our field that may also throw some light on the accuracies and misconceptions of the two most influential currents of Freudian psychoanalysis (Lacanian and object relations theory) as well as placing them in a relationship of checks and balances to one another. With this exercise, I do not intend to prove one true and the other false, although both can function as experimental and alternative hypotheses to each another. Instead, the two forms of psychoanalysis will be appraised as an instantiation of two world systems (S_1 and S_2, respectively) across different fields and phenomena.

In one world system, one theory prevails across different national and gender interests, while the same is true for the other world system. Anglo American feminism eliminates sexual differences (confusing them with gender oppression and gender roles) while Latin, Continental, and Eastern thought upholds them. While eliminating sexual difference with an egalitarian ethos, the former risks the pathologies of a matriarchal system presided over by a dominant mother and a disavowed, subjugated, and contested father. Conversely, by upholding sexual difference, the second group risks not only gender stereotypes but devolving into a patriarchal system presided over by a domineering father and a degraded and subjugated mother.

Unfortunately for human beings, there are division, misrecognition, and miscommunication between the two world systems that generate fault lines and fractures in the structure that sustains human existence. The two world systems need to be placed in a relationship to one another, as seen in Lacan's formulation of the paternal/parental metaphor. It is a question of the relationship between mother and father, nature and the desire of the mother, and culture or the NoF and the structure of signification and jouissance.

In the case of a problem with being able to live independently, for example, we look for evidence that could prove or disprove hypotheses A and B. Hypothesis A is that a problem with independence or separation was caused by a failure of good-enough mothering or a deficit of maternal desire for the child, while hypothesis B holds that pampering, overinvestment, fusion between mother and child, and the rejection of the phallic function of symbolic castration caused the difficulty with separation and independence. Evidence supporting either hypothesis would explain the insufficient separation and differentiation between mother and child, self and other.

According to hypothesis A, a subject can't separate or function independently because the lack of good-enough mothering led to a deficit of independent living skills due to insufficient support (deficit of maternal desire and care giving) in childhood. Conversely, the null hypothesis would be that the deficit in independence was caused by an excess of dependence on the mother in childhood. How to decide between the two hypotheses, or a combination of the two, for that matter?

In my opinion, these hypotheses have validity independently from the larger question of whether separation or independence are relevant objective concepts or only culturally relative ones that are dependent on the epistemological and cultural orientation of the analyst. Typically, in our field, one system or theory would defend A, while a second theory would defend B without attempting to logically or empirically rule out one or the other. In one theoretical world, A prevails, while in the other, B prevails, and the two worlds remain at odds with each other. In the Introduction, I characterized the conflict between systems as a conflict between different forms of reason.

An analyst can also test the hypothesis not only on the basis of evidential sayings but also by how the analysand responds to interventions. Do they become more or less independent with more or less support? If the analysand becomes less independent with support, then this would give weight to the hypothesis that the problem with independence was given by excessive fusion and dependence in childhood.

Regarding the possibility that changing combinations between the two hypotheses would best explain the problems at hand, it is important to note that in the actual treatment, any mediating variables could be investigated (or a decision made not to) right there and then. For example, any traumas or forced separations that could impact the hypotheses, or the evidence, would be explored alongside the main questions. In clinical trials research, one would have to isolate the variables and handle them separately, thus artificially removing them from their own natural context.

All this for what purpose? So that we could precisely measure the extent to which the hypothesis determines the problem in question? Mind you that I have already done violence to the theory, and the phenomena it describes, by reducing it to somewhat simplistic categories for purposes of research. Then I could develop two Likert scales to measure the evidence with some questions that test the hypothesis in the light of the evidence. The scores are submitted to statistical analysis of probability that will determine the likelihood that the hypothesis is correct according to the distribution of large samples and numbers.

Researchers will accept margins of significance that are no larger than a flip of a coin (.5). Then supposedly if the margin of correlation is significant, I can proceed to construct a "scientific theory" with the two reduced and simplistic constructs that have been empirically proven by the research "artifice" and a flip of coin. Here the principle that the simplest theory is the best theory does not apply, given that simplicity is an artifice of the method. The theory here is simplistic rather than simple, given that it does not adequately reflect the complexity of the actual state of affairs.

Coming back to the question of decidability or being able to decide which hypothesis is true or false, I recognize that the phenomena in question varies case by case: in some cases, A may be true and B false, while in others, the reverse may be true. In addition, there are three criteria by which we can decide which hypothesis is correct on a case-by-case basis. The first criterion is subjective: the analysand experiences the ring of truth or truth-effects in their own experience, regardless of whether they feel understood according to their preferred conscious narratives or way of seeing things. Second, there are memories and fantasies revealed in key significant signifiers and speech that will provide confirmation of one hypothesis and not the other. This point is important because psychoanalytic data here is not anecdotal, as is often claimed in simplistic and vulgarized versions of empiricism. Anecdotal refers to storytelling or a social narrative but not to the unconscious signifying chain.

In psychoanalysis, speech statements (data) proceed according to the laws of signification and language that generate at least three levels of the conscious and unconscious signifying chain, as explained in Chapter 2 on the signifying chain. Third and finally, the correct hypothesis will lead to the analysand's increased independence as a function of the treatment. The three probative criteria provide accurate explanations and resolutions rather than the probability that one or the other hypothesis may be the case. Given the impracticality and ethical questions raised by the impossibility of using large random samples from actual clinical practice, rational explanation using levels of logic and reason to sort out the evidence are superior to establishing the probabilities for entire populations, as can be done with eye color, height, age, dates, types of blood, or blood pressure readings, for example.

Probability starts with a coin toss with a 50% chance of heads or tails, yes or no, true or false. Can we say that there is a .5 chance that children will be desired and cared for by their mothers and a .5 chance that they won't? In fact, this may not be the case, and the actual numbers may be quite different, since there are many more variables than a simple binary choice. We would have to toss the coin many times to find and assess many cases to determine the exact numbers in the group distribution.

Do we need an experiment or large random samples to test the hypotheses that lack of support or too much support could result in difficulties with separation/independence? The hypothesis could be established as a premise, to be confirmed by the singular evidence provided by specific memories/fantasies/dreams described by narratives and key words/signifiers, by examining patterns in relationships, and by the retroactive confirmation provided by the analysand becoming increasingly independent and able to tolerate being away from a loved one as a function of the evidence, the hypotheses, and interventions.

In this case, the probative value of a hypothesis cannot be established by the ratio between the relative probability that one or the other hypothesis could lead to independence. For most evidence, obtaining the figures necessary for computing the likelihood ratio is problematic. There is no a priori way of determining the correct reference class. Different reference classes may produce very different likelihood ratios. Any choice of reference group is contestable in principle. The reference class composed of mothers who have children but either desire them or not (as objects or subjects) has to be established by evidential reasoning where context, concept, logical argument, and judgment play fundamental roles.

P is the probability that a subject cannot function independently due to the evidence adduced in the course of treatment supporting the hypotheses that either persistent dyadic fusion with the mother or a deficit or breach of maternal desire and duty of care is the case. The utility of the hypotheses being true is much greater than the disutility that the hypotheses and interventions may be incorrect. The treatment will at least produce a placebo effect, and the intervention itself may facilitate the subject's independence regardless of the evidence and hypotheses. Thus, understanding standards of proof in terms of mathematical probabilities is indeed very controversial.

That one or the other hypothesis represents forms of either environmental family failure or psychical structural failure, and that this harmed the capacity of the subject to function independently, is something that will be intuitively clear and convincing and therefore useful in practice and consistent with analytic knowledge and tradition. In fact, this is an example of how Lacan's theory bridges both hypotheses despite the concept of the NoF that appears to represent only one of the hypothesis (how something appears is not the structure of what appears). What Lacan calls the paternal metaphor includes two factors: the desire of the mother and the Name of the father. The desire of the mother is a signified for the NoF as a signifier, or the NoF is a signifier for the desire of the mother as a signified.

This theoretical formulation can be translated into the terms of the hypotheses discussed. For example, not enough maternal desire/support already indicates a libidinal disinvestment in the child in such a way that the child does not become first an object that can be latter ratified as a subject by the NoF. In some cases, the father in the family (rather than the function) may intervene despite the failure of maternal desire to shore up the child as a subject, but the first damage has already been done. A father's disinterest in the mother's disinterest in the child would also indicate a disinterest in his descendancy. In either case, such a damaged paternal metaphor would fail to establish the subjective structure in the child necessary for a new independent subject to thrive.

On the other hand, if the mother's desire is in fact established, meaning that the child is established as an object of the mother's desire, then the NoF as a function (not the father as a family member) needs to symbolically castrate this object, helping separate the subject from the mother in the process. The symbolic mother facilitates this process by relinquishing her object to the father and the symbolic order.

If the mother fails to collaborate in this process, the imaginary mother is stronger than the symbolic mother, and the father is a contested father, then the NoF will be compromised in the capacity to break up the fusion between mother and child at the point that it has outlived its usefulness. This also indicates a failure in the symbolic mother to love the child as a subject beyond herself. Even if the biological father is a 'deadbeat dad,' the symbolic mother needs to avow the symbolic function, or the symbolic father, to generate subjective structure in the child even in the absence of the biological father.

In addition, regardless of the hypotheses, there is a coherent relation between evidential statements/speech, the two hypotheses, and the interventions of the analyst. Another factor is the strength of the theory (best available explanation of the evidence rather than its probability) and its logical levels of articulation, the extent to which the researchers are convinced by the reasonableness of the hypotheses, and the extent to which the hypotheses are warranted by the evidence provided by the subject's speech.

Psychoanalysis relies on theory emerging from Western and Eastern intellectual traditions, as well as science, and thus is not based on prejudicial beliefs lacking theoretical argumentation or logical analysis. Psychoanalytic theory is not based on beliefs that represent preferred opinion, cultural prejudice, wishful thinking, and/or national or gender bias. Finally, a treatment will typically have many sessions in which the hypotheses can be tested or challenged.

Dissemination bias regarding the ineffectiveness of psychoanalysis as a treatment method

Freudian psychoanalysis became taboo within the clinic of evidence-based practices. There are many reasons for this being the case, despite the fact that a close cousin of psychoanalysis, psychodynamic psychotherapy, has been shown to be efficacious in evidence-based controlled studies (Schedler, 2010). Meta-analysis by Leichsenring and Rabung (2009) showed that long-term psychodynamic psychotherapy (LTPP) showed significantly higher outcomes in overall effectiveness, target problems, and personality functioning than shorter forms of psychotherapy. It also showed that LTPP patients with complex mental disorders on average were better off than 96% of the patients in the comparison groups ($P = .002$). Thus, within the psychodynamic field widely construed, there are many who consider psychodynamic psychotherapy a more efficient treatment than psychoanalysis.

When it comes to psychoanalysis, the situation is even worse, and subsequently, we will discuss how psychoanalysis has had a big role to play in this being the case. There seems to be an interesting dissemination bias that considers psychoanalysis an outdated form of treatment that is rarely used mostly because of its lack of efficacy. This conviction is being repeated like a gospel not only between health care professionals but also between health care policy makers and researchers.

In addition to LTPP, there are a number of studies that prove the contrary. For example, a study performed by Busch, Milrod and Sandberg (2013) not only demonstrated the efficacy of psychoanalytic treatment for panic disorder but also provided guidelines on ways psychoanalysis could be introduced into the era of evidence-based medicine. There is also empirical evidence that psychoanalysis, as a long-term psychotherapeutic treatment, produces more robust results and outcomes over time. The relapse rates of short-term treatments such as CBT (cognitive behavior therapy) or medications tend to increase over time, while the after-termination results of psychoanalysis indicate that patients get better over time, and the analysis tends to continue producing effects post-termination. The evidence for these results comes from controlled studies and not only from consumer-reported studies of outcome (Levy, 2011).

Since its inception, psychoanalysis has not relied on statistical sampling methods and control groups but has operated according to the single clinical case study method as a point of articulation between theory and clinical practice. In addition, there is a practical problem in presenting the empirical evidence revealed in the practice of psychoanalysis as a treatment method.

The problem is social, ethical, and legal in nature. People often complain that Lacan never spoke about cases, and this is contrasted to Freud's presentation of famous case histories. However, despite Freud's attempts to disguise and protect the identity of his patients, one by one, historians eventually revealed the identities of most if not all of his analysands. Nowadays extensive psychoanalytic case histories cannot be published without written consent from the patients. Statistically based studies using experimental and control groups also require prior consent, but the material reported in these studies differs greatly from the unconscious material disclosed in analytical sessions. The latter typically contains much more sensitive and confidential information.

Psychologists or psychiatrists who use experimental designs rarely engage the kind of material that analysands speak to their analyst during the course of an analysis, so their data invariably remains within the normal socially acceptable narrative that people could share about themselves with anyone. In addition, empirically based theories are also constructed on the basis of surface constructs that match the conscious narratives and concerns of people. In this regard, and as shown in the graph of desire in the previous chapter, statistically validated psychotherapy remains within the narrative floor of the graph of desire.

Then measures are constructed on the basis of such constructs where the questions asked from research subjects are entirely based on the conscious narratives of patients. Conscious narratives and words can be analyzed and counted in various ways, and there have been empirical studies doing precisely this (Pennebaker, 1995, 1997). However, these studies are limited to disclosures of traumatic experiences or to such things as determining hidden motivations in the texts written by terrorists or determining a subject's health status by analyzing their use of causal words or personal pronouns.

Some psychoanalysts (Langs, Baladamenti and Thomson, 1996) have used statistical models to discover the most efficient process to be used in the analytical environment. They start out from the phenomenological or empirical point of view that communication between individuals is a form of storytelling that follows certain laws implicit in language that lead to 'communicative adaptation' and 'co-constructed' speech. However, the problem is that this unit of analysis is entirely within the conscious social narrative level of the signifying chain that simply represents conformity and adaptation to the values of contemporary normative society. This may be psychotherapy, but it is not psychoanalysis. Langs (1998) understands that the surface or manifest level of narratives are an unreliable basis for assessing psychical structural material or the analyst's interventions. Coding themes in the social narrative of a patient, although meaningful, does not represent truth at the level of the Ucs. in which the symptom is lodged.

Finally, the empirical subjects used in empirical or evidence-based behavioral practice (EBP) are often university students that differ greatly from the populations seen in clinical practice. Thus, clinical experience may be wider than the evidence produced in statistical research and not only vice versa. What works in the clinic may not be proven by controlled studies, and what is proven efficient in academic studies may not work in the clinic. Most university researchers are not clinicians, as well as vice versa. In fact, when EBP is used in the clinic, the rates of clinical effectiveness are not greater than that of clinicians not using EBP. The two aspects of clinical experience and the singularity of each subject have been the hallmarks of the psychoanalytic observational and scientific method since Freud.

As stated previously regarding Einstein's epistemology, theory and practice do not form two complementary pieces of a whole or directly translate or correspond to one another. There is no bi-univocal one-to-one correspondence between the totality of a theory and a practice. Either one or the other tends to be excluded in the process. Either an excess of theory eclipses the possibility of thinking about patients and interventions, or focusing on patients and interventions makes for a more restricted theory. Theory and practice cannot be substituted for one another without a loss of truth. The correspondence between theory and practice is artificial or made up. The substitution of theory for practice or practice for theory leads to a reduplication of the field of truth. Where there was one truth, now there are two.

The reason for this being the case, according to Lacanian theory, is that truth can only be half said, and, therefore, there is always a truth that remains unsaid interacting with a relative truth that has been said. These two truths are neither one nor two. Whatever you say, in the relative 'fictional' side of truth, always has another side not being said, and the trick is to leave it unsaid, or say it in a saying rather than a statement, to avoid being falsely misled by the promise of another substitution that also will not be "It."

The Real in Lacan is a dimension of experience that lies beyond words or images, although its "interior" aspect can manifest in poetic language, the creative imagination, jouissance, and topology. Except for the case of psychoses, where the NoF has been foreclosed, the Real unconscious is to be distinguished from the repressed unconscious because the Real unconscious has nothing repressed in it (images or words) but is an aspect of experience that is beyond or outside representation. Lacan makes a clear differentiation between the Real and his two other registers: Imaginary and Symbolic. However, at the same time, he claims that his mathemes (symbolic formulas that are not arithmetical in nature) help us in approaching the Real. In Badiou's (2014) words:

> the Real of the subject is unsymbolizable. As a result, Lacan goes as far as possible in formalization in order to experience a fundamental impasse. At some point, the integral formalization should break down because it no longer has a hold on the very thing it is trying to grasp. This is the moment when we touch on the real point of the subject.
>
> (p. 50)

A good way to conceptualize the conundrum of the Real is to use the example of some of the findings of modern physics. Take, for example, the uncertainty principle formulated by Heisenberg. Heisenberg showed that position and velocity cannot both be measured at the same time. Any attempt to measure precisely the velocity of a subatomic particle, such as an electron, will alter its course in such an unpredictable way that it renders the results invalid.

The impossibility of the measurement is closely related to the connection between particles and waves in the subatomic realm, and it has nothing to do with lack of equipment or flaws in observation techniques. When waves are measured, they become particles and lose their superposition, or the ability to manifest in more than one place at a time. Einstein had trouble accepting the results of quantum theory and commented that " matter must have a separate reality independent of the measurements. That is, an electron has spin, location and so forth even when it is not being measured. I like to think that the moon is there even if I am not looking at it" (cited by O'Conner, 1999, p. 41). But the independent reality of the particle is the wave, not the particle itself. What the moon itself is in the Real without the observation or the finger pointing at it, we cannot say for a fact.

It is true that the moon is there even when we are not looking at it; however, we should not mistake the moon with our finger pointing at it. In other words, reality is not the Real. On the other hand, we would not know anything of it without the observation or the finger pointing at it. Thus, the Real is known through what is Real within the Symbolic. The wave is also the particle.

Finally, when discussing cases, from an ethical/practical point of view, the clinician/analyst will have to continue to disguise and modify clinical material in order to say the truth about truth. It is important to remember that the challenge that we are facing is not only a question of protecting patients' privacy but also the impossibility to describe, measure, or scale every aspect of psychoanalytic sessions. Even the best, most accurate description of it will not stand for the 'real thing.'

An interesting relationship exists between practical reason and *techne*, method, or technique. Practice means that the singular individual has to be directly engaged in a Real practice or specific type of activity rather than simply being treated as a number or a constituent of a set, category, or experiment. The treatment method of free association, for example, constitutes ways of unchaining thoughts and feelings or truth from pre-determined chains of thinking, knowledge, or prejudice and ideology. The theory or the first principles orient us towards the Real of a practice but do not constitute it or absorb it into the closed circularity of established discourse. This way, the theory can change the practice and the practice inform the theory but without either one being reduced to each other. Both the Real of the theory and the Real of the practice have to remain open or unsaturated as well as related to one another.

Hans Steiner (1977) has pointed out that when faced with the question of the scientific status of psychoanalysis, one is bewildered by the array of opinions, both theoretical and research based. Despite a great degree of accumulation of research data showing that psychoanalysis or psychoanalytic psychotherapy is an evidence-based practice, many detractors continue to affirm that psychoanalysis is not an empirical or evidence-based practice that has been objectively tested.

Steiner then asks why is psychoanalysis still an object of controversy despite all the evidence already established? Can this be explained as something more than the simple resistance to the unconscious and to the socially inconvenient truths of desire that need to be quickly brushed aside and hidden under the proverbial carpet? Steiner cites Freud when he stated that although experimental confirmations of psychoanalysis do no harm, psychoanalysis already provides a wealth of reliable observations that are independent from experimental validation. Thus Freud appears to have restricted: "the process of observation and validation to the analytic situation" (p. 518).

If psychoanalysis is already an empirically derived practice, why would it need validation and testing from the outside by people who are not intrinsically involved with the theory and the practice and who have not been analyzed? Would this not be a setup to become a victim of the defenses against unconscious desire and sexuality?

Conversely, if only practicing psychoanalysts can validate the theory, does this make psychoanalysis function like a sect that needs to be validated from the inside only? The answer to this question obviously refers to the need for epistemological critique and the free exercise of critical reason as an indispensable aspect of the scientific method. But what about the need for large samples, random sampling, and quantification, which are necessary ingredients of scientific research within natural science in general? The problem with this aspect of the scientific method is that the propensities discovered by the repetition of the experiment on many subjects may be an artifice of the assumptions and the 'setup' of the experiment. In addition, psychoanalytic truths leading to the development and dissipation of symptomatology cannot be discovered or changed without the involvement of subjective experience. There is a dimension of reality (what Lacan calls the Real) that only yields its secrets in the singular case and in an actual practice and not in an experiment. The experiment and finite frequentism in statistics only engages two types of reason (episteme and techne), while nous, dialectical, and practical reason are also required for the study of the singular case.

This explains why Freud would say that for the singular case, the observations produced in the case of a singular analysis and a single session are sufficient. The singular case observation does constitute a test and an evaluation of the theory and the practice, although it may not produce the propensities and probabilities of a random sample and statistical testing. What is important here is not the obstinate or dogmatic insistence on the psychoanalytic method but the logical argument regarding the import of the singular case for the study of human subjectivity and the existence of different types of rationality.

On the other hand, psychoanalysts are also responsible for the fate of their profession. For years, many health care providers saw them as arrogant and ignorant of the 'real world' realities of public and insurance-based mental health services. In addition, when we look at the textbooks for trainees, we notice that they usually contain a very simplistic look at Freud's ideas, which makes them appear silly and outlandish.

After the height of its powers in the 1950s, one by one, most clinical settings and training hospitals in the United States ceased to be psychoanalytic. However, despite the rise of statistical research in psychology, in large part, this change can be attributed to psychoanalysis itself. Most psychoanalysts under the regulation of the International Psychoanalytic Association (IPS) took a kind of 'all or nothing' or 'take it or leave it' attitude. The new generation of political 'powers that be' and administrators chose the 'nothing' or 'leave it' option, resulting in the inevitable decline of psychoanalysis.

Even some Lacanian analysts would rather predict and accept the end and demise of psychoanalysis than have to bend it or stretch it to meet changing circumstances and populations (while topologically preserving its structure). I remember that after I managed to establish Lacanian clinical practice and formation within a public outpatient clinic in San Francisco at a time of maximum rejection of Freudian psychoanalysis, and I invited Lacanian analysts from Europe or Latin American, I was surprised to hear that they too, like the American psychoanalytic establishment, would rather witness the disappearance of psychoanalysis than address the external criticisms to the field or literature outside their own.

If Lacanian psychoanalysis is like a coffee cup, then the coffee cup still preserves the structure of the doughnut that represents Freudian psychoanalysis. There is no sense in mourning the loss of the doughnut (Freudian psychoanalysis) when the doughnut is preserved in the form of a cup of coffee (Lacanian psychoanalysis). By the same token, there is no sense in mourning the loss of Lacanian psychoanalysis if Lacanian psychoanalysis engages other discourses within contemporary culture.

If Lacanians from abroad merely attempt to take advantage of the growth of Lacanian analysis in the United States to promote their own national interests and local agendas elsewhere, and in disregard of the battles hard won by local efforts and of the characteristics of the local culture, then in the end, Lacanian analysis will suffer the same fate as Freudian analysis. The practices of citation, and the scansion of speech and session, support the function of free association as a method leading to the manifestation of the unconscious signifying chain. Thus Lacanian psychoanalysis both advances Freudian psychoanalysis and at the same time addresses the external critique of the field without compromising its internal structure.

There are many reasons for the decline of psychoanalysis, but we will only focus on a few. First we will examine reasons internal to psychoanalysis itself that we will associate with a dogmatic epistemological position. This dogmatic position is not only directly associated with the theory but also, and more importantly, with the frame of psychoanalysis.

Prior to inventing psychoanalysis (the 'talking cure'), Freud experimented with many treatment methods available at that time such as hypnosis and suggestion. In passing, it is important to note that these methods are still being used today both within and outside psychoanalysis. This is not the place to argue this point, but it is enough to say that suggestion is an integral part of both research and cognitive behavioral therapy. In systematic desensitization, it has been shown that muscle relaxation and the hierarchy of stimulus items are not the key curative factors. Jaffe (1968) showed how induced expectation of success (i.e. suggestion) was more powerful than the treatment itself. The placebo group with the expectation of success fared better than the treatment group without the expectation of success.

The invention of what later came to be called the standard frame for the practice of psychoanalysis evolved out of slowly trying different clinical methods over time. This contrasts sharply with the structured teaching for the general population that follows after the death of the founding intellect. Consequent generations are not exposed to the original teachings and in addition may not have the same motivation or capacities than those that were formed closely after the original invention.

So the standard treatment, like standardized testing in general education, is a way of transmitting and disseminating a theory and a practice (as well as information) to a wider population. Here an inverse relation can be observed between professional education and clinical practice. The standard frame allows for structured training for a larger group of specialized clinicians who may have a more technical and less intellectual focus in their cognitive orientation. At the same time, as already mentioned, a standard treatment also makes it more difficult to shape the theory and the practice to changing times, populations, and settings. In general education, we also have the example of Finland, where they eliminated all standardized testing in education and saw a rise in educational outcomes for their student population. Rather than study the logic of the test established by researchers who only function with limited forms of rationality and memorize or guess answers to multiple-choice questions, students had to know and be able to explain the answers to questions.

There is an inherent conflict or contradiction between invention or innovation and tradition, the individual leader and the group, and between invention and practice according to the standard operating procedures outlined by manuals and handbooks. Furthermore, institutionalized practices that come to be identified with the tradition may come to oppose the spirit of the original teachings or invention. Institutions are privileged sites to access and study unconscious mental structures that are operative in groups. On the other hand, Winnicott was right when he said, "it is not possible to be original except on a basis of tradition." In this sense, the non-standard frame is the source of the standard frame rather than the other way around. In addition, creative individuals will always experiment and practice beyond the limits set by current standard practices because otherwise science and knowledge would not evolve.

Standard and non-standard frames

Freud invented a standard treatment out of prior practices that did not conform to the new standards he developed, yet continued to use the new method in non-standard ways. Nonetheless, Freud did not have a framework to account for the contradictions between the standard and non-standard ways within his practice.

However, as argued by many in the philosophy of science, mainstream science always needs to tolerate rogue elements in its midst because new ideas could not evolve otherwise that could be consequently proven to be true within the framework of science.

The theoretization of the non-standard frame was, essentially, Lacan's contribution to the practice and effectiveness of psychoanalysis. Lacan wrote "Variations on the Standard Treatment" back in 1953 (Lacan, 1966/2006). In this paper, he stated: "A psychoanalysis, whether standard or not, is the treatment one expects from a psychoanalyst" (p. 274).

The standard treatment was further developed and institutionalized under the IPA and the leadership of Anna Freud to protect the legacy of Freud and in the process made the standard treatment the official statement regarding the practice of psychoanalysis. While establishing the standard treatment, the IPA intended to be "more Freudian than Freud" and treated Freud's unorthodox or non-standard methods as Freud's idiosyncrasies, lack of a personal analysis, and being the first analyst. By the same token, they crystallized and froze Freud's actual idiosyncrasies into the rigid structure of an international organization.

Institutions, as sociologists have pointed out, often gain a life of their own and have a self-preservation drive, operating according to the prescriptions of their leaders but in the process rigidifying and distorting the qualities that their leaders possess. Freud was well aware of this fact and is reported to have said, "My pupils are more orthodox than I" (cited by Roazen, p. 401). Although this feature of organizations is quite common, it is also a key characteristic of obsessional neurosis (being more Freudian than Freud, or papist than the Pope). This is what makes obsessional dynamics have a normal flare (where the behavior of the majority of people is found) or the flare of a normal neurosis associated with civilization.

Although many analysts in every generation have practiced in non-standard ways, such non-standard methods remain uninvestigated and have rarely been reported. I realize that there are many historical nuances regarding the standard treatment that historians might dispute, but I believe that the distinction between standard and non-standard holds across time and not only has heuristic value but is also a very important axis or vertex from which to examine the question of psychoanalytic practice in both public and private settings.

Octave Mannoni in France gave a famous example regarding what he called the Procrustean couch: if someone does not fit into the frame, then you cut off an arm, then a leg, and so on. This is how many analysts from IPA institutes are perceived outside psychoanalysis. Analysts are perceived as only wanting to help patients that are good candidates for psychoanalysis or work with diagnoses that fit into the psychoanalytic frame. Although this may be relevant for private practice with a less disturbed population, it severely handicaps psychoanalytic work within institutions and with minorities.

In addition, the distinction between standard and non-standard treatment differs from the distinction often made between psychoanalysis and psychotherapy. Although psychoanalytic psychotherapy is often perceived as having wider applicability than psychoanalysis, the former is still perceived as only appropriate for a less disturbed and higher-functioning population. In this sense, the notion of a non-standard treatment or a multiform criterion for the practice of psychoanalysis is directly related to the need to apply psychoanalysis to a wider range of clinical populations.

Clinical examples

Winnicott is known to have worked with analysands with more severe forms of psychopathology. He also gave more emphasis to environmental failures in a child's development that, according to the object relations perspective, are pre-oedipal in nature. Thus, once an analysand said to Winnicott (1971/2011, p. 124): "All I have got is what I have not got." She later added "And what will you do about it?" As Winnicott remained silent, she said, "Oh, I see." Thereupon, Winnicott made a comment full of humanity and humility: "I am silent because I don't know what to say." In relation to what the analysand said, Winnicott disclosed his own lack rather than indicating that he had the object that the analysand was demanding. On several occasions, Winnicott did not hide what he did not know, and he thought it was important for the analyst not to remain in a position of omnipotence.

However, in this example, there is a difference between lack in the analyst and the analysand. Winnicott accepts his lack or 'not-having' anything to say, while the analysand demands that the analyst fill the lack as presented by the analysand. The analysand is conveying her fundamental fantasy that the Other is lacking as a structural condition rather than as an environmental defect or failure while thinking that Winnicott is not a good-enough mother/analyst. The deficit in the analysand's case that Winnicott is presenting refers to the environment mother. Apparently this analysand had sustained early losses that were traumatic beyond the normal loss associated with separation, the loss of the breast in weaning, of feces, or the 'not-having' the imaginary phallus that takes place in normal neurosis.

One could read this case as either a case of contemporary hysteria or a borderline condition, as the analysand wanting the analyst to repair or fill the hole left by the real (small r) absence of a symbolic object (privation of the breast/maternal environment), or as the analysand wanting the analyst to give her something that neither she nor the analyst has (symbolic castration) and that the analyst can only promise to give under false pretenses (the father's imaginary phallus). This is an inevitable and necessary absence or lack (symbolic castration) that has to be accepted rather than filled or treated as a defect. Since the latter is an inevitable existential condition that no adequate environment will ever prevent, this is a form of suffering any subject will have to endure. The analysand accepts this when faced with Winnicott's lack of response.

The questions regarding the diagnosis and the cause of the suffering, jouissance, or symptom are important regarding the treatment, because if one assumes that there are developmental defects or deficits in the person's childhood environment, then treating the lack as Imaginary could cause the analysand to be confused with respect to their experience. On the other hand, if the analyst treats the lack as a defect and provides support with regard to a real symbolic deficit that the analysand experienced in childhood, then this perspective leaves oedipal structure unaddressed and unchanged.

If the deficit were real (in the sense of external social reality), and the analyst is in the place where the mother should have been, then according to object relations theory or ego psychology, the borderline analysand would eventually graduate to an oedipal phase/face of development, where instead of borderline misery, they would experience ordinary neurotic suffering. The problem with this view is that the person's suffering will inevitably change after a therapeutic process. In the case of the borderline condition, after having received empathy from a predictably secure and good-enough therapeutic environment, object relations theory would say that the analysand has improved in their capacity for trust and object relations.

However, this approach neglects the fact that after treatment, the analysand will still be faced with clinging or attachment issues associated with desire, as well as problems with separation in relationships, not because of the borderline condition but for the same reasons that any so-called 'normal neurotic' encounters the same problem. Any merger is with the *objet a*/imaginary phallus as the object of fantasy, and separation and loss refer to an imaginary object that must be symbolized and relinquished rather than repaired or reacquired. In Seminar V, Lacan (1957–1958, p. 152) distinguishes between the 'normal' father with respect to oedipal structure and the 'normative father' in the family structure who may be nice or nasty. That the environmental or historical family father may have been nice or overbearing, present or absent in the family, may have different effects in the family narrative, but the fundamental question for neurosis is whether the father functioned as a metaphor leading to identification with the NoF and the use of the phallus once it has been marked with the certificate of symbolic castration.

During treatment, an analyst will consider any early environmental deficits, particular historical circumstances, or traumatic events in the analysand's upbringing within the context of Oedipal structure and the paternal metaphor. If structure is not examined, then structural questions will continue to haunt the psyche of the analysand despite the efforts of the good-enough analyst.

Another example further illustrates the difference between developmental traumas, normative social narratives, and structural symptoms linked to an unconscious signifying chain. An analysand reported two related dreams. In the first, he is hiding in the dark corner of a shed from men that are searching for him while mocking him at the same time. In the second dream, he is under siege by an army of men. In his associations with the dreams, he made reference to the father figure in a TV show meant to convey an ideal father. In contrast, he referred to himself as a weak version of that. He also noted that he had many dreams where he is being attacked or he is attacking other men, often violently.

The conventional historical narrative provided by the analysand described a history of family violence exemplified in the event in which the mother used a shotgun to put a bullet through the father's hand. The father was a drunk and a poor provider, and the analysand was a good boy and son of the mother, who told him he should not be anything like the father. Yet the analysand turned out to have had vocational and work-related problems, as well as two accidents that disabled him from being able to be a good provider for his family. He was often understated and non-aggressive yet wished to be more aggressive, especially towards other men by whom he felt overpowered.

The third association with the dream points to both a trauma and the upper floor of the graph of desire. He reported being told at some point by his parents that a neighbor sexually abused his sister. The neighbor would take him and his sister to his house after school, because his parents were still at work or busy. The sexual abuse of the sister happened in a shed behind the house. The analysand denied having survivor's guilt or feeling responsible for not preventing the sister's abuse from taking place. He said he was too young to know anything about it.

The symbolic work of analysis is to invent and discover links between random associations the analysand produces within the psychoanalytic session. In this case, he is linking weak father with a weak man under attack and more remotely with an identification with his sister being sexually assaulted in a shed. The word shed provides the link between the dream image, between shed and she, and what happened to the sister in a shed in his childhood. What is repressed is that the signification of 'weak' man in relationship to aggressive men is being equated to being a small girl under sexual attack by an older man and that he is considering himself a girl like his sister. 'Weak' girl is being unconsciously equated to weak man or father.

In terms of technique, the analyst simply asks the analysand to associate to the dream putting him in the position of his sister. If the analysand is not ready or balks at the content of the material, the analyst would be content with waiting until the analysand is ready to shed defenses or his unconscious produces more material to this effect. Finally, the symbolic work of analysis represents something of the psychical, beyond the necessary telling of a traumatic experience. The difficult telling or reporting of sexual abuse, for example, takes place on a different level of narration acceptable to and consistent with social norms.

Lacanian theory explains that the analysand's unconscious is equating femininity with an imaginary form of 'weakness' (both males and females are feminine in this instance) and strong masculinity with an imaginary form of masculine strength or domination (in males or females). Both forms of weakness are victims of imaginary castration, while strength and aggressiveness are linked to an unbarred and uncastrated form of masculinity. In the analysand's mind, there is no category for symbolically castrated masculinity or femininity. The men or the mother are either violently aggressive, or the sister, women, and men are 'weak' victims to more 'powerful' masculine predators, whether male or female.

New names and words will have to be discovered or invented to symbolize something about a productive form of symbolic femininity and a Real femininity beyond symbolic castration. The same can be said about men and the father. There will be no Real sexed femininity for a man in the Symbolic register, but a man may access the Real in other ways that are also available to women (jouissance of meaning or of the mystic, for example).

For a woman, and femininity in the Real and the Symbolic, the *sinthome* will be found in the ways that a woman makes do with the lack of a signifier for femininity. For example, one female analysand may have identified with a masculine signifier such as wearing men's hiking or military boots. Since, as a female, she is not entirely comfortable wearing men's boots (a symptom of her rejection of femininity), because they put her at odds with her gender, she also has bins full of women's shoes that point to some signifier of femininity that she also is not entirely comfortable with. The latter experimentation will become her *sinthome*.

The process of symbolization and nomination will invent something new at the site of the symptom in the analysand's psyche to repair the damage done by the failures of the paternal or parental metaphor (the father's irresponsibility and drunkenness and the mother's aggressiveness). The normative environmental father failed to be sober, and this led to a failure in the normal oedipal function. Structural failures, errors, or slips will appear as mistakes within the family story or narrative that the analysand offers within the treatment. As the analysand tells their family story, structural elements of the signifying chain will appear in patient's speech. Structural elements of the unconscious signifying chain refer to the normal elements of oedipal structure more than the normative narrative regarding the family.

Conclusion

The multiform criterion for the practice of analysis represents an operational mode that recognizes the evanescent pulsation of the unconscious (opening and closing during sessions) within a different temporal dimension of speech that breaks the homogeneity of the well-known family story line and points to facts of the structure. The non-standard frame privileges the manifestation of the unconscious signifying chain rather than repairing the normative and environmental failures of the parents within a better holding environment. The latter is more likely to happen within a standard frame that provides a predictable and stable environment for reparenting the analysand. The unconscious, instead, manifests in the here and now of a session and within the singularity of the frame for each treatment. On a case-by-case basis, each treatment may have a variable length and frequency of sessions and treatment.

Although in general, the analyst speaks less than the analysand, sometimes the analyst will speak more and sometimes speak less, sometimes ask the right questions, or make necessary and contraposing citations of the analysand, and sometimes let the analysand speak freely without interruption. The telling of the normative family story, and the manifest content of speech as far as the structure is concerned, is favored by the analyst remaining silent in the session, session after session. Sometimes the analyst may focus on conscious material if this is all the analysand may speak about, but this is a strategy within the transference to help bring out unconscious material. The analyst must meet the analysand where the unconscious manifests or slips rather than always staying silent and waiting for the analysand to speak about something that they may never speak about or they may never know that they knew without the help of the analyst.

Paradoxically, many Lacanians who have not had the experience of control analysis will inadvertently fall into the stereotype of the silent, passive analyst associated not with Freud but with ego psychology and the standard frame. In such cases, because of the absence of clinical experience and control analysis, the new theory is practiced according to stereotypes that the media and society associate with traditional psychoanalysis (standard frame). The new theory is not a better justification for the standard frame that otherwise should remain unchanged.

Standardization is problematic because it leads to the false conclusion that it contains the origin of a scientific discovery or remains true to it, when, in fact, it may not. Lacan's use of the Real as an act, and the scansion of speech and session, was his way of re-establishing the Real of the unconscious within a Symbolic series rather than simply replacing Real unconscious experience for a standard or normative Symbolic that eventually becomes Imaginary.

In general, this book argues that the non-standard frame is needed to reinvent psychoanalysis past its current slumbers and decline. Except for the very wealthy, most people don't have the time or the money for four or five sessions a week for ten or more years. Standardizing the length of the session and passive listening (not the same as active hearing or *J'ouis-sense*) without citation or scansion of the analysand's speech, or of the time of the session, leads to analyses conducted entirely on the basis of the narrative or manifest content level of speech or on the basis of the analyst's wild interpretations of the analysand's behavior or body language. Interpreting the patient's actions or speech on the basis of material that has not appeared in the analysand's speech leads to the analysand either submitting to the treatment without real change or to warning the analysand's unconscious defenses to know what to avoid talking about in the future. Both of these conditions result in drawn-out, boring (without desire or the Other), unproductive, and interminable analyses.

The two systems of non-standard and standard analysis (S_1 and S_2) are represented in Table 3.1.

Lacanians bet on the idea that the scansion of speech and session increases the effectiveness of the session and prevents stalemates and idle repetitive speech in analysis. In contrast, the standard frame often leads to stalemates, impasses, or interminable analyses. However, to be consistent, the non-standard frame has to include a standard frame as a possible variation in the treatment. Otherwise, the non-standard frame paradoxically becomes a standard frame. Conversely, a standard frame that allows for the variations of a non-standard analysis can no longer be said to be a standard analysis, although the latter could still be practiced depending on the singular analysand and the context.

To summarize, I would like to use the basic schema of Lacan's graph of desire to represent the different categories used in this chapter. I am only using three of the overall lines included in the graph. In addition, the mathemes at the edges (both inside and outside the circles) are ignored as not being relevant for the current purposes. For a more detailed exposition of the graph of desire, please refer to the previous chapter.

Lacanian psychoanalysis encompasses the three horizontal vectors used: one vertical and two horizontal, plus the short circuit between i(a) and m.

Table 3.1 Table of Non-Standard and Standard Analysis

Non-Standard Analysis	*Standard Analysis*
Transference analysis and interventions within the transference	Transference interpretations
No fixed length of session	45- to 50-minute length of session
No fixed length of treatment	Exceedingly long length of treatment
No fixed sitting arrangement	Exclusive use of the couch
Possible variation in the location of the treatment (i.e. use of phone, online video sessions, etc.)	Exclusive use of the private office
Scansion of speech and session	Free association
Going from the Unknown to the Unknown	Going from the Unknown to the Known
Personal Analysis	

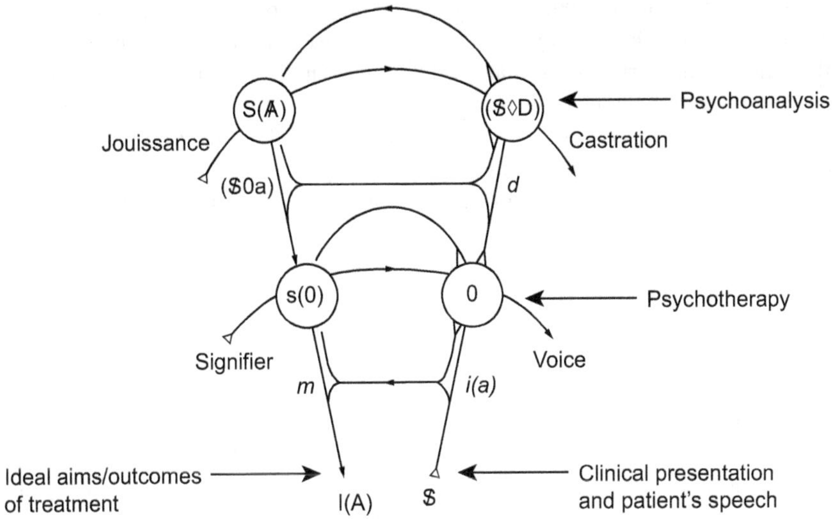

Figure 3.1 Differences between psychotherapy and psychoanalysis shown in the full graph (of desire).

The vertical vector (of desire) begins with the clinical problem presentation and the patient or analysand's speech and ends in the outcome expected from applied psychoanalysis. The symbols that Lacan uses for the vertical vector are the divided subject or $ (clinical problem) and the ego ideal or I[A] (the ideal aims or outcomes of treatment). Pure psychoanalysis represents the upper floor horizontal vector going from left to right and associated with free association and interventions on the unconscious signifying chain (from the signifier of lack in the unconscious to the demands of the drive and the questions of jouissance and desire).

The lower level represents the manifest narratives and problems/statements addressed by the psychotherapist and most commonly associated with psychotherapy. The 'short circuit' or 'shortcut' below the narrative level represents the involvement of the speaker's ego in the narrative or how the narrative reinforces the analysand's narcissistic defenses. In the example used previously, the symbolization of the sister's trauma and story would represent the lower level signifying chain, while the signifying chain linking the shed with issues of 'sexuation' or conflicting gender identifications and the question of a weak or strong father, and aggressiveness in relationships, are part of the upper level of the signifying chain.

The standard and non-standard treatment for the practice of psychoanalysis may take place in either of the two levels and may or may not achieve the aims of applied psychoanalysis. However, the standard frame carries the serious risk that standardization of the frame will reduce psychoanalysis to the normative narrative about loving objects and secure attachments.

Finally, non-psychoanalytic psychotherapy would entirely exclude and bypass the upper floor of the graph. Although both psychoanalysis and psychotherapy may reach the applied end point of the vertical vector, psychoanalysis leads to self-knowledge and to unknown knowing or unconscious knowing, an expanded awareness or psychical state, and conscious knowledge of the unconscious. But then the question arises as to what the difference is in the outcome when the upper level of the signifying chain is reached or included, if both signifying chains can lead to positive outcomes in terms of symptom resolution. Does pure psychoanalysis (in standard or non-standard formats) lead to more long-lasting results and lower relapse rates but through what Lacan calls the identification with the *sinthome*?

What Lacan calls identification with the *sinthome* at the end of analysis for our purposes may be simply defined as a modification of the psychical and characterological structure of the subject as a result of the work with the symptom in treatment. The change in characterological structure leads to the subject taking responsibility for the symptoms which in the process become *sinthomes* rather than simple symptoms. The *sinthome* becomes a source of unconscious knowing. There is a different qualitative relationship to the symptom instead of the symptom being quantitatively eradicated. Difficult characterological traits may still be there but are now ego-dystonic and a source of ongoing jouissance and change for the subject.

According to Lacanian theory, the post-treatment effects of analysis refer not to the identification with the analyst as a good object, as termination is understood within object relations theory. The analysand may identify and want to be like the analyst as an ego ideal, but this form of identity will be a form of idealization of the good analyst or a compliance with the treatment as opposed to representing a form of 'unbeing' in the Real subject. The nomination process and jouissance associated with the *sinthome* will support the function of the *sinthome* as a source of unconscious knowledge. This is more fundamental than internalizing the ego of the analyst as a good object.

The work with the *sinthome* continues after analysis in the self-analysis and would explain lower relapse rates post-termination. Knowing how to work with the *sinthome*, or caring for the *sinthome* in the service of personal development, is a very different thing than thinking that you are cured or enlightened once and for all. The latter, in fact, is a fantasy caused by our gaining ideas, ideas of self-improvement, and in general the instrumental and humanistic culture of contemporary society. In the latter case, humanism fails to humanize the subject, creating instead an imaginary ego with a humanistic façade.

References

APA Presidential Task Force. (2006). Evidence-Based Practice in Psychology. *American Psychologist*, May–June.

Badiou, A. (2014). *Jacques Lacan, Past and Present: A Dialogue*. New York: Columbia University Press. Kindle Edition.

Einstein, A. (1944). *The Collected Papers of Albert Einstein*. Princeton, NJ: Princeton University Press, 1986-present).

Etchegoyen, H. (2005). *Fundamentals of Psychoanalytic Technique*. London: Karnac.

Fonagy, P. (2003). Psychoanalysis Today. *World Psychiatry*, 2, 2 June.
Freud, S. (1918). From the History of an Infantile Neurosis. *SE*, 17, 1–123, 1914.
Hicks, R. D. (1907). *Aristotle De Anima with Translation, Introduction, and Notes*. London: Cambridge University Press.
Hock Lai, H. (2015). The Legal Concept of Evidence. In: *The Stanford Encyclopedia of Philosophy* (Winter 2015 Edition). Edited by E. N. Zalta. https://plato.stanford.edu/archives/win2015/entries/evidence-legal/.
Howard, D. (2017). Einstein's Philosophy of Science. In: *The Stanford Encyclopedia of Philosophy* (Fall 2017 Edition). Edited by E. N. Zalta. https://plato.stanford.edu/archives/fall2017/entries/einstein-philscience/.
Jaffe, L. W. (1968). *Non-Specific Treatment Factors and Deconditioning in Fear Reduction*, University of Southern California. Unpublished doctoral dissertation.
Lacan, J. (1957–1958). *The Formations of the Unconscious: Book V: The Seminar of Jacques Lacan*. Edited by J.-A. Miller and Translated by R. Grigg. London: Polity Press.
Lacan, J. (1966). *Ecrits*. Translated by B. Fink. New York: W.W. Norton & Company, 2006.
Langs, R. (1998a). *Current Theories of Psychoanalysis*. Madison, CT: International University Press.
Langs, R. (1998b). *Ground Rules in Psychotherapy and Counselling*. London: Karnac Books.
Langs, R., Baladamenti, A. and Thomson, L. (1996). *The Cosmic Cycle: The Unification of Mind, Matter, and Energy*. Brooklyn, NY: Alliance.
Leichsenring, F. and Rabung, S. (2008). Effectiveness of Long-Term Psychodynamic Psychotherapy: A Meta-Analysis. *Journal of the American Medical Association.*, 300, 1551–1565.
Leichsenring, F. and Rabung, S. (2009). Analyzing Effectiveness of Long-Term Psychodynamic Psychotherapy Reply. *J Am Med Assoc.*, 301, 932–933.
Levy, R. A., Ablon, J. S. and Kächele, H. (2011). *Psychodynamic Psychotherapy Research: Evidence-Based Practice and Practice-Based Evidence*. Springer, Kindle Edition.
Miller, J. A. (2015). Pure Psychoanalysis, Applied Psychoanalysis, and Psychotherapy. www.lacan.com/lacinkXX2.htm. Accessed February 2015.
Moncayo, R. (2017). *Lalangue, Sinthome, Jouissance, and Nomination: A Reading Companion and Commentary on Lacan's Seminar XXIII*. London: Karnac.
Moncayo, R. and Romanowicz, M. (2015). *The Real Jouissance of Uncountable Numbers: The Philosophy of Science within Lacanian Psychoanalysis*. London: Karnac.
O'Conner, P. (1999). *Words Fail Me*. New York: Houghton Harcourt Publishing.
Pennebaker, J. (1995). *Emotion, Disclosure, and Health*. Washington, DC: American Psychological Association.
Pennebaker, J. (1997). *Opening up: The Healing Power of Confiding in Others*. New York: Guilford.
Roazen, P. (1975). *Freud and His Followers*. New York: Knopf.
Romanowicz, M. and Moncayo, R. (2015). Going Beyond Castration in the Graph of Desire. *The Letter (The Irish Journal for Lacanian Psychoanalysis)*, (58), Spring, 31–58.
Schedler, J. (2010). The Efficacy of Psychodynamic Psychotherapy. *American Psychologist*, February–March.
Steiner, H. (1977). Freud Against Himself. *Perspectives in Biology and Medicine*, Summer.
Winnicott, D. (1971). Transitional Objects and Transitional Phenomena. In: *Reading Winnicott*. London: Routledge, 2011.

4 Preliminary sessions and considerations

The question of the setting or best site for practice is intrinsically related to the question of the first phase of transference, or at least how transference appears at the beginning of treatment. People go to a private practitioner or to a clinic that houses clinicians licensed to practice under government auspices. A clinician is supposed to know something or to have undergone training leading to a license. However, so-called clinical consumers of mental health services that are not themselves knowledgeable about the field will simply go to a licensed clinician for help without knowing anything about their orientation.

I have certainly had my share of referrals of people who come to see me simply to get help for their symptoms. Although this is not a demand for analysis, a request for help with symptoms and suffering was precisely what Lacan considered necessary to begin an analysis. Those who come to learn about themselves or analysis were not accepted into analysis by Lacan. However true this may be, the fact remains that many requests for Lacanian analysis comes from people already interested in Lacan due to an interest in psychoanalysis or because of having studied Lacan in the university, and therefore they choose this orientation to speak about their personal problems.

The interest in the theory, however, does not predict how analyzable the analysand may be. I have worked with analysands on the "autistic spectrum," who have obsessional structures (with autistic symptoms in this case) and who are not so good candidates for analysis. Although such analysands display a deficit or poverty of verbal associations, they nonetheless are able to use their symptoms as signifiers and display a willingness to work on interpersonal problems. Despite the infrequent manifestation of the unconscious signifying chain in the treatment (often making the analysis less interesting), Lacanian analysis can still help such analysands achieve a marked decrease in symptomatology and increased social functioning.

The setting is an office, whether private, public, or online. The difference between the first two options again subdivides into differences between economic and subjective factors. Typically, in a public clinic, where services are free or low cost, the demand for treatment is due to symptoms, just like in analysis in private practice, but a clinic patient may or may not be interested in their symptoms or personal analysis.

In a public clinic, the subject itself may be a symptom for others and to the public Other, but the subject may only be interested in economic help and general health care. Under such circumstances, pure psychoanalysis is impossible, whether standard or non-standard. However, psychoanalytic principles could still be applied to the understanding of the patient, the relationship to the patient, and the understanding of group dynamics and work relationships among the mental health professionals of a clinic.

Countries with economic resources are able to provide public psychotherapy to citizens without economic resources and without private insurance but who can take care of their minimal economic needs and are interested in psychotherapeutic help for their symptoms. In such cases, pure psychoanalysis could take place in a non-standard format as a variation of analysis. However, a public clinic always raises privacy and confidentiality questions and the involvement of 'governmental' institutions.

Private practice is the natural format for pure psychoanalysis, if only because in institutions for various reasons (some rational, some irrational, ideological, or based on prejudice) not of concern to us right now, a couch cannot be used. Private insurance used to reimburse analysands for analysis from the 1950s to the early 1980s. More recently, in the last ten years, PPOs (not HMOs) have begun reimbursing analysands once again for their analysis. The analysand pays the analyst, and the analyst provides a weekly bill for the sessions. Only big corporations and government institutions are able to offer PPO health insurance to their workers.

In addition, private in the case of analysis also means increased confidentiality of the material discussed in analytical sessions, and this is confirmed by the absence of contact between the analyst and an insurance company or an institution. Such practice is also consistent with the Freudian approach to healing that temporarily, or initially, at least, gets the big Other off the back of the subject.

It is well known that preliminary analytical sessions are used to clarify the demand for a personal analysis. In cases where the clinical presentation is more urgent and immediate, intensive treatment several times a week may be needed, and this may differ from what ordinarily is understood as preliminary or pretreatment. The transition between intensive treatment or applied psychoanalysis and pure analysis or analysis proper may be less noticeable in these cases other than what is discussed in the treatment about the difference between eliminating symptoms and doing the work of free association. Typically, these two forms of intervention have in common that the analysand is sitting up rather than lying down on the couch. That the analysand is sitting up does not mean that the session is face to face unless otherwise stipulated and prescribed. In general, if the analysand is not on the couch, it works better to have analyst and analysand sit in perpendicular chairs or sitting arrangements.

The clarification of the demand for analysis also involves determining whether the analytic pair is a good match as far as the collaboration between the parties that analysis requires. Within the preliminary sessions, several things can be tested: the capacity to free associate; to use and tolerate citations and interpretations; to modulate affect, experience, and signifiers; to consider the relationship between fantasy and reality, and among fantasy, trauma, and symptom. In addition, the preliminary sessions can also be used to differentiate psychotherapy from psychoanalysis. This refers to the frequency of sessions; the length of sessions; how the cancellation of sessions, vacations, and payment are handled; and an estimation of the length of treatment. We don't provide guarantees regarding the length of treatment, but if an estimate has to be given, the numbers given randomly coincide with the logic of the Borromean knot: three or four years with a frequency of no less than two sessions a week. It is a matter of a singular analysis, with a frequency of two to three sessions a week for a rough estimate of three to four years.

The fee is something that has to be discussed right at the beginning of the treatment. I have a fee for analysis, and if analysands have financial limitations, then I give them the lowest fee I can charge, and they propose a fee they can afford within that range. If the analysand cancels, then if my schedule allows, I offer them a make-up session, and if none can be found, then they are responsible for the fee. The only exception is if they are obviously physically ill at the time of the session, in which case the session can be rescheduled for another time.

The variable length of a Lacanian session is also explained, with the caveat that the fee is per session, not per length of time. I don't do very short sessions of 5 or 10 minutes. In general, I don't consider such very short sessions useful or therapeutic, although there can be exceptions to the rule. I tell prospective analysands that the sessions last anywhere from 20 to 45 minutes. In cases of analytical intensity, I may go beyond 45 minutes, since I schedule analysands on the hour (some Lacanians schedule them every 30 minutes). Lacan's use of the *very* short session was not a method, in my opinion, but idiosyncratic to him and practical given the number of people waiting to see him in the waiting room.

How sessions end is also explained: the analyst will indicate a time to stop (is this a good time to stop, or let's stop here, or was there anything else you wanted to say today?). The analysand then has a chance to agree or disagree. If they wish to continue, they are asked what they would like to speak about, and once this is clarified and some work done to this effect, the analyst again indicates the end of the session, this time without giving the option to continue.

During the preliminary sessions, we evaluate symptoms, risk factors, and history of treatment but do not engage in a detailed psychosocial history given that this will eventually emerge during the course of the analysis. If shorter treatment is indicated by the financial restrictions of public institutions, then this criterion has to be reconsidered, and a psychosocial history may need to be taken at the beginning of treatment.

Finally, a few words are in order regarding doing analysis online. Just like in the office, the session begins face to face in front of the screen. Once greetings have taken place and any practical question discussed, the analysand proceeds to lie down on a couch in a private and confidential room and to place the computer behind him or her. If the connection is poor, as it often is, the video portion can be closed and reopened to say goodbye once the session has ended. Either way, the body can be found in the virtual meeting room. The only difference between two bodies in the office and in the virtual meeting room is that online, the two bodies cannot merge. At the same time that a virtual medium could facilitate fantasy material, the fact that it is taking place remotely or at a distance favors the mediations associated with the symbolic function.

5 The singular frame, logical time, and the scansion of sessions

Lacan's analytical practice needs to be contrasted with the post-Freudian classical notion of an analytical contract. The latter implies a series of quasi-legislative standard norms that define a 'proper' analytical frame. Such attempts at strict uniformity and conformity constitute what Octave Mannoni called a Procrustean couch: if someone does not fit into the frame, then you cut off an arm, then a leg, and so on.

Lacan insisted that the question of the frame be considered on a case-by-case basis and not in standard fashion. The standard-length session, for example, is only one of the clinical tools available to a psychoanalyst and in fact may be more appropriate for once-a-week psychotherapy than psychoanalysis. I call the standard frame post-Freudian because Freud practiced in many different ways with his patients. He did pieces of analytical work walking, on horseback, and in cafés. I do not advise conducting analyses in this fashion, but such examples help to highlight the elasticity of analytic technique as practiced by its founder.

Theoretical differences will inevitably lead to different ways of practicing analysis, no matter how much one attempts to maintain the homogeneity of a standard clinical frame. This perspective differs from that of the IPA, which accepts theoretical differences among psychoanalysts so long as the standard frame stays the same across different schools. Theory and practice cannot be dissociated. For example, if the differences between the first phase of Oedipus (the pre-oedipal for other schools) with the mother and the second phase of Oedipus (Oedipus proper) with the father are collapsed, the result will not only be a confusion between registers and levels, but this will have a direct impact on the nature of the therapeutic relationship and the kind of material that is evoked and worked through in the session.

Often the Other of the unconscious will be reduced to the other of an interpersonal relationship and to issues taking place in the imaginary ego-to-ego relationship between analyst and analysand. One of the main things that will get excluded in the process early on is the question of sexuality. The interpersonal refers to personal experience, while the deciphering of the unconscious as a text, indicative of various forms of jouissance, is a 'transubjective' or 'transindividual' experience. The difference between the two is that the personal (mask) also includes the egoic narrative that leads to false forms of intimacy without the extimacy of the Unconscious that is 'in the subject' rather than the subject.

In other schools, there are entire analyses carried out mostly focused on issues of trust and attachment. "The analytic setting is a medium for personal growth not exclusively the provision of a convincing translation of the unconscious" (Philipps, 1988, p. 140). The clinical validity of this approach to analysis stems from the fact that there are psychotherapy clients where these questions figure prominently. These are psychotherapy clients who report receiving inadequate maternal or parental support and where, therefore, the questions of desire and sexuality are obscured and appear secondary to fixations to the first phase of Oedipus.

Nevertheless, what Philipps calls a convincing translation of the unconscious, in a hermeneutic sense, stays only at the level of a signifying text, as if there were nothing outside the text. But, in fact, with the later Lacan, we know that the signifier also has a relationship to the body and to the Real of jouissance. Psychic structure, in fact, can be affected by psychoanalysis, and this implies a transformation of character and subjective experience (i.e. 'personal growth,' or in less 'rosy' humanistic language: "the 'unbeing' of the Real subject"). One can refer to such transformations as emotional maturation if you prefer, but it would represent a simplified substitutive way of representing a complex structure.

The clinical validity of treating the borderline condition around questions of trust and attachment stems from the fact that there are psychotherapy clients where these questions figure prominently. This would be a specialized approach for some patients, but specialists often don't stop at that. For example, the borderline diagnosis is generalized to the overall clinical population to justify an approach to psychoanalysis without an emphasis on Oedipal structure, the father, or the questions of the phallus and sexual difference. Specialists want to overturn the theory constructed by the rare 'truth-seekers.' I believe that Lacan called the pre-oedipal the first phase of Oedipus in order to prevent this kind of split between the preoedipal and the oedipal proper. In the first phase of Oedipus, the unconscious object is the *objet a*, but, as shown in previous chapters, the *objet a* has a structural relationship to the phallus.

Finally, it is a common phenomenon of the early phase of analysis that analysands report feeling unloved by a parent, as if this indicated a lack of maternal desire for a child, when in fact the apparent lack of love often represents an imaginary way of interpreting an Oedipal rejection. In this case, maternal rejection refers to the child not being the end all and be all of the mother, either due to the mother's own narcissism or the mother's desire for the Other (partner, work, education, etc.).

From this perspective, it is possible to argue that the Freudian unconscious has all but disappeared from both the conceptual and clinical horizon of such schools as object relations and self-psychology despite the strict observance of a classical analytic frame. The standard frame only gives the formal appearance of continuity between the practices of contemporary schools of psychoanalysis and the tradition of Freudian analysis. In reality, the former widely diverge from the latter at both theoretical and practical levels.

The scansion of the session, as a capital point in the Lacanian clinic, is closely related to Lacan's unconventional definition of the analytical frame. This is difficult to write about in the United States because of the prevailing object-relations view regarding the analytic frame as a holding environment and because Lacan was expelled from the IPA for the introduction of this practice.

Lacan (1966) established a difference between what he called logical and chronological time. Logical time is composed of the following interrelated elements: 1) an instant of seeing, 2) a time for understanding, and 3) a moment of concluding. This conceptual tool was used to establish an operational mode that would address the evanescent pulsation of the unconscious according to a different temporal dimension than that of the ego-consciousness associated with ordinary speech.

The instant of seeing refers to the surprising opening and closing of the unconscious, as revealed, for example, in a disruptive slip of the tongue or parapraxis. In this respect, Lacan teaches that the moment of concluding retroactively precipitates the time for understanding. The unconscious has to open and close before the time for understanding can begin. What is at stake is to reproduce, during an analytical session, an operation that would have the same effect of precipitating the time for understanding both within and outside the session, for the session does not end when it ends.

Through the act of ending a session, the analyst is betting on the moment of understanding. To be sure, such a bet involves the risk that the analyst may have chosen a mistaken moment to end a session. Nevertheless, the advantages derived from this practice far outweigh the negative consequences that could arise from a mistake at this level. Conversely, the advantage of neutralizing such risk with the standard length of a session is small in comparison to the risk of a stagnated analysis under a standard frame.

The scansion of the session, as a way of punctuating an unconscious knowing that has erupted in the discourse of the *analysand*, like a lapsus or a parapraxis, reaffirms the meaning that the message has come from the Other (and not from the ego defenses of the analyst). As an act, the cutting of the session does not abandon the analytical scene or situation (this is how acting out is commonly defined) but points rather to the discourse of the Other. In addition, through a personal analysis, the analyst has come to know his/her own subjective state in order to sufficiently distinguish a defensive reaction from a responsive act in accordance with the unconscious (of the analysand).

In the scansion of a session, the question becomes one of elevating an act to the dignity of a silent interpretation and of utilizing an act in the same way that an unconscious formation can be revealed through an act (bundled actions) and not only through a word or group of words. The scansion of a session manifests the opening and closing of the unconscious at the level of an act. Moreover, just as the analyst does not know what he/she has said or whether the interpretation will be effective until an interpretation has been uttered and received by the analysand, so the pertinence of the act of cutting a session is only known *a posteriori*.

In addition, and among other things on a more practical level, the standard 50 minutes produces in the analyst a feeling of boredom if not outright sleepiness. Especially with obsessive, ruminating analysands, the analyst often is looking at a watch waiting for the end of the session. Thus, many analysts who work this way end up burned out, tired, and bored. With the standard session, an analyst can almost predict how all the sessions will go in any given workday. Someone may say, "Oh! Here he/she comes to speak about this, and I will say this other, they will respond with that," and so on.

All of this eliminates something decisive about analysis: the element of surprise. Without the element of surprise, all that remains is a stagnated situation that leads nowhere. In this regard, Lacan argues that a chronometrical halt ignores what transpires within the session. Instead, what he purported to do was to cut in accordance with the content and process of a session. Thus, each session acquires a singular characteristic. In addition, in accord with the non-linear synchronic time of the unconscious, a session, as a piece of psychical work, cannot be measured on a linear time scale. Incidentally, the same applies to the analyst's fees. The analysand is not paying for a linear accumulation of minutes that are owed to him/her but for the psychical work accomplished in each session regardless of the time taken to do so.

Thus, this line of thought makes it important not to dilute or minimize a significant point reached in a session by continuing to work on something else. Moreover, such an analytical tool is used to differentiate between what Lacan called empty and full speech. Perhaps "empty" is not the happiest expression for this context, since it conveys only a negative view of emptiness, whereas Lacan also used this term to describe *das Ding* (the Thing or 'no-thing') as a dignified void at the center of the Real.

In 1953, during seminar I, Lacan spoke of the full speech, which he considered true speech regarding desire. However, towards the end of his work (1976–77), the values are reversed, and full speech becomes imaginary meaning, while the Real of jouissance becomes more closely linked to empty speech. I submit that imaginary meaning is also of two kinds: the first is fantasized or conventional and the second is the fullness of meaning of a riddle for example, where the signifying elements do not exhaust the meaning of the riddle. The second form of imaginary meaning is found in the jouissance of meaning as a form of the Third jouissance.

In the first form of imaginary meaning, we find signification versus empty formal significance and the full word versus the parrot's empty speech. Already at this point, empty speech has the ambiguity of being idle parrot speech (imitating and speaking a lot without saying anything) and a speech that only has a formal significance that sometimes he calls signification without meaning. Meaning is full and imaginary. Signification is symbolic and refers to the signifier, while significance is empty speech or signification in the sense of meaning without double meaning or too much meaning.

This development was already anticipated in Seminar V (Lacan, 1957–1958, p. 120), where he defined full speech as a function of the square constituted by four edges within the graph of desire (the message, the Other, the ego, and the metonymic object). The square of full speech involves the short circuit of the ego of narcissism (a demand for ego satisfaction) and excludes altogether the unconscious signifying chain proper in the upper part of the graph of desire. He mentions statements such "You are my master," or "You are my man," and "The woman of the man." The second statement refers to the possession of the fantasy woman that a woman wants to be and that a man lacks and wants to possess. The first and last statements refer to the virile man that a woman depends on and that he always wants to show that he is. These are imaginary constructions that attempt to close and 'fulfill' the gap in the ego or divided subject. The later notion of empty speech is built around senseless signifiers belonging to the upper signifying chain that would debunk and deconstruct these statements into the vicissitudes of the *objet a*/phallus.

The analysand often "believes" that his or her well-rehearsed and rationalized, psychotherapeutic story line or problem presentation is very meaningful indeed. However, analysis as the discourse of the unconscious is concerned with unfolding not so much the well-known story line but rather the often-ignored phantasms or unconscious core fantasies. Thus, it behooves an analyst to discern between the false or idle, but maybe meaningful, ordered and rational speech and the true, senseless speech regarding the phantasm. Session cutting may be used for just such a purpose.

A common objection to the scansion of the session is that it represents an abusive, arbitrary, autocratic, or authoritarian and sadistic action on the part of the analyst perpetrated on a masochistic and submissive analysand. It is true that there are patients, particularly in psychotherapy, who will not tolerate or even need the variable length session. The point here is that the scansion of the session can also be introduced gently and in consensual fashion. The analyst may say, "Is this a good place to stop?" or "Shall we stop or stay here?" or "Is there anything else you would like to speak about today?" If the analysand wishes to continue on to something else that proves to be productive and meaningful, then at the end of that associative or signifying chain, and the working through of the effects thereof, the analyst once again introduces the cut to end the session.

There will be times when the analyst also ends the session in an abrupt way to underscore and punctuate the emergence of something significant within the analysis. Lacan did five-minute sessions, but this was greatly, if not entirely, due to the number of patients waiting to be seen. At some point, due to the high demand for his services, Lacan stopped giving appointments. People simply gathered in his waiting room and waited to be signaled into his office.

The following example derived from clinical practice helps to illustrate the rationale behind the scansion of a session. A Spanish-speaking analysand with obsessive and procrastinating characteristics came into a session describing his conflict over deciding whether to mail a letter he had written to his mother for the purpose of disclosing his sexual orientation. The analysand felt very indecisive and afraid, understandably so, of sending such a letter. During the session, the analysand made a repeated slip of the tongue. In Spanish, the correct translation for postal letter is *carta*, but instead the analysand used the word *letra* that corresponds to letter of the alphabet in English. In association with *letra*, a childhood memory came to mind of a grandfather having given the analysand an 'ink-pen.' The analysand interpreted this memory as one of momentarily getting from a grandfather the 'recognition' (and phallus) he did not get or rejected from his father.

In addition, the slip also indicated that the English language, which this bilingual analysand was using in his daily life, was also involved in the articulation of the signifying chain (postal letter translated as *letra* instead of *carta*). Thus, "not mail" stood for "not male," which is what he feared communicating to his mother. The difficulty in sending the letter signified his own difficulty with knowing something about (homo) sexuality and sexual difference (not male) and not only the fear about how the mother would respond to knowing something different about his sexual orientation (this is something he had talked about at length in previous sessions).

At this point, the analyst rose from the chair and signaled the end of the session. Rather than to intellectualize, dilute, or add anything redundant or extra to the analysand's own knowing of the unconscious, the ending of the session at this point produced a punctuation that supported a change in psychical structure. Therefore, scanding the time of the session after an important knowing has occurred may very well be an important overall criterion to observe as a way of focusing, punctuating, and promoting the working through of significant material. Finally, after the aforementioned session, the analysand sent the letter and was surprised to discover, sometime later, that his mother responded rather positively to his disclosure.

In relation to the act of cutting of a session, Lacan introduces another clinical notion: that of the "horror of the act." When Lacan says that the analyst has a horror of his/her act, he is referring to the act of interpretation. Every analyst can recognize this phenomenon in his/her own subjectivity when a doubt arises in the form of: 'Should I tell him/her this or not; and if I tell him/her what will happen; how will the person react; will there be anger, will I have to apologize or placate?' Therefore, the horror of the act (of cutting a session) has an important role to play in determining a strict and rigid observance of the 50-minute hour.

In addition, the observance of the 50-minute session is also related to the aforementioned concept of analytic "holding" and the maternal influence embedded in this notion. However, the decisive point that Lacan is introducing has to do with the function of the symbolic father as the agent of the phallic function of symbolic castration, which, according to Lacan, is the function that establishes and supports a system of *symbolic* exchange known as the Symbolic order. This function of the father needs to be differentiated from any patriarchal role that solely refers to the imaginary father. In fact, if the function of the father is thrown out with the bathwater of the imaginary father, the result will be either social anarchy and postmodern chaos or a fascist political organization that in the end are the two sides of a same coin.

The North American New Left borrowed their political analysis from Reich (1942) and others in the Freudian Left (Deleuze and Guattari [1972], for example), who were only following Engels (1884) when he argued that the patriarchal organization is the same as the structure of capitalism (Deleuze and Guattari argued that Oedipal structure was the same as the structure of capitalism).

Soon after the communist revolutions, it became clear that communism had not abandoned patriarchy or domination, and in fact the Frankfurt School (Jeffries,

2017), who also influenced the New Left, argued early on that the so-called nuclear family, or better the paternal metaphor, as we now call it after Lacan, was a point of resistance to fascism. They noted how much totalitarian states abandon the function of the father and mother in raising children and force parents to surrender the education of their children to the state.

The police, for example, can become more and more involved in family disputes as a result of the loss of parental/paternal authority and parental permissiveness. In fascist governments, the state urges children to report parents if they do not obey the fascist leader and betray a fascist totalitarian ideology. The fascist leader becomes the imaginary father. In what could be called neo-liberal forms of fascism, the liberal state intervenes in the family supposedly to protect a child from abuse (necessary in many cases), but this may have the deleterious side effect of undermining the parents' capacity to discipline their children. Something similar happened to the socialist Israeli Kibbutz experience, where, although not fascistic, the experiment to have children housed and raised separately from their parents did not succeed.

Braunstein (2012) has also argued that the change from the master's discourse, linked to the traditional super ego and societies of discipline presided over by a dominant patriarch, to the capitalist discourse of late capitalism is characterized by a disavowal of symbolic castration and the NoF. Although I am not sure that the master's discourse arising from the middle ages is the same as the early phase of capitalism linked to the protestant ethic (both are linked to discipline societies), the capitalist discourse, or what Braunstein calls the discourse of the markets, is characterized by an adherence to identifications to new gang leaders, autocrats, radical forms of fundamentalism, and so on. Demands arising from objects of consumption become demands of the drive to enjoy and the demands of the *objet a* are misrecognized for the demands of an unbarred primal father.

The symbolic function of castration, far from being arbitrary, is what enables the analyst to distinguish between empty and full speech. This law is also closely associated with the fundamental rule of free association: say anything or please speak. To be precise, speak so the analyst may see how much weed may need to be cut so that something of the register and ring of truth may remain within the speech and experience of the analysand. If the analyst encourages the analysand to speak something foolish, it is not for the sake of foolishness per se but rather so that they may arrive at the core of their being.

From a Lacanian perspective, the desire of the mother is at play in the love dimension of the fundamental rule of free association. In reference to Plato's "Symposium," Lacan (1960–1961) states that in the initial phase of analysis, the analyst is in the position of *Erastes* or lover and the analysand in that of being lovable or *Eromenos*. It is as if the analyst were saying to the analysand: you can say anything silly or foolish and you will still be loved. Even the most incoherent and ungrammatical of sentences will be accepted in analysis. Thus, the rule of free association can be seen as a declaration of unconditional love.

Moreover, the scansion of the time of the session and the scansion of speech create and organize a range of possible modifications with regard to the practice of analysis associated with what I call a multiform criterion for the practice of analysis. For example, when there is a moment of analytical intensity, an additional analytical session may be scheduled. This breaks with the stability of schedules, as it occurs in the standard analytical frame mode. In other cases, the sessions may need to be distanced from one another. This illustrates why Lacan insisted that the question of the frame had to be considered on a case-by-case basis and not in standard fashion. The direction of the cure will be different for every analysand. Modifications and transformations need to be considered in relation to the analysand's demand and aimed at preventing, in relation to the time frame, the analyst falling into the imaginary role of a mother who is unconditionally available to the analysand. Otherwise, in the transference, the analyst will appear as yet another symptom. Being in analysis becomes the analysand's neurosis.

In a similar vein, one cannot think of session frequency in a linear fashion. Such thinking, which is so frequent in many psychoanalytic circles, leads to the kind of logic that says once a week is counseling, two or three times a week is psychotherapy, and only four or five times a week is psychoanalysis. Not only is this impractical, especially nowadays, but it is also methodologically flawed. If the analysis is conducted five times a week but from the position of the Master, in horror of the act and without any regard for the singularity of the frame in each and every case, such analysis might be spinning wheels and going nowhere session after session.

Conversely, if the position and discourse of the analyst are maintained, if the frame is always being fine-tuned with regard to the changing metabolism of the analysand's demand, and the sessions are being cut accordingly, even one session a week could be considered psychoanalysis. Moreover, the position of the analyst is fundamentally more of a psychical position than a physical one. Although psychoanalysis began on the couch and the couch will always remain our analytical field of investigation, an analysis can also be conducted from a chair, although not necessarily in a face-to-face setup.

When using a chair, at times it may be especially important to be able to avoid eye contact, since, as Freud pointed out, analysands usually communicate their fantasies with a sense of shame and embarrassment. In addition, many analysands are prone to developing very intense transference reactions from very early on in the analysis. Therefore, strictly speaking, what differentiates psychotherapy from psychoanalysis is neither the couch nor the frequency of sessions but rather the psychical position and desire of the analyst and the senseless speech regarding the fantasy.

Having said this, it is also true that, for the most part, it is important to differentiate at the beginning of a treatment if the treatment will be psychotherapy or if it constitutes a request/demand for analysis. Here the difference between the two can be the explicitly defined length of the treatment (at least three years in duration for an analysis) and the frequency of the sessions (two, three, or four sessions a week for analysis). On the other hand, I have conducted once-a-week treatments of several years that in the end also led to significant analytical material and a working through of a transference neurosis resulting in structural psychical and characterological transformations.

Difference between advice giving within the context of the transference versus advice in disregard of the transference

Not to give advice is not a rule on the order of the golden rule of free association. Although the prescription not to give advice is commonly known as what differentiates psychoanalysis from other forms of treatment, most analysts give advice in one form or another. This leads many to think that analysts say one thing in the theory but then do another in practice. This in turn leads to a push for treatments by manual where clinicians follow the letter of the law with regard to a treatment practice.

An alternative approach is to reconcile the theory and the practice by understanding the difference between advice within and outside the transference. Advice works within the transference to knowledge or to the 'subject supposed to know(ing).' In psychoanalysis, we believe that potentially transformative personal knowledge is contained within the analysand rather than the analyst, though, at the outset of analysis, it is the analysand's perception of the analyst as the one who knows that initiates the transference relation. We work with the transference in such a way that unconscious knowing of fantasy life is brought to bear on symptoms, character traits, and relationships. But so long as the path of transference analysis lays wide open, and the clinician can move back and forth between their knowledge and the analysand's own knowing, then advice could also be used as an ancillary or supplemental tool of the treatment.

Freud (1913) established a distinction between advice (*Ratschlage*) and rule (*Regel*). With respect to the direction of the cure, two different factors are discernible. First, a series of variables (counsel, advice) that allows a certain margin of uncertainty, indefiniteness, and creativity. Second, the formulation of what is non-negotiable and constitutes the foundation of psychoanalysis: the rule of free association. If this distinction is read retroactively, one discovers that advice does not acquire the character of being fundamental. What is fundamental? The term not only indicates that something is important but also clearly connotes a reference to the foundation of a structure. Contrary to indications or varied forms of advice which may or may not be more or less negotiable, the rule of free association constitutes the founding rock of psychoanalysis.

Having said this, it is also important to note that Lacan did in fact contribute a new method to psychoanalysis that supplements the rule of free association, namely the scansion of speech and of the time of the session. Free association was in need of a correction, because, as many both inside and outside psychoanalysis have noticed, free association sometimes can lead to idle or defensive speech when analysands freely associate themselves away from repressed and otherwise unsettling material.

Although analysts want their analysands to speak about themselves, and not only speak about themselves but speak about themselves to their analyst, the analyst does not ask the analysand to speak about themselves but simply to speak openly without holding anything back. When analysands can speak like this, then they will in fact be closer to themselves, to the so-called language of the heart, jouissance or lalangue, although these may be 'extimate' to their ego. By freely speaking as a necessity, any foolishness that comes to mind could be explored without risking injury or offense to the Other. Analysis creates an original situation where foolishness (*bêtises*) may be neither criticized nor made marginal. Here we find the equivocal genuine trap of the analyst: speak foolishly, because through foolishness, the core of your being will be revealed. What is fundamental arises not out of a conscious intention but out of whatever speech element may break the homogeneity of the conscious ego. The fundamental rule establishes an analysis as the practice of listening for the "*J'ouis-sance*" that speaks between the spaces of what the prattle is intending to communicate.

References

Braunstein, N. (2012). *El Inconsciente, la Tecnica y el Discurso Capitalista*. Mexico: Siglo Veintiuno.

Deleuze, G. and Guattari, F. (1972). *Anti-Oedipus*. Translated by R. Hurley, M. Seem and H. R. Lane. London and New York: Continuum, 2004.

Engels, F. (1884). *The Origin of the Family, Private Property and the State*. London: Penguin Classics.

Freud, S. (1913). On Beginning the Treatment. *SE*, 12, p. 121–144.

Freud, S. (1959). *Group Psychology and the Analysis of the Ego*. New York: Norton, 1922.

Freud, S. (1965). *The Interpretation of Dreams*. New York: Avon Books, 1900.

Freud, S. (1965). *The Psychopathology of Everyday Life*. New York: Norton, 1901.

Jeffries, S. (2017). *Grand Hotel Abyss: The Lives of the Frankfurt School*. London: Verso.

Lacan, J. (1957–1958). *Formations of the Unconscious: The Seminar of Jacques Lacan*. Book V. Translated by R. Grigg. London: Polity Press.

Lacan, J. (1960–1961). *The Seminar of Jacques Lacan*. Book VIII. Edited by J.-A. Miller and Translated by B. Fink. London: Polity Press, 2015.

Lacan, J. (1966). Logical Time and the Assertion of Anticipated Certainty. In: *Ecrits*. Translated by B. Fink. New York: Norton, 2006.

Philipps, A. (1988). *Winnicott*. Cambridge: Harvard University Press.

Reich, W. (1942). *The Mass Psychology of Fascism*. New York: Farrar, Straus & Giroux.

6 The subject supposed to know(ing), love and hate, and the question of the negative transference

Lacan redefines the classical psychoanalytic concept of transference around the question of knowing (*savoir* in French or *saber* in Spanish). Knowing is not knowledge (*conocimiento* in Spanish and *connaissance* in French), because Lacan makes a distinction between the referential knowledge of science and a textual knowing in the psychoanalytic situation regarding the text of the unconscious.

However, this early hermeneutic perspective needs to be distinguished from the later Lacan, where the text of the unconscious also has a reference to the Real of jouissance rather than only the reality of the signifier. The earlier view appears to be hermeneutic, since there does not seem to be anything outside the text. Signifiers simply lead to other signifiers within the Symbolic or are embedded in the images of the Imaginary. From the point of view of knowledge, the ego is a mis-*connaissance*, while the subject represents a moment of unconscious knowing. Mis-*connaissance* is a form of 'me-*connaissance*' or a kind of self-centered knowledge rather than self-knowledge in the usual more objective sense.

In formulating this conception of the transference, Lacan is redefining classical concepts derived from Freud's (1915) Metapsychological papers. There Freud insists that unconscious feelings do not exist. Feelings can be displaced but always remain capable of consciousness. Instead, the unconscious has to do with an associative chain of representations that convey a knowing about sexuality apparently ignored by the ego. The analysand does not know that he/she knows. Thus, Lacan can be understood when he says that analysis is about a searching for a knowing that is not based on book knowledge. In other words, in every session, the analysand is looking for an "unknown knowing" (*L'insu qui sait*). This is a serious game and not just mere word play. How does 'unknown-knowing' take place in the transference? The analysand often says: "I do not *know* what is wrong with me." The analysand knows that the symptom means something, although this something is unknown.

To begin to approach the relationship between knowledge and ignorance, it is first necessary to clarify and define what is meant by knowing or knowledge and ignorance or not knowing or even non-knowing. There are forms of knowledge that represent ignorance and forms of ignorance that represent knowledge. Knowledge can transform into ignorance and ignorance into knowledge. As Bion (1963) stated, the desire to know (K link) becomes the desire not to know (-K link).

Knowledge, ignorance, knowing, not-knowing and non-knowing are often confused in the literature, although Lacan left many clues to establish precise differences among them.

> *Inscitia* is brute ignorance, whereas *inscientia* is non-knowing constituted as such, as empty, as appeal of the emptiness at the centre of knowledge.
>
> (Lacan, Seminar VIII. Session 11: February 8, 1961. Translated by Cormac Gallagher)

Brute ignorance is not wanting to know anything (passion for ignorance) about unconscious knowing or non-knowing (Lacan's *l'nsu qui sait*, or the unknown that knows or unknowingly knows without conscious deliberation). In this sense, *inscitia* or sheer ignorance can be equivalent to knowledge, or what Lacan called *connaisance*, while *inscientia* coincides with savoir as a learned or doctoral ignorance (to distinguish it from sheer ignorance). *Inscientia* selectively ignores defensive knowledge in self or others, or the doctor's own packaged knowledge, to remain surprised by unconscious knowing. The proud expert or specialist may passionately ignore the unconscious and be derisive of the ignorance of others.

Within object relations psychoanalysis, Bion (1970) also proposed the related notion of negative capability (borrowed from Keats) as the patience, or the scientific faith (or doubt, for that matter) that grants the mental ability to tolerate the frustration and bewilderment of not knowing or of not understanding ambiguous texts, conversations, situations, and emotions. This negative capability stands in sharp contrast to a full proof and unfalsifiable knowledge (whether factual or theoretical).

Lacan and Bion, in their own ways, distinguished between purely intellectual, cognitive, or discursive understanding and an experiential or intuitive understanding of speech that also constitutes a form of emotional working through and realization: the "I don't know" of unknown or unconscious knowing. The ego has to be able to say I don't know or suspend saturated textbook knowledge and meaning in order to access 'unknown-knowing' or the treasure chest of signification and significance ('signifierness' according to Fink's [2007] translation) within the dimension of the Real and jouissance. Knowledge and experiential knowing are also related, since unconscious knowing manifests within the gaps, holes, and omissions in the ego's comprehension of reality. Conscious ego comprehension works on behalf of the ego's self-interest and builds an imaginary sense of a complete and non-lacking narcissistic "whole" self.

In Plato's Banquet (Symposium), Socrates said to Alcibiades something like: "There where you see or know something in me, I am nothing" or "I know emptiness," which is a variation of the classical "I only know that I don't know." "Don't know mind" is what allows the subject to know something unconscious or fundamental as an after-effect of the admission of not-knowing or ignorance. But once the ego's level of comprehension has been suspended and unconscious knowing has been revealed, the subject still has to appropriate and take responsibility for the understanding contained within the Symbolic and have the courage to speak in their own words and name. Humility would constitute a form of false modesty at this point. The knowledge of the Other has to become the knowing of the One to prevent a simple regression from the false comprehension of the ego to the prepossession in favor of traditional authorities.

The question of knowing in psychoanalysis is related to transference phenomena but also to the phenomena of repression. Repressed knowing comes back from repression in the form of the transference to the analyst. Freud (1909, p. 54) considers two forms of repression at work in hysteria and obsessive neurosis, respectively, and both have a relationship to knowledge. The two forms are childhood amnesia or the lacuna of speech, failures of memory or recollection in the recent or remote past, and the robbing of a memory or a representation of its unconscious significance. What is missing in speech or in memory does not cease from being written by an unconscious form of ciphering/coding, and at the same time, the unconscious signification of words is in a state of constant erasure. According to Freud, the obsessive both knows and does not know his/her unconscious traumas and fantasies. The more he/she knows via intellectualization, the more he/she can doubt the same subject-matter of thoughts.

Here two kinds of knowing and not knowing can be distinguished: 1) not knowing in the case of ignoring repressed thoughts and 2) not knowing in the sense of doubting the significance of a conflict. These two forms of knowing and not knowing are also examples or derivatives of the larger division or splitting of consciousness and subjectivity. A subject is both aware and blind with regard to painful or censored experiences. At one point, an analysand may act surprised by the material, and at other times, and in a different signifying context, they are, of course, acquainted with the material. This phenomenon happens at least on two levels. The defensive ego does not know the unconscious significance of certain psychical material, or of the unconscious attempts to defend against such material, and at the same time, the ego knows about things that he/she wants to conceal from the Other. In the latter case, the ego appears not to know, but in fact knows, and what they appear to know, in fact they do not know. In the case of disavowal, denial specifically refers to the difference between the sexes.

The phenomenon known as doctoral ignorance provides a further example of two types of knowing and not-knowing. The term doctoral or learned ignorance was introduced by German medieval Christian philosopher and theologian Nicholas of Cusa (1444): "The more he knows that he is unknowing, the more learned he will be" (p. 6). Doctoral ignorance, or what Lacan called *inscientia* to distinguish it from brute ignorance or *inscitia*, commonly refers to an attitude of openness to the unknown common to both the mystic and the scientific attitude. In addition, phenomenologists link the *èpoge* (the method of bracketing anything that is not essential to a phenomenon) to the attitude of the Greek skeptics that had roots in the Socratic statement that he only knew that he did not know. In contrast to this, ignorance, period, refers not only to a knowledge deficit but to an active refusal and disinterest in knowing or knowledge.

Here doctoral ignorance has a double significance. On the side of the subject, and on the one hand, doctoral ignorance corresponds to the imaginary ego that claims to know and ignores the signifying chain as well as the subject of the Real or of the unknown. In this case, a learned individual may also reject, dismiss, or have contempt for the uneducated public or class or for opinions different from their own. On the other hand, doctoral ignorance can refer to savoir, knowing, or truth and its seekers being ignored by the specialists of university discourse. As I said earlier, specialists can reject the truth-seeker and theoretician. On the other hand, doctoral knowledge and scholars can also be ignored and rejected by the people: 'So what that you wrote books, books are good for nothing, they are all going to the trash bin of history, and the sooner the better.' Ph.D. stands for shit piled high and deep. The passion for ignorance actively rejects the passion for knowledge or wisdom.

At the level of the Symbolic and the subject, doctoral ignorance can be understood as a constructive non-knowing that points to the subject that withstands mainstream (university) discourse and its prejudices yet is not discouraged, nonetheless, in the search for true knowledge and the permutation of known discourse. At the level of the Real, non-knowing refers to unknown knowing of the lack and the savoir of emptiness that is transmitted outside the university. Symbolic doctoral non-knowing can be used as a name for analytic knowing, savoir, or the experience of the unconscious contained and transmitted within a school of psychoanalysis.

Not-knowing also refers to the desire not to know inconvenient knowledge and therefore is intrinsically linked to negation as a key ego defense. Negation and not-knowing here function as denial, or defensive rather than creative negation. The ego says, 'I rather or I don't want to talk about that, and if you insist, I can make life very unpleasant for you.' The patient routinely avoids talking about certain subjects (topics and people) to the point where the analyst finally gives up asking and begins to collude with the patient's defenses. This leads to stagnation and interrupted or partially successful/unsuccessful treatments.

For Freud (1925), denial, as a defense, and as a form of negation, was not unconscious. Unconscious repression utilizes denial, and denial is a form of the negative, but in denial, the repressed is intellectually accepted and unconsciously negated at the same time. The ego can recognize his/her division and the existence of repression but deny that it applies to the ego at a particular circumstance. In denial, negation is not unconscious, since it requires a deliberate action/decision, a judgment or choice by the subject. The ego says: 'I am fine, I am not lacking anything, have not lost anything or anybody, I am not "less than," and I don't want anything that I can't have.'

Negation can be both a form of logic or discourse and at the same time function as an intellectual form of psychical defense. The intellectual defense corresponds to the imaginary ego or Other. The ego or the imaginary Other knows there may be something there in the phenomenon that could be understood further, but the first impulse is to deny it. 'That is not an issue and I will in fact ignore it.' In the Symbolic, the subject pays with his or her person and proceeds to explore what may be there despite the risk of appearing in a negative light.

An example of negation is provided by a female analysand who had a dream that she was a man penetrating a woman. When asked for associations, she says that she believes in fluidity between male and female, man and woman, and that she does not have a problem with the dream. Nobody had said there was a problem or that she had a problem, but she is defending herself against perceiving the analysis of the dream as a form of criticism. This is an example of denial of sexual difference as a formal negation in the form of an intellectual argument or judgment. One could certainly say that the analysand's response to the dream reflects social mores or rigid gender roles, but, time and time again, analytic experience has shown that the subjective super-ego, as a faculty of self-criticism, is not an exact photocopy of external social values and often may contradict them. Values and jouissance can contradict each other and manifest in different areas of the psyche/knot.

Following, I asked her, "How did you think or feel as a child about being a girl or a boy, male or female?" The analysand replied: I did not think about that; it was an issue for my mother but not for me: she wanted me to play with dolls and be a girl. "So, you must have accepted that or rejected it," I said after a moment's wait. The analysand replied that both she did not think about it and that she remembers playing with dolls (she does not want to acknowledge that she accepted that). She then continued saying that at ten she was drawn to a woman that dressed as a man, in response to which I said, "That is a female who wants to dress as a man or identify with masculinity. Perhaps that is what you thought when your mother spoke to you about being a girl." I understand that these are not easy questions to ask within the culture, especially if the culture discriminates against homosexuality or masculine traits in females and/or feminine traits in males. The question of hysteria, 'Are you a man or a woman?' or 'What is a man or a woman?' is often answered through the body politic either in the form of a political activism for the right to choose your gender or in the form of a conformist and rigid gender binary. Psychoanalysis is an alternative to both.

In psychoanalysis, the analyst's stance of non-knowing helps an 'enunciating subject' to put forth true or 'senseless' constitutive speech regarding desire.

> It would be necessary to grasp that the subject supposed to know is reduced at the end of analysis to the same "not being there", which is characteristic of the unconscious itself, and that this discovery forms part of the same "truth-operation". . . . The subject supposed to know involves an unconscious knowledge without a subject in search for a subject supposed to know.
>
> (Lacan, 1967–1968. Session of January 17, 1968, VI 4)

The analysand looks for knowing, all the while expecting something from the analyst. Lacan has coined the expression "subject supposed to knowing" to account for the crucial place of knowing in the analytic situation. This is my translation of Lacan's *sujet supposé savoir* (the S.s.S. position). Alan Sheridan (Lacan, 1966; Sheridan, 1975) has translated it as the subject who is supposed to know. However, such translation does not underscore the fact that the subject is not the source of "knowing"; rather it is the subject who is being attributed to knowing.

> Namely: that through the transference the subject is attributed to the knowledge that gives him his consistency as subject of the unconscious, and it is

> that which is transferred onto the analyst, namely, this knowledge inasmuch as it does not think, or calculate, or judge, but carries with it nonetheless the work-effect.
>
> (Lacan, 1974, p. 29)

The subject and knowing can be confounded because the subject can appropriate the agency of unconscious knowledge and filter out any form of inconvenient or censored knowledge. Thus, for therapeutic purposes, it is incumbent for the analytical process to undo this process. Sheridan's translation emphasizes the imaginary ego that is expected to know something (subject supposed to know); mine (subject supposed to knowing) emphasizes the subject who is secondary to knowing and a vehicle for the unconscious and the Symbolic order. As in the case of the English word 'understanding,' the subject is standing under this unknown knowing. Lacan distinguishes between what he calls the referential knowledge of science and what can be called the contextual 'knowing' in the analytic situation. Finally, in Lacan's later work, contextual knowing is also related to a jouissance in the Real.

From this vantage point, the credibility of the analyst is based on two elements: 1) the fact that the psychical symptom is something unknown and uncontrolled by the subject and 2) the fact that the patient attributes knowledge to the doctor regarding the symptom. For Lacanians, these elements are understood as the basis for a positive transference relationship. The latter is what functions as a structural basis for the perceived credibility of the analyst and constitutes a basis for a therapeutic alliance. As such, it provides the initial immediate gratification (benefit) needed to engage an individual in a treatment relationship. In fact, a reduction in symptomatology is often reported in the very early phase of analysis. Within the psychoanalytic field, this phenomenon is known as a "transference cure."

Thus, on the one hand, the analyst-therapist needs to establish his or her credibility on the basis of knowledge regarding psychopathology, psychical/developmental structures and psychotherapeutic processes. This is the basis for a positive transference and for a working alliance with the subject/analyst supposed to know something. On the other hand, analysis proper is regulated by the desire of the analyst as a desire for lack, for emptiness, and non-knowing. In the transference, the desire of the analyst manifests as a desire not to be idealized or desired/loved as a subject supposed to know. In some cases, especially with the severely clinically depressed who lack desire, the analyst has to express a desire for the analysand to continue coming to appointments and speaking.

But if the desire of the analyst is defined according to the desire of the analyst that the analysand continue the analysis, then, as Freud warned, the analysand will infer that the analyst wants something for themselves out of the analysis or wants them to get better. This could also lead the analysand to staying in analysis past the point of being symbolically ready to end it. This in turn leads to interminable analysis, to infantile dependences on the analyst, and to the analyst keeping the analysand in analysis due to the financial needs of the analyst.

The desire of the analyst represents a subjective fruit of the personal analysis, a transformation of jouissance, and not an objective form of neutrality, abstinence, and anonymity. By virtue of the desire of the analyst, the therapist/analyst does not use the power and privilege given to him/her by educational, class, and professional differences as well as the transference of the analysand. Here the curative factor comes not from the knowledge of the analyst (the master's and university discourse) but from an unconscious knowing not based on formal education that the suffering subject (the client or analysand) does not know that he/she knows.

Now the analyst is a subject to whom the analysand has attributed his/her own unconscious knowing. When the analyst desires unconscious knowing about jouissance and relinquishes the ego knowledge or expertise of the master's discourse, he/she functions out of an attitude of not knowing and becomes a vehicle for the non-repressed "unknown-knowing" and understanding contained within the Symbolic, or what Lacan calls the treasure chest of the signifier.

"Unknown-knowing" here includes both the repressed signifying chain of the analysand and the participation of the analyst in the larger unknown (unconscious in a descriptive sense) structure of language and the Symbolic. On this side of the dialectic, credibility is achieved by a symbolic suspension of the ego-based authority of the analyst-psychotherapist in favor of the transformative power of the unconscious.

Redefining the transference on the basis of knowing clarifies the problem of how the transference can be resolved so there can be both a direction to the cure and an end to analysis. If the analyst remains in a position of being the 'subject supposed to know,' then, again, we would be faced with the discourse of a Master who comes to 'own' (ownership is an essential characteristic of lordship or mastery in the Hegelian sense of the term) the analysand for life. Interminable analyses that last 20 and 25 years would be such an example. The subject remains dependent on the knowledge or the love of the analyst rather than ending the analysis by virtue of the textual power of their 'own' unknown knowing. An exception to this principle would be the treatment of psychoses that in many cases could be lifelong.

The transference to the authority of the doctor on the basis of the 'subject supposed to know' functions as a resistance to recover unconscious knowing about experiences of lack and of loss, whether real, imagined, or symbolic: privation, frustration, and castration. By not believing in the attribution of knowledge, or the tribute to his/her knowledge, the analyst can successfully work with knowledge within the transference. The analyst is one step ahead of the analysand because he/she knows that he does not know. The analyst is enlightened about his/her own ignorance and therefore can help the analysand discover what they know within themselves.

However, although standardization or objective evaluation of analysis is ultimately impossible, there are criteria by which to determine if an analysis is taking place in the proper sense of the term. For example, with regard to the transference to the 'subject supposed to knowing' (*sujet suppose savoir*), two things need to take place: 1) a positive transference needs to be established, and 2) the analyst has to remove himself/herself from the position of the subject supposed to know without losing the positive transference that allows the Ucs. of the analysand to manifest.

When the positive transference is established, the analyst says very little to the analysand and approves most of what they say, except in extraordinary circumstances, of course. The analyst accepts the defenses that the ego uses to describe their problems and hears the saying that emerges in the space between words and within the narrative statement (the said).

The positive transference cannot be described as a desire of the analyst to be liked, because otherwise this would be transference and something that the analyst had to work out in his/her own analysis. In fact, the desire of the analyst not to be idealized in the transference supports the strength of the positive transference and can be considered a fruit of the personal analysis. The positive transference is not a response to the desire to be liked and loved but rather to a strategy of savoir and a question of correct method. The desire to be liked and admired is a characteristic of the hysterical master in the formula for the master's discourse:

$$\frac{S_1}{\$} \rightarrow \frac{S_2}{a}$$

The ruler or social master's lack demands that subjects/servants locate the *objet a* in them, but by the same token, they remain divided.

Instead the analyst accepts the leadership of the position but uses it in a different way. This different use is the relinquishing of the position of SsS, a veritable symbolic castration of the position of the master that transforms the position of the analyst from a master position to an analytical position. This is the democratic principle that Lacan envisioned. A free association that permits the Unconscious or the unconscious signifying chain and the Real to emerge. The analyst is an S_0 instead of the S_1 of the master. The S_0 is the *objet a* in the place of the agent in the formula for the analyst's discourse. The analyst moves from the position of the beloved imaginary object (*a*/phallus) to the position of the absence or emptiness of the *objet a*.

The negative transference

We also know that with respect to the vicissitudes of the *objet a*, Lacan (1964/1981) has said "I love you, I mutilate you." So, how does the *objet a* function with respect to the negative transference and hate and destructiveness within the transference? For Winnicott (1968), for example, an analyst must carry an analysand from object relation to object usage, and he adds the twist that in object usage, the object is destroyed and, paradoxically, the object survives the destruction. In Winnicott's theory, object relation means the relationship to fantasy objects and not to reality 'whole' objects that in Lacanian theory actually represent the Other.

Object relations thinking often confuses two types of objects and misses the fact that for Winnicott, the reality object, far from being objective, must be destroyed in fantasy and both the object and the subject must survive the object's destruction. The child says then to the destroyed object that survived the destruction:

"I destroyed you; I love you" (the reverse of Lacan's [1964/1981] "I love you; I mutilate you" referring to the *objet a*). Winnicott's thesis has the surprising effect of proposing that objectivity or the objective object is discovered or created through its destruction.

Winnicott (1947) classifies transference phenomena of the analyst into three types (Etchegoyen, 1991, p. 300): 1) unresolved transference of the analyst; 2) the 'normal' personal subjective experience of the analyst; and 3) 'objective-subjective' responses of love and hate to the actions, speech, and character of the analysand. For Winnicott, the analyst has to have a necessary ability to hate the analysand objectively. When a disturbed child provoked a feeling of anger and hate in him, Winnicott told the child about his hate, and this allowed Winnicott to carry on with the treatment of the child.

Working with functional adults is different because the focus will be in speech and not in play or actions during the session. The equivalent of the objective feeling of anger that Winnicott mentions would be the frustrations that the analyst experiences in listening to idle talk or storytelling far removed from the core of the subject's experience in the unconscious signifying chain. The objective feeling of anger goes along with the patience that the analyst has to uphold in the analytical position.

In Lacanian analysis, hate in the transference, or the de-supposition of the Other/analyst as the 'subject supposed to know,' is not the same as the analyst in analysis no longer occupying the position of the subject supposed to know. In other words, the analyst not relying on the 'subject supposed to know' has to be differentiated from the analysand's attempt in the negative transference to challenge and contest the knowledge of the analyst. Because the analyst does not hold onto the subject supposed to know, he/she is in a position to listen to the disavowal of the very knowledge (by the analysand) that they have suspended. So, here is a formulation: the negative transference disavows both the analyst's savoir and the analysand's own 'unknown knowing' and instead sets up the analysand's conscious rationalizations in the place where their unconscious knowing or savoir would be.

The negative transference and the analyst's suspension of their expert authority have very different consequences. If the analysand actively disavows what the analyst knows and presents their conscious knowledge as the relevant material for the sessions, then this conscious ego knowledge of the analysand is definitely not the liberating 'unknown-knowing' of the analysand's unconscious. Conversely, if the analysand does not reject the analyst or what they know precisely because the analyst suspends what they know, then the analysand's speech will reveal the subject's own 'unknown knowing.'

When the latter happens, unconscious knowing is located on the side of the unconscious of the analysand. The Lacanian view represents a working through the love transference more than the negative transference. Lacanians don't recommend working through the negative transference ("A negative transference . . . must be dispensed with as soon as possible," Verhague, 2001, p. 38).

Since at the end of a Lacanian analysis, the analyst must become dispensable, or the analysand may be said to have had enough of the analyst, it can be argued that in an analysis, the analysis ends thanks to the negative transference, even if and despite the negative transference not having been interpreted in the course of the analysis. Negative transference refers here to the antipathy (hate would be too strong of a word in this context) that may arise associated with the difficult work with unconscious lack and symbolic castration.

Such antipathy (Winnicott uses the word hate for this phenomenon) would be Symbolic (reality) in this case, although the Symbolic would also lead to an opening towards the Lacanian Real. Lacan says the Real is an obstacle, and to this extent, the Real would also be engaged in symbolic antipathy. In any case, such understanding of the negative transference as a catalyst for the end of analysis needs to be differentiated from the ordinary conception of the negative transference defined by Lacan as de-supposing the analyst as 'subject supposed to know': 'What do you know, or you are wrong about me, and this analysis is not helping, and so on.'

In Seminar XX (Section VIII on knowledge and truth), Lacan (1972–1973) speaks of what he calls hateloving (*L'hainamoration*) and argues that knowledge about love gives rise to hate as its regular underside. Strife, misunderstanding, or equivocation, as the conflict of opinions and identifications, is not a mere rift, as a division or hate ripped open, but rather the intimacy with which opponents belong to each other. In addition, any interpretation can be interpreted as a devaluing message as if the analyst were saying "you do not know what you are saying" (Miller, 2000, p. 21). The analysand also contributes to their experience of devaluation via the idealizing transference: the more ideal the analyst is perceived, the more the analysand will experience themselves reduced to zero, as if they were nothing compared to the analyst.

Especially in the positive or idealizing transference, and when the analyst is located in the position of the object of fantasy (*objet a*), the analyst is in the place of the fullness of Being or agalma. It is this position that, according to Lacan, can trigger love but also hate in the negative transference. For the analysand in these instances, the analyst represents something that they want, they lack, and that they perceive the analyst having. At this juncture, Being corresponds to the fantasy of absolute knowledge as it refers to a particular concept as an object that could complete the divided subject.

At this point, I need to clarify how I am using the concept of Being and of the One used by Lacan (1971–1972) in Seminar XIX. Obviously, as is well known, the analyst does not have the *summum bonum* (agalma) for the analysand (Being is missing in the Other). The agalma cannot be understood as a positive concept (this would be a fantasy or an imaginary One), since, as Socrates said: "There where you think you see something in me (agalma), I am nothing." Being, from Socrates to Plotinus, to Hegel, Heidegger, and Lacan, has to be understood as the One's own non-being. "The idea that being is and that nonbeing is not, I don't know what that means to you, but personally I find that stupid" (Lacan, 1972–1973, p. 22). It is unclear whether Lacan means stupid in the sense of doctoral ignorance as "non-knowing" or simply stupid as in the sense of 'not-knowing' and common ignorance. The least we can say is that, when it comes to psychoanalysis, he is not satisfied with the first formal level of logic: is and is not.

In the citation, being and nonbeing are in discord rather than accord with each other (being is and not being is not). The definitions of being and nonbeing are different in this case. "Obviously the One that maketh Being is not itself Being. It maketh Being (Lacan, 1971–1972, p. 198). "Ontology is a shame or dishonor," (idem, p. 95). "The One is not" (idem, p. 95).

Lowercase being refers to a hypothesis, for example, and nonbeing refers to the null hypothesis. They cannot both be true. In Seminar XIX, Lacan (1971–1972) speaks of the One's own non-being. The One's own non-being is in accord with Hegel's (1832) statement that pure Being and pure Nothing are the same (p. 59). In addition, 'ek-stasis' in Heidegger represents the empty essence of Being and therefore already combines being and non-being (as 'ek-sistence' or 'ex-sistence') as differentiated from existence, plain and simple. Insofar as 'ek-sistence' pertains to Being, this Being is by definition more than the 'being' that is opposed to 'non-being.' Only in 'ek-stasis' and 'ex-sistence' does the Being of a human being appear as emptiness rather than existence.

> Frege constitutes the notion that the One is the concept equal to naught (p. 46). The One is not (p. 96). Just because the One is not this does not mean it does not pose the question (p. 116). That which exists through not being (p. 117). The empty set leads to the birth of the One. The One only begins with its lack (p. 126). The One, when it is veridical, when it says what it has to say, leads in every case to the total rejection of any relation to Being (p. 162). Being is not-all One Being, for also it is naught/not (Lacan, 1971–1972, p. 218).

The One's own non-being refers to Capital being without signifiers or beyond signifiers of being. The Real aspect of Being outside the signifier is best described as senselessness or emptiness of signification (S_1 without S_2) and/or as a form of jouissance. "I'm speaking of the One as a real, a real that may equally have nothing to do with any reality whatsoever" (idem, p. 121). I observe here that the translator did not capitalize Real to differentiate it from reality, thus continuing the equivocation between the terms. Equivocation here could mean the flexibility to go from one term to the Other or to consider how the two terms are related, but it could also mean to be confused about equally significant differences between the terms.

But if the Real has no sense, then what is the relation of the Real to the true? Does truth depend on sense or non-sense (fiction)? In addition, is truth the same as the true? (see Appendix II on this question). "The true about the Real is that the Real has no sense." It is well known that Lacan has said that the only truth is one that can only be half-said and that only half of it can be said. Finally, Lacan also stated that "Truth has the structure of fiction" (Lacan, 1966a, p. 625). Truth, or *Aletheia* in Greek, can only be half-disclosed or unconcealed. The other half remains concealed or undisclosed as a mystery of jouissance or 'ek-stasis.'

Lacan does not use the term 'fiction' in the sense of a falsehood but in the sense of a scientific construct as an approximation. Fictions for Bentham, the founder of utilitarianism in philosophy, cited by Lacan in Seminar VII, were necessary objects of discourse such as norms, conventions, or social contracts. When Lacan says that truth has the structure of fiction, the reference is to a normative discourse that empiricism would consider objective. This formulation implies that objective truth is a fiction (the signifier is a semblance), as distinct from a non-fictional form of truth that could be subjective or 'transubjective' (truth as jouissance). That subjective truth is not fictional in nature, represents a complete reversal of traditional references. Is there truth outside fiction and language, or is there truth in the Real as a subjective truth that is 'extimate' to the normative ego?

The true as fictional norm is not the same as what is true about the Real or truth in the Real as nonsense. The first presents truth as sense or fiction (I think, therefore I am); the second presents truth as nonsense or nonfiction (I am where I don't think, or I think where I am not because it is not the ego doing the thinking). Nonsense is a form of subjective truth that does not mean random meaninglessness in language, since nonsense can refer to mathematical symbols that are meaningless in language yet function within mathematical systems.

Real truth is nonsense or empty, and the other half-side of truth is the fictional sense of statements and the said. Being as a concept devoid of signification, an S_1 signifier without an S_2 signified, is equivalent to the side of truth that is in the Real of nonsense rather than on the side of narrative fiction or relative truth. Now according to the formulation that truth can only be half-said as a fiction, the half-side of truth that is in the Real of nonsense (truth of truth) cannot be said. Now does this 'cannot be said' mean that it cannot be said in words but can be said in silence, for example? It could also mean that it cannot be said in statements but can be said in equivocal sayings, or an experience of jouissance, or a mathematical symbol or formula. All of these may be true.

Lacan also says that truth is only possible by voiding the Real. We have to ask: Which side of truth does this truth in Lacan's statement refer to? A fiction voids the Real by fictionalizing it as a half-truth, or by saying that the Real 'Is not that.' The void is not fiction, and fiction is not the void despite being purely fictional or empty and without substance. But by fictionalizing the Real, since the negation or voiding of the Real is a negation of something without symbolic or imaginary characteristics, all you get is a half-truth. On the other hand, this could also mean that truth within language voids or conceals the Real through fictional words but is revealed in non-fictional numbers rather than verbal half-fictions. The Symbolic within the Real represents an excess of words that fail to hit the Real. The Real within the Symbolic is when the Real is revealed in pure signifiers and where the signified is in the Real of jouissance.

The fullness of the One's own non being, or of the Real as a vacuum plenum, that grounds unformulated truth as a form of jouissance, and that manifests within the Symbolic as senselessness or a gap in meaning, is misinterpreted in the Imaginary transference as the analyst having the agalma or the phallic *objet a* that the analysand lacks. The analyst as *objet a* in the Imaginary represents a semblance of being. Hate is an interpretant sign (affect) that the analyst is perceived as a complete Being in the place of truth outside signification. Hate, in this case, is what Lacan calls a truth passion. But since Lacan says that there is no Being in the Other, such projected Being as an imaginary One can only be a fantasy that the Other has something that the subject lacks. Real being is the One's own non-being. The subject has to reach its own Being through pure signifiers and the knowing of the One. "I recognize that this One here is but knowledge superior unto the subject, that is, unconscious insofar as it manifests itself as 'ex-sisting'" (1971–1972, p. 218).

Given that love deceives with respect to an altruistic love object that turns out to be the ego's own narcissistic object, at least certain forms of hate may be realistic responses to losses generated by the symbolic function. However, this formulation is not without problems, given that it is indeed difficult to differentiate the hatred associated with the experience of imaginary castration from the hate directed at Real and symbolic obstacles. The only difference is that the Real remains an obstacle past the acceptance of the obstacle associated with the incest prohibition. In other words, even if the subject accepts the symbolic loss associated with the incest prohibition, the subject will inevitably have to deal with both the external world and the Real as an obstacle.

Furthermore, the symbolic and the Real add additional obstacles linked to hate beyond the Imaginary of how the subject defends against symbolic castration with the fantasy. The Real adds another obstacle of incomprehension beyond the rational arguments found within the Symbolic. With respect to symbolic and Real hate, Lacan says that hate is a lucid passion that goes beyond the mask and appearances of the Imaginary and the potential obsessions of the Symbolic.

It is the three forms of hate (in RSI) that are the determining factors for the manifestation of a negative transference. For this reason, Reich was the first disciple of Freud to focus on the negative transference and the analysis of resistance not to build better defensive egos as in ego psychology but to deconstruct the narcissistic aspects of a normal neurotic ego. However, the drives that are released from repression thereby are not revolutionary forms of sexuality that don't exist, nor raw and cruel forms of overt and riotous aggressiveness. When reactive formations are undone, drives are not sublimated towards ego drives that pre-existed life or death drives, but rather, sublimation is realized as a vicissitude of the drive itself rather than an ego formation associated with social ideals.

It is not accurate or enough to merely think of love, kindness, or generosity as aggressive counterpunches or reaction formations; this is only part of the story. Being kind does not preclude being fierce or having a wrathful persona ("*L'a mort*," Lacan would shout to his audience with a dramatic gesture!). In fact, this may be a good characterization of Lacan. A fierce kindness is a facet of the drive and to be distinguished from socialized 'niceness.' In addition, any form of analysis will involve disillusionments with respect to the forbidden love object that eventually the subject will have to relinquish, even if this does not mean, in fact, that the subject has to lose actual relationships.

Clearly any one of these factors could lead to hating and resenting the analyst: inevitable narcissistic injury or forms of ego-loss; the loss of the social façade and hypocrisy associated with being nice as a reaction formation; and the frustrations/castrations associated with external reality, the Other, and the Real. However, there are mitigating factors that make these problems bearable for a subject in analysis. The analyst as a social authority differs from the Other of the Law, family, or government. In addition to free association, in general, any analyst will not be judgmental with respect to a healthy enjoyment of phallic jouissance. This facilitates a positive transference relationship and serves as an antidote against the perception that analysis is a frustrating experience that requires the analysand's subordination to the analyst.

Analysts of the past, including Freud, were disappointed with what they could do or the therapeutic results they could achieve with the words linked to the social narrative of the patient that in many cases remained on the level of idle or parrot speech: the more they speak, the less they say. Faced with this obstacle, analysts thought that the observation of behavior and body language could carry them to the finish line or provide a real means of therapeutic success (body work is another variant of this). This begins a trend in psychoanalysis to interpret any behavior and not just the formations of the unconscious as they appear in speech (although explanation and interpretation in the absence of the analysand's speech may be necessary in regressed or acute states). Lacan instead also moves away from the social narrative but towards a theorization of the Ucs. signifying chain, the voice and the *objet a*, and how the two chains interact, especially in relationship to the Real of jouissance.

Lacan argues that the *unskilled* use of authority and knowledge in the analytic situation generates resistance in the analysand as an iatrogenic effect. Resistance is the resistance of the analyst to relinquish the knowledge that the analysand or the analytical situation attributes to him/her.

In Seminar XX, Lacan says that those who hate him make for better readers of his work, the same way that he declared that Deleuze was his only disciple (who hated the lack and the negative, especially in Hegel). In other words, the better readers of his work will hate him objectively. Many readers, especially when beginning to read stimulating works, will experience a form of hatred towards the thinking articulated in a piece of writing. In this case, hate would be more objective than love, since love ordinarily becomes a slave of narcissistic wishes. Hate is often associated with criticism, since love tends to be more accepting and ingratiating of the other's qualities and speech. Critique and analysis often involve discrimination and the breaking down of symbolic elements into its component parts – an act that not only can take place in the presence of hostility or ambivalent feelings but may be more successful precisely because of that.

This is why dialogue fails despite its illusory promise to bring thinkers and agents to a conversation free of the constraints that ordinary communication or miscommunication places on theoretical discourse. Dialogue fails when discussants are not able to dispose or modulate the aggressivity that is part of knowledge and university discourse. Although this is not the topic under consideration, in passing I will say that paraconsistent and dialogical forms of logic have in fact proposed formal ways to handle the contrariness and hate that emerges in dialogical situations. This, of course, has nothing to do with analytical discourse, since the aggressivity associated with statements and propositions is not handled in the same way in the analytic process.

Nevertheless, the basic point here is that there is a link between knowledge, cognitive discrimination, and hate. Nonetheless, despite the aggressive and disagreeable taste that many academic or theoretical interactions may leave behind, Lacan does not fail to mention that aggressive and even paranoid polemics, or doctrinal sophistries and intellectual entanglements, may cause the advance of knowledge and science. This is a more realistic appraisal of the consideration that conferences can be means of indirect conflict resolution. If anything, hatred and paranoia have to be taken as sinthomes and used to reveal psychical structure. One thing is to praise the folly, madness, and delirium associated with love or what is enlightened about delusion, as Erasmus, Shakespeare, and Baudelaire have done in their literary works that challenged the pieties and hypocrisy of the Catholic Church. Quite another thing is to praise and champion hate, murder, and nihilism for its own sake.

Since human beings have hate towards the external world due to the frustrating characteristics associated with the reality principle, there is a basic mistrust towards the world, even and despite good-enough mothering. This is why Lacan believes that human knowledge has a basic paranoid structure, the principal effect of which is hate, and this explains the connection or regular association between knowledge and hate. Finally, hate also has a relationship to knowledge via the experience of envy and jealousy, or what Lacan calls "*jalouissance*." Envy for someone else's talent, knowledge, or academic accomplishments, if acted out, is always a carrier of hate. Envy is the feeling that the other has something that we want and that we lack in order to reach the ego's own ideal ego.

In analytic discourse, there are exceptions to this when someone candidly or publicly acknowledges their envy ("I am so envious of this or that quality of the Other"). This is not envy anymore because envy has been symbolized. Another thing completely would be to act invidiously in a way that crystallizes and champions the envy. This would be to ignore the illusion that the subject lacks something the Other has, when in reality the demand embedded in envy is rooted in the inevitable lack that all subjects have to reach their own ideal ego. The perfection of the ideal ego in fact refers to the fantasy object of being the *objet a* cause of the mother's desire, which is something impossible. Therefore, there will always be envy, no matter how much a subject achieves, because ultimately the ideal ego is a narcissistic fantasy that has to be relinquished with the acceptance of symbolic castration. Envy is based on the subject's own narcissistic fantasy and not on how much the other has accomplished or realized.

Finally, in Seminar XX, Lacan also discloses that his main passion is not love or hate but contempt. I cannot say for sure how Lacan is using the term, but contempt can always be associated with derision and a sense of intellectual superiority or narcissism. Lacan had contempt for common sense, for scientific principles of exposition, for the middle class, and wanted distinction, wealth, and fame instead (Roudinesco, 1990, p. 104). In this respect, contempt can be considered the near enemy of the desire of the analyst. If the analyst desires to be admired and loved by the analysand as an analyst of distinction, then this certainly could interfere with the analytical function.

Contempt can always be associated with derision and a sense of intellectual superiority or narcissism. In this respect, it is often difficult to differentiate the propositions apprehended by a gifted intellect from the hubris and arrogance of the ego personality. When Salvador Dali was asked what his main focus of study was, he answered that Dali, or his personality, was his main interest. Galileo, Newton, Einstein, and Lacan were all known for their intellectual arrogance at various times. Arrogance in this case represents a form of courage to stand against the dominant false knowledge of the time.

The analyst does not want anything personal (certainly not admiration or idealization, however normal these forms of transference may be) from the analysand other than payment: "You don't have any object of use that I want to take from you." The desire of the analyst is an indication or measure of the relative absence of transference or that transference was successfully analyzed in the personal analysis of the analyst (the analyst passed beyond the rock of castration). The analyst does not demand to be loved, recognized, or desired by the analysand.

Instead, love for the analyst can be transformed into knowledge. However, if the analyst interprets transference love by explaining the transference, and to the extent that knowledge entails a frustration or an acceptance of symbolic castration, the conversion of love into knowledge may give rise to hate as its inevitable companion. Instead love without knowledge, or when the latter functions as savoir ('unknown-knowing') rather than *connaissance* or emerges from the spontaneity of the analysand's own speech, knowing does not give rise to hate.

The relationship between love and knowledge is complex because there are different types of both, so when speaking about these terms, different people may mean different things, leading to confusion and disagreement in the use of the terminology. Since in Lacan's work, love has to be understood within RSI, when people speak about love, unbeknownst to them, one may be speaking about imaginary love while another is speaking about symbolic love, and for this reason, they cannot agree on their definition of love.

The love relationship between a lover and a beloved, or *Erastes* and *Eromemos*, is composed of all the three registers of love. Freud was aware that when speaking about love, the definitions abound on many different levels and dimensions; however, sometimes he himself was confused by the different levels in which love operates. In general, his orientation was to reduce the more sublime or romantic forms of love to the sexual drive and to regard the former as mere illusions or semblances of the drive.

In Lacanian theory, illusory romantic sexual love is imaginary love that ultimately threatens to destroy the bonds between people when it becomes clear that the love is for the narcissistic object of fantasy, not the other. Freud thought that this kind of love was doing an injustice to the Other by reducing the Other to the love object (1930, p. 49). Freud goes astray with respect to the various levels of love because of the confusion surrounding the concept of sublimation as an aim-inhibited drive or as a direct satisfaction of the Other jouissance not ruled by the pleasure principle. For this same reason, he could not appraise the function of the Real and the sublimation intrinsically available to women via feminine jouissance (Freud said that females were not capable of sublimation).

Freudian theory associates Shakespeare's (1982) "illusory-deadly-crazy-love" with the aspect of sexuality linked to the death drive rather than with love, since love, as a manifestation of the life drive, is what creates bonds between people. Lacanian theory instead places the social link between people under the heading of symbolic love. The Law, culture, values, agreements, language rules, and commitments create more lasting bonds between people. However, the bonds of the law and commitment, and the knowledge that they represent, can also generate hate and violence, and in this sense, symbolic love can also function as a semblance of hate.

Freud (1930) disagreed with the biblical injunction to love one's neighbor as oneself, since he was pessimistic about the inevitability of unjustified and random violence associated with animal instincts. Freud also thought that it was not always justified to love one's neighbors, since neighbors and siblings can be even more cruel than strangers. Since Judaism does not proselytize to non-Jews, Jews have been regarded as applying the golden rule only to other Jews. However, Leviticus clearly states the commandment to love the stranger or the non-Jew as oneself. It is this commandment that Christianity universalized and interpreted it as a command to proselytize, when in fact the commandment merely refers to loving those around you or that you come into contact with, whether stranger or Jew, but without an attempt to proselytize and convert. On the other hand, it is also true that Jews proselytize to other Jews, while Christians proselytize to the stranger or non-Christian.

Despite the Christian emphasis on universal brotherly love, the Catholic Church in history at times behaved towards non-Christians with hatred and revenge rather than love (if you don't join us, you are against us). In addition, many contemporary evangelicals believe bigotry or hatred towards non Christians is justified. Why should Freud love the stranger when he had the experience of German gentiles forcing his father into the pavement in order to have exclusive use of the sidewalk? Why should Jews love or forgive the Nazis?

From the point of view of imaginary intersubjectivity, the neighbor or lowercase other triggers aggressiveness, rivalry, and the evil eye of what Lacan called "*jalouissance*" (envy and jealousy towards the other). From the point of view of the Imaginary, "love your neighbor as yourself" makes absolutely no sense. The statement itself is a logical contradiction if by self we mean the ego of narcissism. At most, the golden rule is a reaction formation against the natural imaginary hatred felt towards the sibling or fellow member of the same group (*Homo homini lupus*: man is a wolf to man, or to communities, neighbors, and disciplines with adjoining fences and territories: the narcissism of small differences).

Regarding the further Christian dictum to love thy enemies as thyself, this poses a further challenge, since although difficult, or even ridiculous, it is not like embracing hatred as an ideal could be any kind of a solution either. It is also important to remember that for the primal horde, the primal father was both father and enemy at once, and once they killed him, they converted their hate for the father into guilt and the love of the totem. In addition, hatred is not effective when fighting an enemy, something the martial arts know very well. Self-love, love of an 'inside' group, and love of ideals are what makes a soldier an effective killing machine, more than the hatred of the enemy, because the latter at some point will be converted into its opposite, leading to death, treason, and desertion. There are many examples of people that suffer conversion into the opposite at critical moments: American to Russian; hippies into yuppies; socialists into capitalists; capitalists into socialists; females into men; males into women; cops, government officials, and lawyers into criminals, as well as vice versa, in all possible combinations.

The Christian dictum or precept to love thy enemy as thyself seems to abdicate violence even as a means for the justified end of fighting a despot or an oppressive government. In contrast to this, modernity, the master's discourse (Cesar), the university discourse, and even the analytical discourse at times see violence in human beings as inevitable and in many cases justified.

I mentioned in the introduction that the Frankfurt school was well aware of the contradictions of modern or enlightened reason and how formal reason and techne could pass into violent use and exploitation of others. This critique was applied to both bourgeois "civilized" modernity and Marxist informed communist societies. Neither capitalism nor communism could contain the violent excesses of drives, nor the unjustified and unnecessary ways of exploiting others within society. In his famous paper "Critique of Violence," Benjamin (1921) engaged in a critical examination of violence that, of course, meant a lot more than criticizing violence and extolling the virtues of non-violence as a mode of social organization. In fact, Benjamin believes that "no solution to human problems is possible" (p. 247) if violence is totally ignored as a relevant question for human beings.

Traditionally, as Benjamin points out, violence in history has been seen as something natural that only becomes problematical if violence is used for unjust ends. History does not have too many options besides accepting violence as a natural fact of life, since history, other than the history of ideas and inventions, is the history of a series of violent confrontations between different groups of armed men. Both sides of any conflict felt justified in their use of violence, even though in some cases, violence and domination may have been seen as an end in itself. Both parties to any armed conflict saw their ends as justifying the means to carry them out. The ends would not have to be the preservation of their ideologies or cultural myths but could simply represent the instinctual violence needed for the natural survival of the individual (self-preservation) or of the species (sexual reproduction).

Precisely in humans, mythical themes are the cultural ways of handling animal instincts and transforming animal instincts into symbolically organized human drives. In culture, the natural violence found in instinctual nature cannot be simply justified as a natural disposition needed for survival. People buy needed commodities rather than fighting over them. In this sense, economic exchange represents a sublimation or a super structure of what happens in the natural state.

If people resort to fighting and stealing from others, when better means for both parties are available within the culture, then the means are no longer justified by the end of obtaining or providing the goods necessary for survival. In culture, violence is seen as an unnecessary means of obtaining satisfactions not available or permitted in the culture. At some point, a leader may have been cruel, authoritarian, and unfair, and this remains within the heart of every person, but for the most part nowadays, the leadership position alone becomes sufficient reason for subjects to entertain the fantasy of killing, and perhaps eating, the group leader.

Ordinarily unconscious violence, as a means or an end, that exists even in the absence of physical or sexual abuse, is not justified in any legal or social sense. Precisely the psychoanalytic method is a way of handling the excess of violent jouissance present in human beings. This is why the Frankfurt school was suspicious of the Marxist understanding of violence as a natural means to achieve a just and fair social organization for human beings. Freud's perspective on violence was that violence is not only not justified by law but may be precipitated or caused by the law. According to Freud, not much could be done other than accept the inevitable discontents of civilization.

Although Freud did not think that it was possible or necessary to love the enemy, since hate is justified in the case of an enemy, at the same time, he did not think that hate towards the enemy was always explained or justified by the enemy's intentions or actions. The enemy is always invested with the 'lovehate' originally felt towards the father as a rival, in the same way that the father could be invested with the 'lovehate' felt towards the enemy. From Freud's perspective, the fight against an unfair leader is always fraught, since the difference involved between a leader and a follower is enough to trigger violence and sensations of imaginary castration, regardless of the fairness or unfairness of a leader. The unfairness or perversion of a leader (social master) are additional reasons to want to fight a leader, while in a naïve Marxist view, a fair communist companion raised in a communist society would presumably never experience irrational feelings of violence towards people. This is why Benjamin says that Law or Justice are not enough to produce stable agreements and reduce violence between people.

> We are above all obligated to note that a totally nonviolent resolution of conflicts can never lead to a legal contract. For the latter, however peacefully it may have entered into by the parties, leads finally to possible violence [in cases where the agreement is broken].
>
> (p. 243)

Rather nonviolence, as a state of satisfaction where people can freely exchange or give and obtain needed goods, requires a prior agreement and understanding regarding violence and its subjective conditions. "Nonviolent agreement is possible wherever a civilized outlook allows the use of unalloyed means of agreement" (p. 244). A nonviolent agreement has to be chosen and not arrived at by means of laws, contracts, or signed agreements that can be imposed or broken.

I suggest that Benjamin's 'unalloyed agreement' can be defined as the unalloyed in the sense of a pure unmixed affect. This One enigmatic affect refers to both the Greek mind and Lacan's jouissance, as both pleasure and pain, the lack as absence or loss, and the lack of a signifier for the Real, since jouissance in Lacan refers to the drive and the Real as a dimension or a true hole (*vacuum plenum*) outside symbolic reality. For Benjamin, the unalloyed agreement is characterized by courtesy, lack of agitation, and trust or metanoia as its subjective preconditions.

Finally, Benjamin's unalloyed agreement or accord, considered as a binding quality of jouissance, raises the question of the third form of love in the Borromean knot not yet discussed: Love in the Real.

In 1969, Lacan wrote the following:

> When the subject comes out of analysis . . . he no longer needs the demand of this Other to uphold his own desire. He is satisfied with this emptiness in which he can love his neighbor, because it is in this emptiness that he finds his neighbor as-if in himself and he cannot love him in any other way.
>
> (Lacan, 1969, translated by Marini, p. 217)

Love for the emptiness or inexistence of the Other that the subject finds as-if in himself/herself is the closest that Lacan comes to a definition of love in the Real that bears any similarity to the golden rule of civilization mentioned previously. From the point of view of the Real, we love in our neighbors their emptiness/lack rather than an imaginary fantasy object, because their lack resonates with our own emptiness or lack of being. The original nature of humanity is not just his/her animal instincts but the inanimate void of emptiness from which the instincts arose and that contains jouissance and is an aspect of the symbolic and sublime aspects of the death drive. The death drive represents what is impossible about the Real.

Love in the Real is a form of the Other jouissance that is facilitated by the symbolic phallus or the phallic function. Phallic jouissance is transformed from object enjoyment to the enjoyment of the absence of the object as an index of jouissance. What in the Other is lacking, or the object as the presence of a lack, in the Real signifies a different form of jouissance. "The phallic function is written $\Phi\chi$. It exists . . . as a fact of saying. It's a saying no, and even, I would say a *naysaying* . . . there is at-least-one who *naysays*" (1971–1972, p. 178). Naysaying is a pointer to the Other or Third jouissance.

There is something in a woman that is more than the ideal woman in a man's eye. This more is the more of feminine jouissance that requires the phallic function for its manifestation. Conversely, beyond a man's preoccupation with his virility, there is the symbolic phallus as the inexistence of the imaginary phallus that gives a man access to the Symbolic, to phallic jouissance, and the use of metaphor in language. In this sense, the Third jouissance or the Other jouissance, as a function of a Real tie, can represent a supplemental jouissance for the sexes beyond the battle of the sexes and beyond the battle between the Imaginary and the Symbolic. The ideal woman, who represents the golden number (imaginary phallus) in a man's eye, is replaced by femininity in the Real, and a man is defined not by his virility regarding the imaginary phallus but by the symbolic phallus as an emptiness beyond the phallus that also includes it.

Thus, love in the Real can also be approached through the Other jouissance (Fink, 2009) as an unalloyed agreement that women experience in both feminine jouissance and in the act of lovemaking. Fink's text gives several clinical examples of feminine jouissance as an 'Other jouissance.' Men also have access to the Other jouissance through so-called mystical experience. 'Myst' is a word to describe the emptiness, inexistence, or 'ex-sistence' of Being. In the case of woman, it refers to the emptiness of primary femininity. In the Real, women are loved for their emptiness. This is one of the readings of Lacan's statement that woman is one of the names of the father (in plural and lowercase). The lowercase does not mean that she is one of "The" unbarred forms of the imaginary phallus/primal father that does not exist. The unbarred father is imaginary, while in *sensu strictu*, the primal father is the dead father, or the inexistent imaginary father represented by his name (NoF). In the case of the capitalized NoF, and the NoF associated with the sinthome and the Real of the later Lacan, woman and the Name are senseless and cannot be named in a narrative without a loss of truth at the level of the Real of jouissance.

Love in the Real, as hereby defined, can also be brought into relation with savoir rather than knowledge. Savoir is a form of non-knowing constituted as empty rather than as acquired constituted knowledge. In Real love, knowledge is subsumed under an empty unformulated and incomprehensible truth in the Real. Hate is what arises when knowledge is discriminated as a fiction or a half-truth which is something inevitable, since formulated truth has the structure of fiction.

There is a structural discord, intimacy, and/or lack of rapport between the two halves of truth. Formulated truth will always have an element of fiction that does violence to and conceals the other half of truth that remains unformulated within the Real. For this same reason, one cannot find the other half of the soul in the love object but only in the empty half-side of the heart, that love as a signifier represents. Once the other half of truth that is not a fiction is inevitably formulated as a second fiction, it comes to antagonize the first half-fiction already put forward. Hate is the affect that arises in the ego linked to the second half-fiction that has been drawn from the Real to oppose the first half-fictional formulation presented by an interlocutor.

Although hate borrows its jouissance from the Real, hate does not give access to an unformulated truth in the Real that remains undisclosed. Hate only gives access to a second half-truth that fails to leave the Real outside representation. The half-truth that is not a fiction does not fail from not being said. There is an aspect of true forgetting that supports the side of truth that remains in the Real. "In every entry of being into its habitation in words, there's a margin of forgetting, a *lethe* complementary to every *aletheia*" (Lacan, 1953–54, p. 192). This originary form of repression I have theorized as a second type of primary repression linked to the true hole of Lacan's Seminar XXIII. "And it is this hole that I am aiming at . . . that I recognize in the Uverdrangung itself" (9.12.75. II XVI).

A second half-truth fails to close the gap or pacify the discord between knowledge and truth. For truth to include its non-fictional Real side and bring true peace to the saying, the unsayable or impossible has to be included in a One saying beyond the statement. Love in the Real does not represent a restricted access to truth but rather the unknown that knows without formulated knowledge. Truth in the Real here is "non-knowing" or doctoral ignorance rather than ordinary "not-knowing" or stupidity. As soon as *das Ding* (the 'no-thing' as the thing in itself) is exposed to discriminating thought, it can only be identified with relative difference (half-fictions: metonymic images and objects, and the sliding of the signifier).

There is relative difference between signifiers, and then there is the absolute difference between the signifier and what lies outside representation. "The One qua pure difference (that there is) is what distinguishes it from the notion of the element. The One qua attribute is thus distinct from One of pure difference" (Lacan, 1971–1972, p. 167). Relative marks refer to one another, and then there is the mark of the unmarked that now has been marked. Once the unmarked is marked, an absolute difference emerges between the relative differences between marks and the unmarked that now lies outside of them. In actuality, absolute difference is neither sameness nor difference but the 'same difference' with the unmarked found across all marks. In set-theoretic terms, the empty set is found in all sets.

In this sense, love in the Real, as a love for the emptiness of the subject, correlates with a truth of *savoir* that is not a constituted knowledge. "Must it be stated that we have to know [*connaitre*] other bodies of knowledge [*savoirs*] than that of science when it comes to dealing with the epistemological drive?" (Lacan, 2006a, p. 737). Hate instead correlates with knowledge, *connaissance*, cognitive discrimination, and discursiveness without a link to truth and jouissance in the Real. How is this point related to the relationship between love transference and knowledge? When the analysand loves the analyst for a knowledge attributed to him/her, this does not refer to a specific knowledge within a field but rather to a generalized and empty sense of truth that grounds such knowledge.

In a quote subsequently, Lacan will say that at the end of analysis, the subject (supposed to know) is reduced to not being there, which is a characteristic of the unconscious itself. The dissipation of the S.s.S. and the 'inexistence' of the Unconscious form part of the same 'truth operation.' Such operation of truth takes place between the two sides of truth or two truths: the fictional side and the empty or inexistent side of truth that is in the Real. The fictional side of truth, or the signifier as a semblance, gives way to the "ex-sistence" of jouissance.

Not interpreting transference love (to be differentiated from its analysis in the speech of the analysand when the analysand directly addresses the analyst) with knowledge that has not appeared in the analysand's speech would also help keep this form of hate at bay. Knowledge in this context, even if scientific or proceeding from a rational episteme, can be defined as *connaissance* or cognizing and discriminating rather than as *savoir*. *Savoir* is a form of knowing that does not exist ('ex-sists') or is consistent with non-knowing and Nous as a basis for analytical hearing (*J'oui-sens*). In this definition, *savoir* about love does not give rise to hate as its inevitable pair-wise companion.

For Socrates true love gives access to truth and knowledge. Love of sophia and sophia's love yields knowledge. Truth seeks not only the pleasure of the lover, but a concern for the beloved. Romantic ephemeral love is transformed into a lasting and equal friendship. Love of truth is the true love, that is sought in intellectual and spiritual friendship that gives an added value to every relation. Physical passion makes friendship go away. Analytical friendship, or apprenticeship as some cultures call it, is a life in common, involves reciprocal attention, kindness to one another, shared feelings but this is not a substitute for love, or something that will take over in due time, it is the true love that gives access to truth. Imaginary love blocks the access to truth and eventually leads to hate or indifference. True love is empty of content apart from the mutual and lasting affection of friendship. Truth is sought in its nature, not in its object. Beyond the appearances of the object, love is a relation to truth. The transports of love in time will yield to a reciprocal relation to truth and knowledge. We have to be enamored with truth, and help lead this love to knowledge and friendship. This is the meaning of the master as a love object. The master is moved by the force of true love and the knowing how to truly love the truth that must be loved. The wisdom of emptiness is the object of true love.

The attribution of knowledge to the analyst in the transference is experienced as symbolic castration, since the analyst presumably is the one that knows about lack/emptiness. "The Other that knows about love hates me, and I hate what I perceive that the Other knows about love (and the lack thereof)." The subject hates what the Other knows about the subject's Unconscious that exceeds what they thought they knew. Cephalic *connaissance* (cognition) must be symbolically castrated in order to access unconscious *savoir* in the Real.

When the knowledge *in* the Other, perceived as hate, is accepted, the hate associated with truth will eventually subside or be forgotten. Herein lies the question that Winnicott raises with regard to so-called objective hate that must be survived by analyst and analysand alike. The analyst survives not only the hate of the analysand but their own loss that they had to endure as a consequence of the analysand's attacks. The analyst survives by losing the cephalic consciousness that in turn helps the analysand access their own unconscious knowing regarding the fantasy object that had been located within the analyst. This is what the analyst offers up of himself/herself in the analytical function (payment with one's person).

When the analyst does not abandon the cephalic consciousness of their own ego, then the analyst will be prone to making mistakes with the analysand. However, I disagree with Winnicott (1956) when he says that objective anger on the part of the analysand within the transference is always about the analyst's mistakes. Winnicott comes to this conclusion, I believe, because he does not have a constructive view of the negative (privation, frustration, castration) that is not only a part of the psyche and character structure but also an aspect of the structure of the Symbolic and language. Anyone is prone to experience anger as a result of frustration, but the component of the anger that is inevitable with frustration is not so easily differentiated from anger linked to fantasies associated with frustration.

In analysis, the analysand relinquishes their ordinary way of thinking in favor of free association. The analyst has to do the same with respect to their listening and use of speech in the analytical function. To limit the negative transference, the Lacanian analyst does not interpret the positive transference in the absence of its disclosure by the analysand. Thus, the positive transference develops out of the fact that despite having knowledge of the unconscious, the analyst does not always use this knowledge and instead is more interested in what the analysand's unconscious has to say. Now the analysand feels loved and accepted regardless of ungrammatical or senseless speech. Already being loved for his/her support for the subject's unconscious desire, the analyst becomes an *Erastes* or lover relating to a beloved *Eromemos* or analysand.

Lacan (1960–1961) uses the Greek categories in Seminar VIII on the subject of the transference in order to account for what he calls the metaphor of love as it occurs in the psychoanalytic cure. If I speak of metaphor, I am speaking of substitution with respect to the reciprocal substitution that takes place between analyst and analysand in relation to the places of *Erastes* and *Eromemos*. In other words, the lover must become lovable or beloved (analyst) and the beloved turned into a lover (analysand). The analyst becomes *Erastes* or lover by the prescription of the fundamental rule as if it were a love declaration. But how does one emerge from this situation in order to work in the direction of the end of analysis?

In *Group Psychology and the Analysis of the Ego* (Freud, 1921), Freud establishes a very close link between love and hypnosis. Since the psychoanalytic cure can be viewed as a love story – as genuine and deceptive as any other – how avoidable is the conclusion that hypnosis has an important role to play in such a process? The servitude of love requires that love be demanded just as the hypnotized is begging to be ordered, healed, or satisfied. Thus, one becomes subordinated when elevating the analyst to the place of the master. Such elevation/subordination is the motor for the generation of positive and negative transference alike. Hypnosis, like the proverbial serpent, is a recurring presence that must be mastered in order to avoid being fascinated by its power.

References

Benjamin, W. (1921). *Critique of Violence: Selected Writings: Volume 1, 1913–1926.* Edited by M. Bullock and M. Jennings. Cambridge: Harvard University Press, 1996.

Bion, W. (1963). *Elements of Psychoanalysis.* London: Karnac, 1984.

Bion, W. (1970). *Attention and Interpretation.* New Jersey: Jason Aronson, 1995.

Cusa, N. (1440). *De Docta Ignorantia.* Minneapolis: The Arthur Banning Press, 1981.

Etchegoyen, H. (1991). *The Fundamentals of Psychoanalytic Technique.* London: Karnac.

Fink, B. (2007). *Fundamentals of Psychoanalytic Technique: A Lacanian Approach for Practitioners.* New York: Norton.

Fink, B. (2009). Love and the Real. In: *Sexual Identity and the Unconscious.* Published by the Forum du Champ Lacanien, 2011.

Freud, S. (1909). Notes Upon a Case of Obsessional Neurosis. In: *Three Case Histories.* Edited by P. Rieff. New York: Collier Books, 1963.

Freud, S. (1915). Metapsychological Papers. *SE*, 14, 143–215.

Freud, S. (1921) Group Psychology and the Analysis of the Ego. *SE* 18, 67–143.

Freud, S. (1925). Negation. *SE*, 19, 235–239.

Freud, S. (1930). Civilization and Its Discontents. *SE*, 21, 59–145.

Hegel, W. (1832). *The Science of Logic*. Cambridge: Cambridge University Press, 2010.

Lacan, J. (1953–1954). *The Seminar of Jacques Lacan*. Book I. New York: Norton, 1988.

Lacan, J. (1956/1966). The Function of language in Psychoanalysis. In: *The Language of the Self*. Translated by Alan Sheridan, 1975. Baltimore: John Hopkins University Press.

Lacan, J. (1960–1961). *Transference: The Seminar of Jacques Lacan*. Book VIII. London: Polity Press, 2017.

Lacan, J. (1964). *The Four Fundamental Concepts of Psychoanalysis*. Seminar XI. New York: Norton, 1978.

Lacan, J. (1966a). Science and Truth. In: *Ecrits*. Translated by B. Fink. New York and London: Norton, 2006.

Lacan, J. (1966b). The Youth of Gide, or the Letter and Desire. In: *Ecrits*. New York: Norton, 2006.

Lacan, J. (1967–1968). *The Seminar of Jacques Lacan*. Book XV. The Pschoanalytic Act. Translated by Cormac Gallagher from unedited French manuscripts. http://www.lacaninireland.com/web/translations/seminars. Accessed July 6, 2020.

Lacan, J. (1969). La psychanalyse en ce temps. *Bulletin de l'Association Freudienne*, 4/5, October 1983.

Lacan, J. (1971–1972). *The Seminar of Jacques Lacan*. Book XIX. Edited by J.-A. Miller. Cambridge: Polity Press, 2018.

Lacan, J. (1972–1973). *Encore: The Seminar of Jacques Lacan*. Book XX. London: Norton.

Lacan, J. (1974). *Television*. Edited by J. Copjec. New York: London, 1990.

Marini, M. (1994). Psychoanalysis at That Time. In: *Jacques Lacan: The French Context*. New Jersey: Rutgers University.

Miller, J. A. (2000). *La Transferencia Negativa*. Buenos Aires: Tres Haches.

Roudinesco, E. (1990). *Jacques Lacan & Co.: A History of Psychoanalysis in France, 1925–1985*. London: Free Association Books.

Shakespeare, W. (1982). *A Midsummer Night's Dream*. New York: Penguin Books.

Verhague, P. (2001). *Beyond Gender: From Subject to Drive*. New York: Other Press.

Winnicott, D. (1947). Hate in the Countertransference. *International Journal of Psychoanalysis*, 30, 69–74, 1949.

Winnicott, D. (1956). On Transference. *International Journal of Psychoanalysis*, 37, 386–388.

Winnicott, D. (1968). The Use of an Object and Relating Through Identifications. In: *Reading Winnicott*. Edited by L. Coldwell and A. Joyce. London: Routledge, 2011.

7 The payments of the analyst and the direction of the treatment

Lacan outlined the notion of cure direction in "The Direction of the Treatment and the Principles of its Power" (Lacan, 1958/2006). In Lacanian psychoanalysis, the direction of the treatment is determined by how the analyst uses the power granted to him/her by the analysand's transference. The power of the transference appears to be directed to the professional authority of the analyst (subject supposed to know), or some trait of the analyst, that grants the analyst the authority to conduct the analysis. If the analyst takes this personally, fails to make strategic use of the early phase of the positive transference, and merrily goes along believing in the positive transference to the person of the analyst, the analysis will be aimless and endless. Under these circumstances, the analytical relationship becomes a group of two made up of a leader and a follower that forever remains dependent on the analyst's love and knowledge. To prevent impasses in analyses, and in truth, Lacan argues that it is the power of the unconscious, appearing in the involuntary sayings of the analysand, that directs and orients the treatment. It is the opacity and emptiness of the analyst's desire that facilitates free association and the manifestation of the unconscious and the Real in the analysand's speech.

The unconscious of the analysand knows the truth manifesting through the symptom, but due to repression and concomitant disguises, the subject appears to ignore it. From this place of ignorance, the analysand searches for a master in the analyst. In analysis, the analyst occupies the place of the subject's *objet a* cause of desire, and from this place, he/she induces a lack or a void that facilitates the subject's speech. In Lacanian psychoanalysis, the direction of the treatment means something different than what is indicated by the clinical notion of treatment plans and objectives. One cannot evaluate an analysis in terms of the treatment plans and objectives associated with insurance companies and managed care.

Freud (1922/1959) described the wish of people to look for leaders to hold authority over them. The analysand comes into analysis wanting the analyst to wield a curative power over him/her. Despite the appearance of a therapeutic context, to be effective, the analyst has to relinquish the power of orienting or providing moral counsel to the analysand in terms of contemporary values and prevailing social narratives. Lacan always insisted upon differentiating psychoanalysis from counseling, the direction of souls, or pastoral counseling. Subjected to the demand of the Other, the neurotic cannot tolerate being in a situation where he/she may have to speak with his or her own words rather than with those of the Other. The resistance to change in psychoanalysis is addressed in relationship to impediments to free association rather than interpreting it as a resistance to the authority of the analyst or the health values governing the treatment.

Lacan finds antecedents for the position of the analyst in the Stoics and the Socratic mayeutics. Socrates (2003) went around town engaging people in conversation about different subjects, appearing to know nothing and being willing to learn from everyone who professed to know. Socrates made profession of no knowledge except of his own non-knowing. He believed that people know both less and more than what they think they do. To those who appeared to know, he showed them that they actually did not know; to those who appeared not to know, he showed them that in fact they did know.

In the case of the practice of analysis, the analysand comes either positively or negatively predisposed to a therapeutic encounter/interaction. Entering the analytical field already requires a certain ego-deflation or symbolic castration on the part of the analysand. He/she has to be willing to acknowledge a certain degree of suffering and inability to help himself/herself on his/her own. From this place of suffering, stagnation, and helplessness, the analysand reaches out to the analyst. This is the place of not knowing, of the subject of the unconscious, and of expecting and sometimes demanding that the analyst know something and wield a curative power.

When negatively predisposed, the ego of the analysand will devalue the knowledge of the analyst: "I know who I am, and nobody knows more about myself than me, and in fact you know nothing, and I do not think you can help me, and actually I am not doing so bad after all." This is how Lacan defined the negative transference in relationship to knowledge. I disqualify someone that I hate, or I hate whom I disqualify.

Using Lacanian theory, one can distinguish between the ego and the subject at the onset of the treatment. The ego is the small mind that already knows it all and has nothing to learn from anybody. The ego [i(a) or I[A}], as the ego of ego-identity rather than the I of symbolic non-identity, is at the center of all statements and is represented by the short circuit (square) that appears at the base line of the graph of desire. The ego says, I know, I have attained, and wishes to constitute itself as the object and signifier of what the analyst as Other is missing.

The analyst, in turn, under the desire of the analyst, is attentive to the ways in which the analyst and the analysis become a signifier for the analysand's desire. Under the desire of the analyst, the analyst does not wish to become the object cause of the analysand's desire and rather represents a pure desire in between signifiers and objects. The desire of the analyst is a desire for emptiness or inexistence that holds the place of the agalma, or the splendor of the One's own non-being, for the analysand. It is in this sense that the analyst represents the paternal metaphor, or the empty place of the symbolic function capable of 'wowing' the subject into producing the signifiers of desire (*épater le bourgeois*).

But the subject (S, *Je*, or I), as a pure signifier, is more than the ego or the pre-barred S or imaginary phallus/object of the mother's desire that does not appear in the graph of desire other than as the imaginary *objet a*. In fact, the *objet a* is the first identity that an object affords the pre-subject (unbarred S). The pure signifier is also more than the ego as an organizer/agent of the social statement, and than the divided subject ($) that appears at the beginning of the vertical vector of intentionality in the graph of desire.

The vector of desire goes up to the demands of the drive ($◊D) for the signifier of jouissance that is missing within the Other (S[Ø]). The subject (S), as a pure signifier, mediated by symbolic castration, is used not to represent the *a* as the presence of the object or subject of the drive, but rather to represent the *a* as a missing signifier of jouissance. The signifier for the subject (of jouissance) and the signifier of jouissance are both missing. The *Je* represents incessant symbolic activity within a psychical and linguistic environment or system that continues processing even while the ego sleeps. It is the hole in the symbolic, where a signifier for the subject and jouissance could have been, that causes the sliding of the *Je* within symbolic representation. That the Other is lacking, or the opacity of the Other's desire, is a stand-in for a lost object or signifier that constantly fuels the displacements and repetitions of the signifier in the signifying chain. It is in the absence of a signifier for the analyst's desire that new signifiers will appear in the undetermined immediacy of analytical experience.

If the analysand in the transference asks for a master of knowledge, the analyst should act from the place of non-knowing, the equivalent of Socrates showing people that in fact they did know. The analyst does not wish to be recognized as a person of achievement, or precisely becomes a person of achievement (in the Bionian sense) by paying with their person in relationship to the analysand. The analyst pays with their person when they suspend or relativize their own packaged expert knowledge in relationship to the analysand. The analyst privileges what the analysand unconsciously knows rather than their own conscious knowledge.

Analysts suspend the desire for recognition, although if analysts succeed in establishing themselves in the analytical function in the absence of a desire for recognition, then the unintended result may in fact be a successful analysis. It is the desire of the analyst (or the absence of a desire for recognition), or the payment with one's person, that regulates the countertransference. If the analysand claims to know and that the analyst does not, the analyst still responds – without self-consciousness – from the place of a knowing that does not know that it knows. The analyst needs to acknowledge that the individual knows but point in the direction of unconscious knowing by the subject and not the ego.

The analysand does not only pay the analyst because he or she has knowledge or skills that could be of help to the analysand, the usual conception of a professional or contractual relationship. In the history of psychoanalysis, critics have objected to viewing the intimate and personal help that psychoanalysis provides as something tainted or "soiled" by being paid for with money. The analytical function steers clear of being something spiritual that should not be paid for with money, and at the same time, the analyst is not being paid for providing helpful objective information and "skills" associated with human services and access to social goods. Analysis is not simply a love story, nor is it a form of spiritual or philosophical counseling or friendship. The analyst is not being paid for loving or reparenting the analysand. In addition, analysis is not an exploitative asymmetrical relationship, because an analysis does nothing for the analyst's ego.

The analyst is not being paid with money only because of his/her educational efforts and expertise. Lacan tells us that the analyst is paid for his/her own personal payments that are required as part of the analytical function. The analyst pays not only with their professional qualifications but with something of their own personal and subjective being. This refers to a payment, or a subjective loss or payment with their own person in the performance of the analytical function. The analyst pays by relinquishing their social persona and/or suspending normative characteristics of social interaction and conversation.

Some relational North American analysts have critiqued this notion of the payments of the analyst on the grounds that it represents a form of asceticism or a protestant notion of original sin or an inborn, ingrained, intrinsic, or structural culpability or debt that needs to be punished and paid. This seems strikingly different from positive, loving, intimate, supportive links based on humane and symmetrical relationships. However, truth or positivity cannot authentically appear without the negative. Without the negative, humanistic positivity is purely Imaginary, as in the jouissance of the Other with the mother (the Imaginary One). Relational or humanistic positivity is an appearance that obscures the more difficult aspects of relationships that people know and observe, nonetheless. Humanity requires the loss of the fusion with the Other, as well as the structural loss of the *objet a/imaginary phallus*.

More than being paid for their knowledge and expertise, analysts are in fact paid for strategically losing the position of the subject supposed to know and for the third ear or what Lacan calls *J'ouis-sense* (hearing more than listening). Analysts lose the knowledge that otherwise they would be paid for. They are paid for the loss of the claim to knowledge rather than for its use, although it is also true that the loss of knowledge on the side of the analyst in the analytical relationship is also a strategy of a different kind of knowing (*savoir* rather than *connaissance*) considered necessary for a successful analysis. Teaching skills, knowledge, or information is not the default position of the analyst. The default position of the analyst is *J'ouis-sense* (experience of hearing rather than thinking the sense of things).

In addition, the analyst is paid to put up with the transference and the analysand's idle narrative, which are other ways of paying with one's person (forbearance). In listening and putting up with the idle narrative or defensive speech, the analyst waits to hear key signifiers within the narrative that provide access to more truthful speech regarding desire. When the analyst hears key signifiers linked to jouissance, then at that point, analysts ask questions regarding those signifiers, or the relations between signifiers, and ask the analysand to free-associate to them. These are two aspects of the scansion of speech. The analysand provides the evidence that the analyst has heard correctly and acted accordingly by asking the right questions. The analyst's interventions lead to the analysand's unconscious signifying chain and to an experience of jouissance. When this takes place, the analysand realizes a form of knowing that they did not know that they knew.

To let go of the social ego requires a form of subjective destitution, at least a partial and temporary retreat from social behaviors and conditions, and a letting go of what Jung (1957) called the social mask or persona, our favorite ego-images and verbal platitudes. The analytic or therapeutic relationship is not a social relationship because it differs from professional work relations with peers, superiors, and subordinates, and it differs from relationships with lovers, teachers, family, and friends. It also differs from relationships with priests in that the analyst is not a moral guide or a guru. The analyst, like the Buddha, is no more than an arrow pointing inwards to the analysand's own intrinsic mind as the locus of truth and liberation.

In work relations, a certain measure of success, of goals and objectives, is expected from the ego. The ego is expected to know something under the performance requirements governing work relations. Nothing of this sort is expected in a personal analysis. A personal analysis is the place where the ego can fail miserably, and ego ideals are suspect and subject to deconstruction. Even the most ungrammatical form of language will be accepted in analysis. Moreover, psychoanalysis thrives on mistakes as access points or gateways to the unconscious. A Zen saying describes the life history of a Zen teacher as that of one continuous mistake, or of one mistake after another.

I once organized a lecture for Harari at the Wright Institute in Berkeley. Administrators, not being particularly overjoyed about a visiting Lacanian analyst from Latin America, composed a flyer to promote the event and misspelled Harari's name by homophony. As Lacan said in Seminar XXI, those who are not 'duped' by the NoF or Lacan make more serious mistakes (*Les non-dupes errant: les noms du père*). Instead of Harari, they wrote "Errari" (meaning to 'err'). Roberto was not insulted by this mistake; he did not take it personally, and instead told me: Raul, an analyst is established by his/her mistakes. This of course does not mean that a subject should deliberately make mistakes. The mistakes that establish an analyst are those orchestrated by the unconscious rather than the ego.

In addition, for the analysand, the renunciation of a social relationship suspends the mental defenses operative through social discourse and results in openness to inner experience. In social, sexual, and familiar relations, the ego desires, expects, and even demands things from others. The analyst pays with his person when not using these dispositions in relation to the analysand. To help the analysand, the analyst must ultimately even give up the desire to cure or provide a successful treatment to the patient because this inevitably leads to a narcissistic ambition or wish for personal success on the part of the analyst that will trigger a corresponding wish to fail on the part of the analysand as an integral part of the negative transference.

Not that the analyst is not interested in relieving the symptoms of the analysand, but a direct gain orientation or idea only intensifies the ego-resistance of the patient to the treatment and to the cure. In addition, if the analysand perceives that the ego of the analyst is involved in the success of the treatment, then like a child with a parent, the analysand will unconsciously defeat or oppose the analyst/doctor by compromising his or her own success.

But then what are the gratifications 'permitted' to the analyst? Although money and livelihood are legitimate and explicit needs of an analyst, this should not lead one to think that greediness towards money on the part of the analyst could not become a hindrance to the treatment and the therapeutic relationship. Ultimately the practice of analysis is done for its own sake, while symptom relief for the analysand and payment of the analyst are side benefits or added values of the practice for both parties. Analysis satisfies an inmost request for unconscious knowing and convenient forms of jouissance.

Paying with one's person also requires not using personal values. Does this mean that there are no values implied in the analytical situation? The value of the abstention of judgment implies values of a different order or metavalues. Because psychoanalysis is not moral education, other than the implied health values of the treatment, the analyst does not impose his/her own personal values, although if asked, the analyst may not deny them, either. The analyst accepts the different values of the analysand, although if their values conflict with the Law, rather than correct them, the analyst asks them about their thoughts and feelings regarding their predicament before the Law.

Whenever an analyst encounters homophobia or dislike for homosexuality, or heterophobia or dislike for heterosexuality, sexism or dislike for men or women, addiction to prostitution, or racism and anti-Semitism, it is not fruitful to try to reform the analysand into adopting the correct values. This will only engender argument and ego battles and wreck the therapeutic relationship. Rather, abstaining from preaching one's values will facilitate an exploration of the themes and conflicts that lie at the root of such ethical failures. In the long run, such a method stands a much better chance of preventing problematic social attitudes and values.

I am not advocating a value-free or "objective" scientific approach. As established elsewhere (2008), subjectivity is always implicit in any relationship between a knower and a known. It is not possible to avoid a subjective position. The question becomes one of how to work with our subjectivity in order to realize subjectivity and knowledge without a subject and affect a subjective destitution. Truth, or a truth-operation, is rectified error within the context of a permutation of subjective experience. As aforementioned, psychoanalysis thrives on mistakes as gateways to unconscious truths, and an analyst is, therefore, established by his/her mistakes.

Ego-ideas and ideals, in the sense of ideological or defensive false views that block symbolic understanding, are foregone moment to moment, one piece at a time. To acknowledge being wrong and give up ego attachments to wrong beliefs and assumptions requires a certain humility and sobriety of mind that is a basic subjective characteristic of the scientific attitude. It is this attitude that clears and prepares the mind for new insights to arise.

Finally, while the use of words represents the second payment of the analyst, the third is the payment with the core of one's being. Is there any use in thinking of the practice of interpretation as a personal payment rather than interpretation simply following from the intellectual brilliance of the analyst's cephalic consciousness? The important point here is that there is a discontinuity between ordinary social narratives and the use of speech in analysis. The third payment with the analyst's own-being or non-being is what prepares the ground of Being and language for a differential use of words in relationship to the Real. The last two payments will be addressed in the next two chapters.

References

Freud, S. (1959). *Group Psychology and the Analysis of the Ego*. New York: Norton, 1922.

Jung, C. (1957). *Two Essays in Analytical Psychology: The Collected Works of C. G. Jung*. Edited and Translated by G. Adler & R. F. C. Hull. Princeton, NJ: Princeton University Press.

Lacan, J. (1966). The Direction of the Treatment and the Principles of Its Power. In: *Ecrits*. Translated by B. Fink. New York: Norton, 2006.

Moncayo, R. (2008). *Evolving Lacanian Perspectives for Clinical Psychoanalysis*. London: Karnac.

Plato. *The Last Days of Socrates*. London: Penguin Books, 2003.

8 Interpretation, punctuation, citation, and the scansion of speech

Lacan (1969–1970) stated that an interpretation is somewhere between a citation and an enigma. An analytic interpretation can be defined as the act of substituting an enunciation of the analysand (A) by the same citation of the analysand by the analyst (C) right at the time/moment of the analysand's saying or at a later point in the session (T). The therapeutic property (P) of the interpretation rests not only on the content of the statement but on the analyst having chosen the correct statement (A) and time (T) to cite (C) from the point of view of its links to the unconscious signifying chain (E) and as confirmed by the analysand's response to the citation (R).

If the citation leads the analysand to new material associated with the partial object of the drive and desire, or some form of jouissance is evoked or released, then it is safe to say that the interpretation has successfully reached its destination. Citation evokes enigmatic affects and signifiers. In addition, the analyst needs to have a sense of right timing and that the analysand is ready and able to receive the interpretation, whether consciously or unconsciously.

The analyst cites those signifiers/narrative statements that the analyst infers constitute elements of the unconscious signifying chain that the subject does not know that they know. The ego of the narrative ignores what they are actually saying. As shown earlier in the graph of desire, the descent from the narrative statement [s(O)] towards the ego and aiming towards the ego-ideal acts as a counterforce for the possible ascent from s(O) towards the pure signifier that is always involved in the "technique of the signifier," as Lacan calls it.

The technique of the signifier refers to the citation of key signifiers in the analysand's speech, as well as the scansion, cutting, or segmenting of words and their displacement and condensation into new words. However, there is one additional element of the technique of the signifier that is important for analytical practice, with some qualifications. I have mentioned that there are two signifying chains: one is the social narrative and the other is the unconscious signifying chain that often erupts into the narrative, but not always. Free association as a method facilitates the manifestation of the unconscious signifying chain.

However, sometimes free association just leads to an excess of words and meaning, or idle words that never reach the unconscious signifying chain. Citation can be used if key signifiers appear in the narrative, but at other times, in their absence, the analyst may respond to the analysand's narrative by offering equivocal readings of scenes the narrative has described. Equivocation here works better than explanation. The analysand can then determine whether the shoe fits. These are always tentatively presented and await their confirmation by the analysand. If the Other scene is disconfirmed by the analysand, the analyst is happy to explore a different associative path suggested by the analysand.

Lacan said that to catch the bird of the unconscious, you have to make enough noise for the I of the signifier to fly out of its hiding place. The alluded staging, for example, precisely represents such noise, although at other times the proverbial hmm . . . or cough may also perform that function. It has been said that Freud talked too much during sessions, and although this may be true, since he did not have a personal analysis, one could also wonder whether Freud's talking was the noise that triggered the manifestation of the unconscious in his analysands.

The practice of citation as a form of interpretation is important because it actually represents a scientific moment of psychoanalytic practice. The analyst stays with the evidence, and at the same time, the analysand's statements are used to bring out the unconscious saying within the statement, and this not only has a therapeutic effect but also provides a confirmation of the theory. This is quite a different mode of interpreting than that practiced by the school of ego psychology and Kleinian analysis that will, for example, interpret in the "here and now" the gait of the analysand as they close their door and walk to the couch without any signifiers providing any evidence or confirmation of the interpretation. No wonder that some analysands would have trouble or be disturbed by those interpretations and not because the Unconscious had been evoked. What was evoked was the Imaginary without having the tools to understand its significance in terms of the formations of the Unconscious.

The reason for not interpreting the content of the statement, in the absence of the saying, as an unconscious formation, is that it easily leads to denial or to the analysand hearing it as something that comes from the analyst rather than their own unconscious. The Other of the unconscious is replaced by the otherness of the analyst's interpretation, and the analysand may submit and accept the analyst's interpretation, but the acceptance is superficial and, more importantly, reinforces the analysand defenses and resistances that now know what to avoid speaking about in the future.

Each citation has to be tentatively offered to the analysand, requesting confirmation as to whether the analyst has correctly understood what the analysand said. The theory predicts, and clinical experience confirms, that often the analysand will not recognize their own statement and will attribute it to the intersubjective other instead. In order to work with the defenses of the subject, it is important that the analyst give the analysand the opportunity to reject the citation so that eventually they may recognize it within their own mind. A more advanced analysand will use the subjunctive mode in speech to reflect on their division with respect to their own statements and will use the analyst as a function to work through the contradictions in their speech and experience.

In addition, in contrast to a symmetrical dialogue where somebody talks, and somebody responds, an interpretation, in the analytic sense of the term, means that somebody speaks more, and somebody speaks less, an asymmetrical state of affairs. The asymmetry represented by the fact that the analysand gets to speak more than the analyst balances the asymmetry according to which the analysand discloses their problems and subjective experience and the analyst does not. In addition, the analyst not only has to speak less but also has to speak in a different manner. Citation is one of the ways the analyst speaks in a different manner. Within the psychoanalytic situation, dreams and unconventional linguistic formations, such as slips, puns, jokes, and so on, are matched by the use of interpretative speech (citing the signifiers that have unconscious signification) on the part of the analyst. A skillful use of citation is meant to evoke something different from conventional or ordinary speech as it appears in the upper floor of the graph of desire.

Moreover, interpretative speech is not the communicative speech of ordinary life in two significant respects: 1) in analysis, the analyst needs to allow what is equivocal, paradoxical and ambiguous instead of expecting and utilizing forms of linear directive speech, and 2) as aforementioned, an interpretation should not be a move whose goal is to obtain something. In other words, interpretative speech, like poetical language, needs to be distinguished from any form of instrumental or communicative discourse. Interpretation does not aim at communicating information as a means for something else or to ask someone to do something but rather simply to evoke and invoke a particular signification.

In the example of the technique of the signifier used in the 'famillionaire' lapsus cited by Freud (1905) and Lacan (1957–1958), the lowly task of working on the rich man's feet contradicts the wish to be someone important like the social 'master' (Rothschild) whose feet he is working on. These opposite signifiers are stamped/pressed together in the signifying chain resulting in a fundamental ambiguity of signification.

According to Lacan, *lalangue*, as the text or language of the unconscious, escapes the grammatical or formal logical organization of discourse. The signifying chain is composed of key signifiers which are polyvocal and equivocal in nature. Moreover, what is evoked by a paralogical use of language is the experience of the unconscious expressed by an unconventional use of conventional language. Metaphorical intuitive utterance transgresses and elevates the ordinary meaning of words. To reveal within language a core unconscious experience beyond language and symbolization requires a different use of language from that of formal, grammatical language and the language of science.

A deviant, innovative, and surprising utterance plays with the binary structure of formal language to make it say something that escapes the determining duality of the Symbolic in terms of social language. But from a purely social conventional point of view, such speech constitutes a payment with one's person, because the subject risks being perceived as unusual, peculiar, foolish, and even downright deviant. This is consistent with what Quinet (2018) calls the analyst-semblant of the *objet a*. The analyst is in the place of the *objet a* and often acts the part. Lacan acted like a fool, clown, and wisecracker, often making use of the volume and pitch of the voice and lallation to make his interpretations.

Lacan also made a distinction between empty and full speech. The analysand often wastes time by focusing on trivialities or rationalizations that remain far removed from the causal core of the subject's suffering. Thus, analysis as the discourse of the unconscious is concerned with unfolding not so much the well-known story line but rather the unknown dreams and unconscious core themes and fantasies. These two dimensions of speech are present in various forms throughout Lacan's work.

If we think of the concept of the two chains in terms of the social narrative or story on one line and the unconscious signifying chain on the other, then we can say that at first in Seminar I, Lacan (1953) called the social narrative 'empty speech' and the unconscious signifying chain full speech. Speech on the basis of the unconscious signifying chain leads to true speech regarding desire. However, towards the end of his work, in Seminar 24 (1976–1977), he reversed the significations and the unconscious signifying chain translated into senseless empty speech linked to the Real and jouissance, while the social narrative is speech full of Imaginary meaning. Finally, in *L'etourdit* (1972), he called the two forms of speech the saying and the said. The said statement is the social narrative and the unconscious manifests in the saying. The two chains or two forms of the message are structural categories or concepts, while the saying and the said, and the full and empty speech are forms of temporal speech or events named with words more than with concepts. The words may change or vary, while the concept is invariant.

In listening, the analyst needs to localize in the flux of speech the capital elements or signifiers, the signifying diamonds and nuggets within the coal and dross of ordinary speech. Thus, to pay with words is to elevate the use of words as done by the dream-work. It implies a conversion of being to a more truthful state. But just as the dream-work is constructed or woven by a larger unconscious subjectivity than the ego, so in interpretative speech, the speaking ego or ego statement is relinquished in favor of the enunciation from the place of non-self.

In order to raise the analytical function, the analyst needs to speak from the place of no-self (the unknown knowing subject) where the ego as the enunciator is canceled as much as possible in favor of allowing the power of the signifier to transform and illuminate the subject. The aphanisis (disappearance) of the ego results in the epiphany (appearance) of the subject (true subject is no ego). Thus, the cognitive ego is not the agent of insight, but rather it is the subject who bears witness to the lightening of wit and knowing contained within the treasure chest of the signifier.

In addition, the interpretative saying should be brief and concise, with less emphasis on rational syntaxes and conjunction. One's sayings should be surprising and fresh and imply an enunciation from the place of S or S_1, or the pure signifier, and the corresponding aphanisis or disappearance of the ego.

Thus, the fact that the Lacanian dimension of the Real exists outside language does not mean that we are left in a position of not being able to say anything about the core of our experience. Silence does not necessarily possess more truth-value to reveal the Real – although sometimes it may. By now (and 50 years after the Colloquium of Bonneval [Ey, 1966]), it is well known that Lacan's aphorism – the unconscious is structured like a language – should not be interpreted as meaning that the structure of the unconscious is identical to the structure of social language.

Grammatical structure refers to the rules and principles used for constructing sentences in language. Rules and principles determine what forms are allowed or not allowed for constructing sentences in language. Metaphor and metonymy function within grammatical structure and are usually linked to motivation or what in psychoanalysis we call desire, as articulated in the differences between the sexes.

For Lacanian theory, the unconscious activity of desire is revealed through metaphor and metonymy. Signifiers of desire function as signified for a chain or series of signifiers used in language. Only the signifiers of desire, or the signifiers that represent the lack or absence of the object of desire, concern the unconscious with respect to the structure of language. Language rules, and social laws governing kinship and sexual relations between the sexes, are both Preconscious and/or unconscious in a descriptive sense. The repressed unconscious contains repressed signifiers of desire that are revealed in the preconscious mind through metaphor and metonymy. The larger relation between linguistic and psychical structure is represented by the interlocking relation between signifiers of desire and signifiers organized by grammar rules in language. When I say that the unconscious mind is manifested in speech or language, I am not only referring to a relationship between unconscious desire, motivation, and the forms of language. The unconscious does not represent the "emotional" aspect of the mind but rather the relationship between repressed signifiers of desire and the general Preconscious structure of language in general.

It is very important to understand the function of Mind as something more than the primitive id; reptilian brain; or brain, period. Otherwise, with cognitivism or psycholinguistics, knowledge and cognition are reduced to *technê*, not as an art form but as a form of information processing controlled by the conscious ego and formal analytical reason (a form of rationality shared by humans and machines). What we don't understand is reduced to the irrationality of emotion, as if emotion were not controlled by mathematical structure. As I wrote, and quoted Lacan in the introduction:

> "The fact that the signifying chain continues to unfold and continues to be organized in the Other, whether you know it or not, this is essentially Freud's discovery" (Lacan [1957–1958], p. 132). The small piece of Real enjoyment (S_1) that a subject can drain from the larger unconscious doing that escapes us is what we call an act of wit (l'esprit)."

In this context, the unconscious structured as a language refers not only to the unconscious structure of language (in a Preconscious descriptive sense) but actually to the relations between the Unconscious structured by signifiers of desire (the reach of language into the unconscious structure of the drive and the brain) and the Preconscious structure of language and rules governing human activity within society. Metaphor and metonymy are the language forms that regulate (reveal and conceal) the manifestation of desire within speech and psychical structure.

Only the unconscious in a descriptive sense, or the Preconscious, is structurally related to the formal structure of language. In the conscious and Preconscious signifying chain, signifiers are woven together by metaphor. Metaphor represents things through resemblance or similarity: one thing is described by other things that share a main characteristic, and one form is used to describe another form (fingers for rays of the sun, early bird for people who get up early, etc.). Metonymy replaces the name of one thing for another contiguous name commonly used for it: pen for sword, sail for boat, or greybeard for man, in the case of synecdoche as an example of metonymy. Substitution, as a rhetorical figure shared with repression, is common to both metaphor and metonymy, while contiguity is the criterion for metonymy.

Metaphors and metonymy are used to speak about material reality, but more often than not, material reality is linked to the psychical reality of desire and its representations. Things are seen according to the intentions and desires of the beholder. Metaphor and metonymy can refer to the signifiers of a repressed unconscious object, or a missing signifier, that functions as a hole or gap around which signifiers turn. Chains of signification (S_1–S_2) turn around a hole within which lies a repressed S_1 that is separated (due to repression) from the series circling around the gap. This is the false hole of Freud's repressed unconscious that Lacan articulates in Seminar XXIII. Obviously, this would have to be a case of an S_1 in a Preconscious chain linked to an S_2. However, because of primary repression, such an S_1 is entangled with another S_1 lodged in the repressed unconscious. To use the famous example that Leclaire (1966) gave at the Colloquium of Bonneval (1975), the preconscious signifier unicorn (from Lilly to "*licorn*" [unicorn]) and its associated meanings (S_1–S_2) is the substitute for the primarily repressed signifier of the imaginary phallus as a transitive signifier circulating between mother, child, and imaginary father.

Within the language of jouissance or of the One (lalangue), significance is a function of the association between the phonological elements of speech or between the sounds of a word or signifier and the sounds of another word or signifier. Sounds function as a level of significance beneath words and grammatical structure. For example, pitch as a perceptual property of the sound of the voice differentiates between the voice of a man or a woman regardless of biological gender (a male can have a high pitch, and a female can have a low-pitched voice). In lalangue, sounds do not convey linguistic meaning (like metaphor and metonymy do) and instead reveal desire directly through what could be called the mathematical structure of sound waves.

Lalangue could be defined as the study of sound within speech and yet outside the system of language. Sound is related to desire through the voice that for Lacanian psychoanalysis constitutes a form of the *objet a*, cause of desire. At first a child recognizes their mother's love and desire for them through the cooing sound of her voice more than the actual signifiers used. Sound constitutes the subject as an object of desire, and this refers to the pleasure experienced listening to the

"the sound of music" that represents the desire of and for the mother (as in the classical Julie Andrews movie by the same name). Sound or phonology in lalangue is not concerned with the proper rules governing the pronunciation of words in language but rather with an equivocation in pronunciation, or sound 'equivocality.' Phonemes, as a sound of the voice, say more than the narrative content of statements in language. The sound of the voice (void) is a positivity that reveals what cannot be said in language, or that is said in language in the form of negation: "It's not that" or "but not that."

Both the repressed Freudian unconscious and the Lacanian Real unconscious have the structure of a different kind of language – the language of the unconscious. The language of the unconscious here means two things. First, that repressed signifiers of unconscious desire function as signified for signifiers that, through metaphor and metonymy, are revealed in the Preconscious structure of language. Second, that in the language of the One or jouissance, S_1, as a sound in language, linked to the sound of another word, points to the sound of what is unsayable in the mother's desire with respect to the phallic signifier linked to the NoF. The language of the Other thrives on the metaphorical rather than grammatical or syntactic elements of language, while lalangue, as the language of the One or jouissance, thrives on the homophonic and phonological elements of language.

Herewith are presented two case vignettes as examples of the language of the Unconscious. The first will exemplify the homophonic element and the second the metaphoric, although in the example given, the two cannot be entirely separated. An analysand, whom I will call J., had been struggling over not wanting to have "two sessions a week." He was also in conflict with seeing his struggle as having anything to do with the analyst. At the beginning of the next session, he made a comment regarding the waiting room saying: "your waiting room is 'too weak'." I have said that lalangue appears as a deviant or peculiar predication. Somebody could say, "This must be a grammatical mistake; no English speaker would say your waiting room is too weak!" And yet the fact remains that this was an educated native English speaker. The analyst, or the subject that is me but also an imaginary ego, responded by saying "two a week is too weak." Again, a deviant predication is matched by a peculiar interpretation. In this example, we observe that homophony is being used to challenge the 'rules' of the treatment.

The analysand represented here by the letter J. (the signifier is what represents the subject for another signifier – the analyst) and who was marked and effected/affected by being named after an aunt whom his father envied (the subject appears first in the Other), was caught in an imaginary ego-struggle with the analyst. To the resistance of his imaginary ego, two sessions a week represented an imaginary form of castration. I say imaginary, because he experienced two sessions a week as something being taken from him rather than given to him. Thus, he wanted to tell me in some way that it was not he but I that was weak. The analysand was making an imaginary or ego-defensive use of the symbolic link, whereas the analyst appeals to the aphanisis or disappearance of the imaginary ego and the appearance or epiphany of the metaphoric subject as an effect of the signifier. Once lalangue becomes linked to the Other via the act of interpretation, it is no longer a question of an imaginary ego-to-ego relationship. Now the signifier and the laws of the Symbolic represent the subject once again.

For the second example of lalangue, an analysand reports she is having sleeping problems because she is too excited thinking about presenting for a class. She continues with a dream where she is the teacher of younger students who come to pay her a social visit, and they decide to take a day trip. For the day trip, she will drive a big motorcycle, and the dream ends when one of the younger male students is telling her about his wishes and fears of success and expecting advice from her. She says she feels aroused by this. She explored the associative links between her thoughts before the dream and the thoughts/images in the dream itself. There is her love for a man teacher and her own desire to be a teacher and to be loved by male students. In discussing this and the difference between her thoughts and the dream, she confounded and equivocated the homophony between luck and lack.

She sees male teachers that she loves as lucky and herself as "lacky," with lack being the main signifier of desire as a negative deficit state that diminishes her. The beloved is lucky, and the lover is 'lacky.' A lackey is also someone in a subordinate position, and she would rather be the beloved instead of the lover. The Beloved is complete in her fantasy, and the lover is a 'lacky' lackey. In this sense, in her unconscious, a man is a lover because he has the imaginary phallus, and a woman is the beloved who is the imaginary phallus that a man lacks. It is unclear when she is a beloved of her student whether she is beloved as a woman or as a man-teacher for her knowledge, whether she is beloved for what she is or what she has. She did not have a category or a signifier for a woman of knowledge. Although she wants to be desired for having an attractive feminine body, she also thinks critically of women who are very attractive and lack knowledge. She is also critical of men's 'selfish' drive or desire to have sex with desirable women.

In the 'metaphoric' example, an analysand is telling me how he has been able to be effortless and timely in his current university studies. He makes a joke on me, saying that he is dictating and that I should write down what he is saying. He associates this with being effortless in playing a wind instrument as a young boy until he had to put in effort to match the high notes of another student. Both of these comments served as introductions to his problem of not being able to put any effort into writing and finally finishing his dissertation. Then his associations go to his obsessive thoughts that his parents will die. He grew up in fear that his mother would die and says that his father wants to live forever but that he wants him to die. I interpreted that his efforts are geared towards remaining a child of his mother and not to grow up. If his parents die, then he has to be a man instead of his mother's boy.

Being a man for him means paying a price, such as losing his hair and not having feminine objects of desire. (In prior sessions, the analysand had spoken about his fears and desires to be a grown-up responsible man. He feared losing his hair like his father. He also had a dream where he was pregnant with a boy.) His response to my intervention was to quote a revered figure of his to the effect that being a man means having the baton of the phallus. "That's having something whereas for you being a man has represented not having hair like your father.

Boldness is the baton," I said, and ended the session. Boldness is the baton that represents the symbolic phallus as a resisted absence that nevertheless generates a symbolic consistency and efficacy for the subject. What is being let go is the ego as the imaginary phallus of the mother's desire.

Because free association can lead to defensive or idle speech, free association can be supplemented with the technique of dream analysis, where the analysand is asked to free-associate to different elements of the dream. The flow of speech can be interrupted, and the analysand is asked to say more or what comes to mind about this or that word/phrase. I have extrapolated Freud's method of dream analysis and put it to use in the analysis of speech and the use of citation as an interpretative method. Analysands are regularly asked if they have had dreams and are asked to keep a dream journal. On the other hand, dreams can be ignored or bypassed if the analysand is obsessively focusing on dreams and taking all of the time of the session to give the analyst a minute recounting of various dreams. The focus on dreams can also be defensive.

The analyst employs punctuation and scansion of the analysand's discourse. Pauses that interrupt the flow of speech and open a particular sentence to a different meaning than the meaning that was going to be given by the last word of a sentence are an example of unconscious formations not mentioned by Freud. In this instance, the analyst simply repeats the sentence in scanted form. This allows the analysand to hear its different unconscious signification. Other uses of the resources of language include homophony and the holophrase, or a word that stands for a whole sentence, and using such words for interpretation or free association. In addition, words can be cut and segmented to produce new meaning, and the antithetical meaning of words is explored in both directions. Finally, the meanings of first and last names and pseudonyms are also explored.

Lacan (1953) also linked punctuation to the scansion of the session, which as a concluding moment precipitates the time for understanding between sessions.

> It is, therefore, a propitious punctuation that gives meaning to the subject's discourse. This is why the ending of the session – which current technique makes into an interruption that is purely determined by the clock and, as such, takes no account of the thread of the subject's discourse – plays the part of a scansion which has the full value of an intervention by the analyst that is designed to precipitate concluding moments.
>
> (p. 209)

Explanation as a form of interpretation is usually limited and more prevalent during the pre-treatment assessment phase (preliminary sessions) or in the later phases of the personal analysis of an analyst in formation. According to Lacan's 'renewed technique of interpretation' (Lacan, 1953; Nobus, 2000), the analyst asks questions by using the analysand's words verbatim, while directing the analysand's attention to his/her own speech. The analyst is governed by his/her desire to listen to the signifying chain that determines the development of the analysand's symptomatology.

In interpretation, I distinguish three floors/levels and regard the third as the proper analytical level:

1 *Going from the known to the known.* We do not focus on what an analysand already knows about their problems based on common sense or from what they have acquired from previous therapies, friends, or support groups. During the assessment phase, this information is brought out, and the analysand is asked what they have understood from previous treatment. The assumption is that if they continue to have symptoms, this means that there are dimensions or floors of the unconscious that have not been affected or transformed by prior treatment.

2 *Going from the unknown to the known.* This category falls under what is usually understood as making the unconscious conscious by providing wholesale interpretations or explanations of unconscious conflicts that the analysand will either accept or reject. In this category, the unconscious is reduced to what is already known, to ego processes either in the analyst or the analysand, that become defensive towards the knowledge of the analyst. In Lacanian psychoanalysis, the analyst also limits this type of interpretation in favor of the analysand himself/herself arriving at the interpretation via the exploration of the signifying chain. Lacanian analysts regard this level of interpretation as imaginary and as meaning rather than signification.

   It is similar to when an analysand thinks that dream association is about giving a global interpretation of the meaning of a dream. This level of interpretation also refers to the question of Lacanian analysts analyzing rather than interpreting the transference. If the analysand is talking about feelings or associations they have in relationship to somebody else (the so-called extra-analytical transferences), the Lacanian analyst does not say "and maybe you feel that way about me." The transference is only analyzed when the analysand speaks about it directly. Although it is not easy for many analysands to speak about their thoughts or feelings about the analyst, analysts have other ways to encourage their analysands to verbalize their transference experience. For example, an analyst could ask: "Is it difficult to speak about that?"

3 *Going from the unknown to the unknown.* This is interpretation proper. Lacan said that interpretation is found somewhere in between a quote and an enigma: "The enigma and the citation constitute the two axes of analytic interpretation" (Nobus, 2000). An interpretation is a symbolic reflection or mirroring back of those speech elements where analysands are not aware of what they are saying. "The less you understand, the better you listen" (Lacan, 1954–55). According to Lacan (1966), the analyst must 'forget what he/she knows' when listening and offering interpretations. The aim of interpretations is disrupting meaning and reducing signifiers to their "non-sense" (Lacan, 1954–55; Evans, 1996). Enigmatic sayings point to the subject of the enunciation and to the Real of jouissance (S_1–S_0) of Lacan's later work. They use descriptively unconscious or preconscious speech elements to affect repressed speech elements lodged in the unconscious or in the Real of unconscious experience.

This is a key level of interpretation for the work with unconscious fantasy material.

Returning to the question of the scansion of the session in analysis, Lacan refers to it as being similar to the scansion of verses in poetry. The latter is the action of differentiating verses by their rhythmic components or by the accents and syllables of an expression. From this perspective, one cannot fail to notice the interpenetration of the practice of analysis with the analysis of discourse and with the utilization of available resources within language. In addition, closely associated with scansion is the aforementioned concept of punctuation that should be taken in its usual grammatical sense: namely to locate a period, a comma, an interrogation sign.

The scan and scansion of words within the analysand's discourse constitutes another form of scansion practice. Thus, in the example given previously of the analysand being afraid of mailing a letter disclosing the analysand's sexual orientation to a parent, the analysand said "I cannot mail it," and the analyst responded: "not male." This example also shows how an interpretation that makes conflicts conscious at first glance may not be experienced as something helpful due to the increase in anxiety and anger at the Other for bringing back to awareness a conflict that had been warded off. Interventions that support the analysand's defenses and beliefs are usually experienced favorably by the analysand as something helpful. Thus, a subject could say 'Why do I need a treatment that makes me feel worse or raises anxiety?' The answer, obviously, is that temporary setbacks are justified by long-term changes that may support the subject's functioning.

In passing, and to conclude, it should be noted that the analytic and linguistic practice of deconstructing ordinary language has illustrious precedence in the Jewish Talmud and Kabbalah (Bakan, 1958). There the practices of *notarikon* and *temurah* have to do with dividing, permutating, or rearranging and condensing words. These common devices are used as vehicles for reaching new meaning and releasing the primary libidinal sparks contained within the letters. *Notarikon* makes words by condensing the first or last letters of a word with the last or first letters of another word. *Temurah* changes words by changing the order of the letters. For example, in Hebrew, *oneg* means pleasure and *nega* is associated with the meaning of pain. The letters in a different order describe opposite but interrelated terms. This is precisely the meaning of the Lacanian concept of jouissance (the common root of pleasure and pain).

References

Bakan, D. (1958). *Sigmund Freud and the Jewish Mystical Tradition.* Boston: Beacon Press.

Evans, D. (1996). *An Introductory Dictionary of Lacanian Psychoanalysis.* London and New York: Routledge.

Ey, H. (1966). *El Inconsciente (coloquio de Bonneval).* Buenos Aires: Siglo Veintiuno, 1975.

Freud, S. (1905). Jokes and Their Relation to the Unconscious. *SE,* 8.

Lacan, J. (1953). The Function and Field of Speech and Language in Psychoanalysis. In: *Ecrits.* Translated by B. Fink. New York: Norton, 2006.

Lacan, J. (1954–1955). *The Seminar.* Book II. The Ego in Freud's Theory and in the Technique of Psychoanalysis, 1954–55. Translated by S. Tomaselli and Notes by J. Forrester (p. 141). New York: Norton; Cambridge: Cambridge University Press, 1988.

Lacan, J. (1957–1958). *Seminar V on the Formations of the Unconscious.* Edited by J. A. Miller and Translated by R. Grigg. Cambridge: Polity Press, 2017.

Lacan, J. (1969–1970). *The Other Side of Psychoanalysis: The Seminar of Jacques Lacan.* Book XVII. New York: Norton.

Lacan, J. (1972). L'etourdit. *The Letter*, 41, 31–80, 2009.

Lacan, J. (1976–1977). *L'Insu que Sait . . . (Love Is the Unknown That Knows About the One Mistake): Seminar 24.* Translated by C. Gallagher, unpublished. Lacaninireland.com. Accessed August 24, 2015.

Nobus, D. (2000). *Jacques Lacan and the Freudian Practice of Psychoanalysis.* London: Routledge, p. 174.

Quinet, A. (2018). *Lacan's Clinical Technique: Lack(a)nian Analysis.* London: Routledge.

9 The resistance and desire of the analyst, and the question of the countertransference

The resistance of the analyst

It is important to understand the techniques of punctuation, scansion, and what Lacan calls the problem of "the horror of the act" in order to also understand, in a clinical context, what Lacan meant with the "to impress the bourgeois" (*épater le bourgeois*) aphorism that he borrowed from the French decadent movement. This aphorism points to the Lacanian understanding of resistance. Lacan begins by emphasizing that desire, not the ego, resists. Resistance comes more from desire (id resistance, as Freud [1926] called it) than from ego defenses. Specifically, within the symptom, it is desiring that resists. In this regard, it is important to remember that Freud stated that the sexual life of any psychically distressed subject is found within the symptom.

Therefore, the question arises as to why the symptom insists, persists, and resists – a very different way of formulating the question of resistance than that following from the agency of the ego's defense mechanisms. It is well known that the latter concept implies the existence of a fictional little man or homunculus living inside the subject's psychical habitat for the purpose of directing and managing the development of defensive operations. Moreover, not only does Lacan criticize Anna Freud's (1936) mechanistic and anthropomorphic understanding of defense mechanisms; he also underscores that defensive operations are primarily taking place within language.

The analysand resists because of their defenses, not because of the analyst. And yes, defenses are more a function of an unconscious symbolic code than an ego mechanism. It is the aspect of the resistance of the analysand towards the person of the analyst that Lacan says is actually the resistance of the analyst. The analysand is resisting the normalizing action of the analyst more than their own unconscious. Lacan says that the normalizing action of the analyst is due to the analyst's own resistance to give up the normalizing expert identification. This is what needs to be impressed upon the bourgeois analyst who is proud and attached to their expertise (*épater le bourgeois*).

Usually it is believed that Lacan was opposed to the analysis of resistance and that he considered all resistance to be the resistance of the analyst to give up the position of the subject supposed to know (the place of reality and ego knowledge). Rather than rejecting the analysis of the analysand's resistances, it is important to stress the Lacanian–Freudian differentiation between working with the analysand's resistance to speak about the formations of the unconscious and the question of the resistance to the person (ego or authority) of the analyst. The Lacanian analyst does not interpret the latter (to avoid getting bogged down in the imaginary ego to ego relationship) and instead simply encourages the analysand to continue speaking.

At this juncture, Lacan discovers both a very old and very new discipline: rhetoric. This field can be defined as the study of all the different formations, deformations, and transformations of a discourse in accordance with certain definable forms and figures. Metaphor and metonymy are among the most well-known classical figures within the rhetorical field. Thus, desire is insisting and resisting through the formation of symptoms and substitutive formations. It is important to remember that, within Freudian theory, repression always fails because its sole purpose is to produce a metaphorical substitute of the repressed. Lacan states that repression and the return of the repressed are one and the same thing. The success of repression consists of an ability to generate the production of a substitute. Therefore, repression is the contorted and distorted way in which desire re-appears. Finally, it is precisely because the resistance of desire is the resistance of the symptom, as representative of desire, that it is so difficult for the subject to accept the direction of the cure.

The clinical consequence of this is twofold. First, it provides a tacit foundation for the Lacanian understanding of desire and explains why it is so important to clarify questions of desire, because this has a direct impact on the symptom. Second, the ego should not be believed when it says that it does not want to have anything to do with the symptom. "I want this symptom removed," says the ego. The ego only appears to want to be rid of the symptom. The more he/she tells us this, the more he/she loves the symptom. Freud used to say that psychotics love their delusions as much as they love themselves. The same can be said of neurotics.

When the analysand says they want the symptom removed, they are complying with what the Other is expecting from them and with how the pleasure principle is directing them to avoid the painful jouissance linked to the symptom. However, the jouissance in the symptom does not care about desire or the Other. The painful jouissance is required by the super-ego that demands the subject's jouissance (suffering).

Thus, if the analyst resists understanding that the analysand does not want the symptom removed, despite all assertions to the contrary, then following Lacan, resistance within the analytic situation is primarily the resistance of the analyst to listen and interpret what is at stake in the symptom. Here appears the question of the therapeutic alliance as an ego-to-ego alliance that ends up strengthening the illusion of the symptom as a foreign intrusion. The analysand often describes the symptom as being like a virus from an unconscious of which he/she knows nothing.

The strategy of treating the symptom as a foreign intrusion is something that is used in extreme cases when the subject or a small child may need help coping with a symptom. The patient in those cases accepts the doctor's help in fighting the symptom. The problem with thinking of the symptom as ego dystonic is that it appears to be a better situation than if the symptom is ego syntonic and the subject does not seek or want treatment. But the fact that someone wants treatment and complains about a symptom does not mean that they are ready to relinquish the punishment and jouissance associated with the symptom.

The symptom

Although the existence of a symptom makes someone readier to enter treatment, this does not mean that they want to change or relinquish the symptom. In contrast to an ego-syntonic character trait, a symptom represents a step forward in the revelation of an unconscious truth regarding desire. However, the step forward represented by an involuntary symptom need not deceive us as to the actual imaginary ego-syntonic nature of the rest of the subject's character structure.

The symptom has to become a psychoanalytic symptom or object and be subjectively rectified before a psychoanalytic operation or intervention can succeed in its transformation. This is true of any analysis, although according to some authors, it is especially true of a training analysis that supposedly has to meet the higher standard of character transformation and not only symptom resolution. There is continuity between a symptom and a character trait that may be a problem for others but not for the subject who is identified with it.

If the analyst believes in the symptom, in the conscious storyline or narrative, or in the transference to the subject supposed to know, then the analyst will collude with the resistance of the analysand. This is what Lacan calls resistance, the resistance of the analyst. If the analyst out of sentimental empathy allows himself/herself to become hostage to the presenting symptom of the analysand, although initially the analysand will experience the analyst as empathic, eventually the psychoanalytic symptom proper will appear in acting out outside the session or in boundary violations, countertransference enactments, or inappropriate self-disclosures of the analyst within the session.

The initial belief in and empathy for the symptom and the storyline has to be purely strategic or a strategy within the transference for purposes of establishing a therapeutic alliance. The analyst knows that it is the subject of the unconscious that knows and not the ego of the patient, but for the time being, he/she pretends that the ego of the analysand knows what he/she is talking about. This is the place of the therapeutic alliance that is an alliance with the patient's ego defenses.

Thus, a therapeutic alliance is typically a strategic alliance at best. Otherwise one could say that the analyst is resisting. True empathy has to be reserved for unconscious experience that the analysand usually experiences as unemphatic and ego dystonic. On the other hand, there is always the case of the exceptional analysand or candidate that comes to analysis with a subjectively rectified symptom and in disbelief of their symptom.

The calculated or strategic vacillation of the analyst's neutrality

In other areas, even though Lacan's concept of the desire of the analyst is a novel way of re-formulating the classical themes of abstinence and neutrality, he also introduces some modifications to the practice. One of them he calls the "calculated vacillation of the analyst's neutrality." If there is a calculation, then, in some way, one must know what the outcome may be. Lacan (1966) introduces this concept in his paper "Subversion of the Subject and Dialectic of Desire," and he explains it in the following way. Many times, when working with a hysteric analysand, a calculated vacillation is worth much more than a series of interpretations that lead nowhere.

Only if the analyst is sure that there will be no actual sexual contact between analyst and analysand may the analyst leave ambiguous and open this possibility in relation to the analysand. In other words, the analysand may believe that a sexual relation with the analyst is possible, and although the analyst knows this will never actually take place, he/she does not explicitly or directly say so. What is at stake here is support of the transference in terms of being able to tolerate an erotic transference instead of using a genetic interpretation (it is not me whom you desire but your father) as a stop-gap, to tolerate an erotic transference instead of avoiding it due to the anxiety in the situation.

On the other hand, the previous would be true only with a neurotic analysand. With a structurally psychotic, or perverse, or even an acting-out severely borderline or hysteric patient, this kind of ambiguity with regard to the erotic transference could be counterproductive. A psychotic patient can easily develop a psychotic transference, and a perverse or sociopathic patient could place the analyst at risk. With the psychotic and perverse or sociopathic patient, for the most part (there always are exceptions), the analyst wants to direct the analysis of the erotic transference away from the therapeutic relationship. The reverse is true with the neurotic analysand: the analyst does well to explore the erotic transference *if* it is directly addressed to the analyst.

Exploring the erotic transference could be interpreted as a kind of seduction, thus the relevance of the calculated vacillation of the analyst's neutrality. On the other hand, it is also true that when the neurotic analysand overtly and directly speaks about the erotic transference, this by itself does not mean that the analyst has to address the issue in the way the analysand is raising it. It is important to remember what Freud said about the transference also being a form of resistance. Conscious fantasies can help sustain the exploration of desire but can also be defenses against speaking about the experience of loss within privation, frustration, and castration.

The third payment with the core of one's being: the desire of the analyst and the question of metaethics and the ethics of the real

The third payment is payment with the core of one's being. Lacan takes this expression from Freud's "The Interpretation of Dreams" (1900/1965), where Freud says that desiring or wishing is the core of our being. Therefore, the third payment aims at the question of desire and directly leads to Lacan's notion of the desire of the analyst.

Lacan invents the concept of the desire of the analyst and declares it the nodular point or hub around which the analysis turns. Why? Because Lacan believed that Freud not only created a new discursive situation but also invented a new subjective position or state: that of the analyst.

Lacan (1961–1962) states that the desire of the analyst is something different from the other desire or the desire of the Other, as well as stating that it is neither the vocational desire to be an analyst nor the personal desire of each analyst: it is an impersonal desire of a being towards death, not of dying, but of a second symbolic death. The desire for death or of death differs from the aim of instinctual aggression.

> Every time that we analysts have to deal with this relationship of the subject to the nothing, we slip regularly between two slopes: the common slope that tends towards a nothing of destruction, the shameful interpretation of aggressivity considered as purely reducible to the biological force of aggression, which is in no way sufficient, except in a degraded way, to support the tendency to nothing as it arises at a certain necessary stage of Freudian thinking in the death drive just before he introduces identification.
>
> (Seminar IX, Lesson 15, page 8, Session of 2.28.62)

A desire of death, or a being-towards-death, in the Heideggerian sense, involves not doing what is customary with desire, which is to attempt to be desired. The analyst must first seek to be desired but then procure that the analysand directs this desire toward others. This is the most difficult payment to accept because it requires that the analyst relinquish the ideal (egoic) position in which the analysand has placed him/her. This is what is stoic about the analyst in the sense of auto-inducing or self-introducing a narcissistic wound so as to push narcissism to further degrees of differentiation and transformation. At this juncture, the importance of termination can be clearly discerned.

There is something deadly both in the desire of the analyst and the termination of analysis in the sense of the separation and non-attachment associated with the death drive. This appears to be contrary to Eros that always leans towards union and synthesis. From this vantage point, one can understand why the analyst's desire is a special subjective position requiring a payment with the core of one's being. The analyst must work on something having to do with his/her own desire. This makes it the most decisive and fundamental of the three payments. It is only on the basis of such payment that one can tolerate paying with words and with one's person. Only if the analyst declines to put himself/herself in the position of being desired for life can he/she transform his/her own ego-identity by temporarily leaving aside values, choices, and other narcissistic gratifications. We can see here how resistance is also related to the desire of the analyst. The desire of the analyst is not the common human desire, because in this case such desire would represent a desire to be recognized and desired as a good analyst. Such desire would become the analyst's resistance, as defined by Lacan.

The notion of the third payment with the core of one's being is also related to the question of the ethics of psychoanalysis and the psychoanalytic situation. In her book on the ethics of the Real, Zupanscic (2011) writes that "We escape to the realm of infinite symbolic metonymy in order to avoid the encounter with the

Real of enjoyment . . . as a moment of terror" (p. 235). Desire is not found in wishful thinking and pursuing the metonymical object of desire from image to image, or lien to lien, like monkeys traveling along treetops in hot pursuit of their object. Ethical or non-pathological desire is found in the encounter or mis-encounter with the Real (of the drive).

The ethics of desire refer to acting in accordance with one's desire, even if this involves rectifying that what we think we want is not what we really want. An ethical act is not defined by the morality of duty or obligation but rather by the subject doing something out of principle without calculating the utilitarian cost/benefit ratio of an activity. Although pain may be associated with an ethical act, pain is not the purpose of the activity. It is not that we have to suffer to obtain what we want but that what we want may require a price that may include pain, but pain is not what is sought.

The moral law is not the imperative of desire, as Zizek (Zupanscic, 2011) has argued, because the ethics of desire precisely involve distinguishing between the desire of the Other and the subject's desire. It the end, it may turn out that the desire of the Other is the subject's desire, but the subject did not know this, thinking naively that their desire was opposed to the Other's desire or that the Law is opposed to desire rather than its condition. But the traditional subject that lives to fulfill the Other's desire rather than the subject's own is the very definition of neurosis and not of the ethics of desire.

Does the ethics of desire represent, then, what Zupanscic (2011) calls the "heroism of the lack" (p. 240), or the desire for the lack, more than the phallus? The *objet a* is the nothing that desire wants. Unsatisfied and displaced desire preserves emptiness as the authentic place of enjoyment. To the metonymical displacements of the imaginary phallus, the subject of the Real or of the drive says: "It's not That." The ethics of the Real represent what Lacan called previously the "tendency to the nothing." The first and second jouissance always produce a remainder that is resolved when the Third Other jouissance stops the replication and fracturing of the *objet a*. The first and second forms of jouissance, when either renounced or satisfied, always produce a remainder or reproduce the *objet a*. For the Third jouissance, there still may be something missing, but the Third does not reproduce the *objet a* because the *a* (the 'no-thing') ultimately dissolves in its approach to the Real. As Socrates said: "There where you think or see me as something, I am nothing."

The tendency to the nothing corresponds to a sublimated death drive or to a death drive that in the end (of aims) crosses over to the other side, the side of Eros. Regarding so-called health values, the Buddha, like Freud, is known to have used the well-known parable of the surgeon. In order to help someone who has been shot with an arrow (of love, perhaps) the doctor has to extract the arrow from the body by cutting, opening up the wound, and temporarily causing more pain, in order for the wound and the body to heal and live. The practice of session cutting, separating, or emptying are all Real acts of an analyst that require the ethical courage of an act done in good faith but without knowing whether the act will be beneficial. An ethical act invokes a sublime reach of the death drive, or what Zupanscic called the heroism of the lack.

The same can be said with respect to paying with one's person as a form of negation of personal values. The abstention of judgment implies values of a different order or metaethics rather than the analyst becoming an immoral or amoral subject. The super ego and the law, far from repressing desire, compel the subject to pursue forbidden desires. Freud (1900, p. 365), following Nietszche (1844), spoke of the transvaluation of psychical values in reference to the workings of repression: what was pleasant becomes unpleasant and vice versa.

The moral good replaces the good of pleasure by turning the latter into something bad and the bad of frustration into something good. The practice of analysis reverses this process: the moral good or super ego becomes suspect, and the bad of desire becomes once again something good and acceptable to the analyst. But since psychoanalysis is not hedonism, this cannot be the end of the story. Becoming intimate with one's desire is not equivalent to the fulfillment of human desire, which is something impossible. The subject can only ask: "Is this what I really want? or 'It's not that' because there are more fundamental desires than this one." But the question for the ethics of desire is not so much whether there are better desires or objects of desire but the fact that 'It's not that' in fact points to the drive as a tendency or push for emptiness or the nothing rather than for a better object of desire.

Finally, it can also be argued that the desire of the analyst produces what Maslow (1968) named a B-cognition or a knowing of the One's own non being (Bion's [1984] transformations in O) which is 'transindividual' and without human desire (the desire to be desired). The desire of the analyst bestows the ability to perceive the ineffable, or a discourse without words. Freud's free-floating attention, Bion's negative capability (the capacity of the analyst to be without memory or desire), or the desire of the analyst are different ways of talking about paying with one's person in terms of not using personal values and preferences and paying with the core of one's being (the One's own non being).

The desire of the analyst and the question of the countertransference

Finally, a few words are in order with respect to Lacan's critique of the concept of countertransference. Clearly, what Lacan had in mind with the concept of the desire of the analyst is not what is usually considered countertransference. Additionally, Lacan points out that the notion of countertransference is fraught with the danger of reducing the experience of the analyst to an imaginary idiosyncratic "felt-experience" lacking the conditions of transmissibility. In contrast to such a notion, the concept of the signifier provides a more objective reference (mediated by the Other) for understanding the analyst's experience.

The subject as signifier is Winnicott's (1971) objective subject that, according to Lacan, is the result of the subject becoming alienated in and represented by the signifier. A paramount example of such would be Freud's paper on "the forgetting of proper names," offered as the first chapter of *The Psychopathology of Everyday Life* (1965). Here Freud self-discloses to the public and to future analysts something of his personal experience with the signifier. The purpose of the self-disclosure is nothing more or less than the transmission of psychoanalysis.

The forgetting of a proper name occurs together with the return of mistaken names. Freud forgot the name of the painter Signorelli and instead produced the names Botticelli and Boltrafio.

> The last half of the name, '-elli', is the remnant of Signorelli, rendered incomplete by the fact that the 'Signor' has been forgotten. 'Bo' is the incomplete remnant of 'Bosnia-Herzegovina', 'Herr having been repressed. It's this same repression that explains that 'Boltrafio' connects the 'Bo' of 'Bosnia-Herzegovina' with 'Trafoi', the name of the locality in which Freud had learned that one of his patients had committed suicide because of sexual impotence.
>
> (Lacan, 1957–1958, p. 31)

Freud develops a schema of the movement of signifiers within a structural understanding of the unconscious (schema subsequently). This example shows the scansion, cutting, or segmenting of words and their displacement and condensation into new words. Moreover, it also shows that substitutions do not appear by mere chance. The painters Botticelli and Boltrafio were not chosen for being painters per se but because association linked them given the context of the signifying situation. The repressed thoughts that were associated with a signifying situation located in Bosnia-Herzegovina had to do with death and sexuality (a patient of Freud committed suicide because of sexual impotence) and ultimately with the father (Signor and Herr).

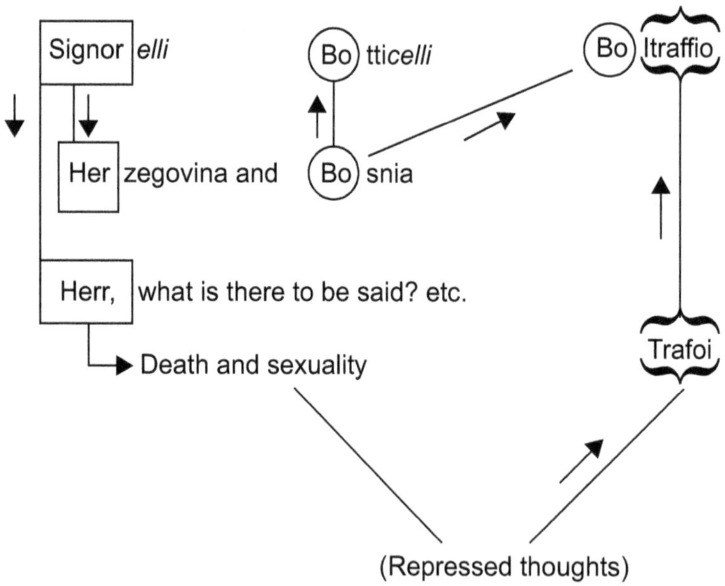

Figure 9.1 Schema of the movement of signifiers.

Source: Freud 1904, p. 5. The drawing is mine.

Nonetheless, the important point is how Freud indicates the way in which something of his own subjective experience is transmissible across time from analyst to analyst beyond the immanence or idiosyncrasies of imaginary subjective experience. With the later Lacan, we would not say that the signifier is objective, because this would amount to a contradiction in terms. The signifier refers to the subject and where the subject and the signifier represent an objective form of subjectivity or a form of knowledge without a subject. But where would truth be in this case, since, for Lacan, subjective truth differs both from emotions and objective knowledge?

Lacan uses the concepts of signifier and subject interchangeably. In addition, the signifier has a relationship to truth in the Real and not only to other signifiers (S_1–S_0 and not only S_1–S_2), and the Real is beyond the Symbolic and the signifier. With the later Lacan, subjective truth is found in the Real of jouissance rather than at the level of the objectivity of the signifier as a form of knowledge without a subject. Without a subject here means without an ego, since the subject of the pure signifier is a shifter, and with the later Lacan, there is also a subject in the Real of jouissance. The Real is the hole of senselessness (without imaginary meaning) around which signifiers turn. The Real and jouissance are transubjective or transindividual more than objective and/or represent subjective truth more than an emotional truth or an objective form of knowledge without a subject. At the same time, the subject is embedded in the signifying network, while the ego represents self-centered and imaginary forms of subjectivism and knowledge.

Feeling or affect, for example, is the subjective experience evoked or effected by the words and actions of the other, while the signified or meaning of affect is not the actual words or events but their jouissance value for the subject. Feelings are triggered by the Other, but what the subject experiences is their own drive and jouissance. Jouissance is of the Real subject and not of the Other. Thus, the analyst cannot be responsible (through projective identification) for the analysand's jouissance in the transference, nor can the analysand be responsible for the jouissance experienced by the analyst as a result of the words or actions of the analysand. The feelings or affect both parties experience are interdependent, but the jouissance is not. Jouissance is the subject's own. Jouissance is what determines if an affect will be pleasant, unpleasant, neutral, or a varying combination of the three.

An analyst cannot confuse their own jouissance or subjective experience as a subject with what the Other projects unto them. The object relations analyst, in the case of the projective identification phenomenon, does not take responsibility for their own experience (or personal analysis) and attribute their experience to the analysand as the source of the unconscious knowledge projected unto the analyst. With the notion of the countertransference as projective identification, for example, the transmission of the signifier beyond the immanence of subjective experience is lost because, despite all assertions to the contrary, there is more and more the unilateral belief that all that happens to the analyst in the analytical situation reaches him/her by way of the analysand.

The key point for our current purposes is that, over time, it is the signifier that holds the key to both transference and countertransference, as well as to the transmission of psychoanalysis, although in the later Lacan, the Real, and jouissance and its transformations, are also involved in the transmission of psychoanalysis. Unconscious knowing or savoir, and the language of the unconscious or lalangue, are linked to the experience of jouissance and its transformations: beginning with the object of desire that the individual is for the Other.

This point raises the question as to why Lacan uses intersubjective concepts (jouissance of the Other and Other jouissance) to formulate jouissance, despite the fact that jouissance is something the subject alone has to take responsibility for. What object or jouissance do I represent for the Other, and what object or jouissance does the Other represent for me? The Other represents the experience of satisfaction (or frustration) and the fact that the child is an object that has a narcissistic value for the mother. The mother gets off on the child as her object, but this is the mother's jouissance, not the child's. In turn, the child experiences satisfaction at the breast regardless of what kind of object the child may represent for the mother at that moment. From then on, the child will have to take responsibility for their own experience of satisfaction or frustration, independently of how this factor interacts with the actions and fantasies of the Other.

It is the signifier that objectifies the object of desire, beyond the immanence of subjective experience, or imaginary idiosyncratic subjectivism, and at the same time, the object, the signifier, and jouissance all belong to different registers of experience. The object is imaginary and metonymical, while jouissance belongs to the Real. Phallic jouissance seeks the signifiers of the phallus more than fusion with the Other (the signifying units more than the unifying imaginary unity). However, the phallus cannot be objectified, not only because the imaginary phallus does not exist, but because the phallus is not a privileged metonymical object but rather the signifier of a lack (symbolic phallus). Because the phallus is not an object, nor a privileged transcendental presence, the signifier of a lack (the missing symbolic phallus) appears in the place of the null set or the lack of a signifier to represent the Real of jouissance.

To conclude, the desire of the analyst is the desire not to remain in the position of a beloved master of knowledge or the subject supposed to know. The more the analyst tries to give to the analysand, either love or knowledge, to please or be loved by the analysand, the more countertransference obstacles he/she will experience and the more the analyst could end up developing a transference neurosis towards his/her analysand. The countertransference needs to be handled through a personal analysis or disclosed to other professionals but not to the analyst's analysand.

On the other hand, this should not lead one to believe that the analyst should never make reference to his/her own subjective experience. Winnicott pointed out that the analyst should not attempt to hide his/her personal failings or mistakes. This is consistent with the Lacanian notion that the analysand needs to come to terms with the lack in the Other, in this case of the analyst. This is particularly true of idealizing transferences or of masochistic analysands who always tend to blame themselves for everything and to raise the analyst to a pedestal of perfection.

References

Bion, W. R. (1984). *Transformations*. London: Karnac.
Freud, A. (1936). *The Ego and the Mechanisms of Defense*. London: Karnac.
Freud, S. (1900). *The Interpretation of Dreams*. New York: Avon Books, 1965.
Freud, S. (1904). *The Psychopathology of Everyday Life*. New York: Norton, 1965.
Freud, S. (1905). Jokes and Their Relation to the Unconscious. *SE*, 8.
Freud, S. (1926). Inhibitions, Symptoms and Anxiety. *SE*, 20, 77–174.
Lacan, J. (1956–1957). *El Seminario. Libro 4. La Relacion de Objeto*. Buenos Aires: Paidos.
Lacan, J. (1957–1958). *Formations of the Unconscious: The Seminar of Jacques Lacan*. Book V. Translated by R. Grigg. London: Polity Press.
Lacan, J. (1961–1962). *Identification*. Book IX. Unedited translation by C. Gallagher. London: Karnac.
Lacan, J. (1966). The Subversion of the Subject and the Dialectic of Desire in the Freudian Unconscious. In: *Ecrits*. Translated by B. Fink. New York: Norton, 2006.
Maslow, A. (1968). *Toward a Psychology of Being*. New York: Van Nostrand Reinhold.
Moncayo, R. (2018). *Knowing, Not-Knowing, and Jouissance: Levels, Symbols, and Codes of Experience in Psychoanalysis*. London: Palgrave McMillan.
Nietszche, F. (1844). *The Essential Nietzsche*. New York: Chartwell Books, 2017.
Winnicott, D. (1971). Creativity and Its Origins. In: *Playing and Reality*, London: Routledge, 1991.
Zupanscic, A. (2011). *Ethics of the Real: Kant and Lacan*. London: Verso.

10 The function of the One in sexual difference and the question of feminine jouissance

Symptom, fantasy, and sexual difference

The notion of the phantasm in Lacan ($\$\lozenge\underline{a}$) dates back to Freud's (1915, 1916–17; Laplanche and Pontalis, 1973) protofantasies or "primal fantasies," which included the question of the origins: the origins of sexuality or the seduction fantasy; the question of castration, or the origin of sexual differences; and the primal scene, or the origin of human life. According to Freud (1915, 1916–17), these universal structures exist in a fantasy dimension and are irreducible to personal individual experience. According to Lacan (1956–57), unconscious fantasy both sustains desire and defends against castration. "What is prohibited is always present in the actual formation of the wish" (Laplanche and Pontalis, 1973). The crossing of the phantasm or fantasy involves elaborating on these two aspects of the fantasy: how the fantasy sustains desire and at the same time defends against symbolic castration.

For Lacan, the symptom is necessary to access unconscious fantasies. Fantasy is an image set in a repressed and unconscious signifying structure. Fantasies may be repressed, acted out, or perceived as elements of the external world. In addition, fantasies veil the lack or the desire of and in the Other (not the desire for the Other). Although fantasies have common elements, they are always singular formations of the subject. Fantasies also often come in contradictory pairs that in the case of hysteria are exemplified by bisexuality and the question of hysteria, according to Lacan: "Am I a man or a woman, am I both a man and a woman, or neither (three possible rational/logical levels)." In addition, the fantasy, or phantasm, as Lacan called it, is staged in the choice of one or two simultaneous and contradictory partners of the different or same sex. For Lacan hysteria since Freud has always been two.

Bisexuality (i.e. Am I a man or a woman?) and the choice of two partners (often one real and one fantasized) are at play in love relations, including transference love in analysis. Love transference to the analyst is fed by the hysterical fantasy of two partners. In this case, the analyst can become the fantasized partner. In the case of two partners, the actual partner will be the 'weak,' less desirable partner (lacking Other), while the fantasized partner is the phallic, 'strong' desirable partner. The analysand typically does not desire the 'weak' (-phi) partner and fantasizes about a 'strong' (phi or +phi) partner instead.

For example, a female analysand did not want to be 'strong' like her mother, who had the 'pants' (imaginary phallus) in the family, and instead wanted the father to be strong, but then chose a husband whom she described as 'weak' like her father and for whom she was 'strong' like her mother. Stereotypically, she thinks that men are strong and women weak, but then she wants to be a female who has a strong personality like a man with opinions (a 'mansplainer' who is always right and likes to give directions) and thinks that her husband is weak like a female with a small penis. She had a dream where her husband was a weak man flying in a plane full of holes and she was a weak woman cooking pancakes with holes in them. The flying phallus 'plane' is 'full' of holes, and the 'pancake' (*lamella/ objet a*) has holes in it.

Then she fantasizes being with a 'strong' man like her analyst, but when she thinks of her analyst as a man and herself as a woman, she then starts thinking of all the flaws of her analyst, and he very quickly becomes a 'weak' man in her eyes. His constructed weakness or imaginary castration is in direct relation to her experiencing imaginary castration or weakness as a woman. In either case, whether she is strong and the man weak, or whether she is weak and the man strong, both instances lead to a lack of sexual rapport between the sexes as formulated by Lacan.

The structural fantasy of two partners, composed of a committed partner and a fantasized lover, does not resolve in a recommitment to a wife or husband or leaving a partner for a new successful relationship to a lover. In either case, the lack of sexual rapport between sexes will be the norm. Although having a relationship may represent so-called healthy functioning, psychoanalysis cannot resolve the predicament that Lacan calls the lack of sexual rapport between the sexes.

As I have written elsewhere (Moncayo, 2017), Lacan's thesis that there is no sexual rapport between the sexes signifies that ancient and classical ideals no longer hold. With the biological maturity of the sexual drive in adolescence, tradition hopes that love would subsume sex under marriage Law. This is a myth that supports a norm but is not consistent with the reality of the unconscious or married/ couple life, for that matter. This is another example of how the two levels of the signifying chain diverge and do not coincide. There is no ideal or better arrangement for relationships among the sexes, because the lack of rapport is structural, although it can be transformed into a sinthome.

From this perspective, the sinthome is the 'know-how-to-make-do' (*savoir-faire*) or how to bear the unbearable lack of rapport in relationships, not only between the sexes but also between love and sexuality (humans eventually are prone not to have sex with those they love and not to love those they have sex with).

Lacan (1971–1972) borrows from Parmenides the notion that the One, as the thing-in-itself, says itself in a saying: there is the One's own non-being. For this reason, in an anti-ontological moment, Lacan thinks that the One as zero or emptiness is the opposite of Being rather than its essence or lack thereof. When One is separated from zero or One is external to zero, then positive imaginary narcissism represents One (of the Imaginary), and zero is equal to negative narcissism in the sense of self-destruction or the self being reduced to a 'nothing' of absence or annihilation (Green, 2001). It is important not to confuse the One of the Imaginary with the One of the Real and not to fail to realize the link between the One and the 'no-thing' of presence in the form of the One's own non-being.

Lacan says that there is no rapport or sexual relation as such between the sexes, because the two sexes are two Ones that don't need each other because they are both the same One. The subject is 'All-alone' at the place where a relationship could have been spoken and lied about or the relation could have been said, revealing thereby, in the saying, the lack of sexual rapport between the sexes or the truth that their actual partner is a third-party fantasy object.

When Lacan says that a woman is not entirely under the phallic function ($\overline{\forall}\mathbf{x}\Phi\mathbf{x}$), ambiguously, this means not only that a woman's sexuality cannot be reduced to phallic jouissance but also that a woman is not entirely under the phallic function of symbolic castration. Despite the function of negating the imaginary phallus, there is no signified there, or there is nothing there that could be negated. The negated signifier refers to a signified that does not exist. The -1 is a structural rather than accidental loss. Its absence refers to an imaginary number ($-1=-\sqrt{-1}$) that does not exist. Instead of a loss of a real penis (-1 as a real number), -1 here is an imaginary number that does not exist (i).

The phallic function represents a unary rather than a binary form negation. Symbolic castration would represent a binary form of negation if the imaginary phallus first existed as a penile object and then was denied (-1). But since what is being denied did not exist to begin with, then the negated signifier (-1) is a no-object. The imaginary phallus is an inexistent signified for the NoF and the desire of the mother, and the object it represents is missing. Under the phallic function, the imaginary phallus becomes an empty place without a signified that facilitates the movement of metonymy and signification in language.

When the imaginary phallus has no signified (no penis or any other object for that matter), or its signified is inexistent with respect to femininity, the imaginary phallus, or the -1 in this case, becomes an imaginary number representative of femininity. An imaginary number designates a place for inexistence or for what of femininity is not within a system of phallic signifiers. Femininity is already 'not that' that can be affirmed in language.

Both sexes are forms of the One that don't need each other, as the other sex qua sex, and although they can 'interbe' and have sexual intimacy, there is no lasting sexual rapport between them. There are 'One sayings,' but not dialogue per se. According to Lacan, it's only when one of the Ones turns the Other into something other than a circle (Moncayo, 2017, p. 84) that the subject can desire its object in the Other, and now there is sex and a relationship. The *objet a* is only a semblance, parceled out by the signifier, of being the very Being of the subject within the Other. Thus, the *objet a* cannot represent a foundation for rapport between the sexes, because the other can only temporarily represent the object that will restore the Being that is missing within the subject. A subject cannot find its Being in the Other but only in their own One's non-being.

With respect to the contradictory pairs at work in bisexuality and the choice of two partners, one male, one female, an analysand reported wanting to have sex with a man, but the only way she could experience orgasm was to imagine that a beautiful woman was looking at her and her lover. She elaborates that since she hates her body and feels disgusted by herself, the only way she could accept a man's desire was by first being 'accepted' by an ideal woman. This seems to be pointing to a hypothesis that she is relating to woman as an object of fantasy, but from the point of view of feminine identification. Somehow it allows her to be a part of the class of beautiful women that 'are' rather than 'have' the phallus. In turn, it compensates for or defends against the representation of imaginary femininity (feeling unattractive/defective). Just like men may fantasize about another woman when having sex with a woman, a woman may fantasize that she is another ideal woman the man is having sex with. Men's and women's fantasies are not symmetrical.

The ideal woman is the one that 'is' the phallus and wants to be loved and desired by men and envied by women, but she herself has no desire and no lack. Ragland (2004) has said that "the Freudian woman does not love men, but that she is nothing without the love of men and that when she loves, she loves as a mother" (pp. 87–88). She adds a very interesting conclusion, "any woman who loves a man in the masquerade, by making herself the object he lacks, by trying to be what she thinks he wants, has given up on her desire" (idem). Her desire precisely is to constitute herself as the object of a man's lack and the agent of his castration, but a woman has no independent desire of her own for what she wants/lacks and wants to receive from a man other than his desire for her. Desire is denied in favor of constituting herself as an object rather than a subject of desire.

Ragland (2004) describes what she calls the Freudian woman as someone who sacrifices her own desire to being-for-another. "Such totalizing love – trying to be the phallus the partner lacks – can only stifle the particularity of desire and keep a woman from loving from the place of feminine sexuality" (p. 88). Looking closer at what is happening in such an Imaginary relationship with a woman's desire is that she only needs a man to give her a fantasy of herself, but this fantasy has phallic overtones in terms of woman as object cause of a man's desire. Ragland comments that such

> Love can only be Imaginary, then, based, as it is, on idealized 'fantasy' picture of the one she hopes he thinks she is, aiming at closure. Of course, such a picture is far from desire. Insofar as a woman already does not love a man qua man, qua father, nor qua possessor of the phallus, but loves in him, rather, the fantasy he gives her of herself.
>
> (p. 88)

In the case of imaginary masculinity, a man is interested in a woman only to the extent that she can provide a confirmation of his virility. A woman wants to be recognized that she is the beautiful phallic object that could confirm a man's virility in the sense that he has the phallus; however, such recognition provides illusive, if not impossible, for both parties. In confirming each other, they both disappear and cancel each other. If she is the *objet a*, then a man's virility is compromised (she is it, and he loses what he has), and if he has the imaginary phallus, then she loses the 'agalmic' quality of her body.

The fantasy that the phallus or sex with a man gave the analysand of herself was this image of being another beautiful woman. She also reported a dream where a strong man would flatter himself, thinking she was in love with him, but she was not. Instead both were in love with his 'monumental' wife, who was an artist. Everybody loved her and brought her gifts. She badly wanted to be the artist. 'The Artist' was not in love and did not care about anyone. She was cold and detached. She seemed to be proud of not wanting anything from anyone. The artist represents the ice queen or *belle indifference*.

The man's wife is clearly 'The' (phallic) woman who 'has it all,' and so she has no lack in comparison to a man who wants her and needs her to complete himself. To have desire for a man, a woman has to risk lack, and this is something that she may experience as 'weakness' or an imaginary castration that she does not accept. Sometimes the experience may be triggered by a derogatory or devaluating comment of the other. But even in the absence of any environmental or sociological gender factor, the pure difference between the sexes can be experienced as an imaginary form of castration that ultimately can trigger murder and the literal castration of the Other.

In such extreme cases, it is most likely that both structural and environmental factors were involved. This fantasy can be seen in the dream of an analysand who dreamt she was a serial killer woman who wore a strange yellow suit and would ask men if she was beautiful, and if they said no, she would kill them. In the case of the movie *Kill Bill*, the hero is seeking revenge for earlier violence and abuse, but the action could also be triggered for purely structural reasons. In the more recent example of the movie Mulan, she fights just as a skillfully with the sword, but she fights to restore the honor of the NoF and her community. This would be an example of symbolic femininity, while Kill Bill represents imaginary masculinity in a female.

In another example, a female analysand reported a dream in which she had a protective membrane, or external vagina over her genitals, like an external membrane spread over the entire vulva instead of the vaginal hole. Between the membrane and her internal vagina, there was an external vagina with no crease, ridge, or rim. Lack of rim made the vagina look damaged.

In her associations, she said her hymen was torn while giving birth. In response to this, she said she acted at the time like nothing had happened, as if femininity and maternity had no impact on her body. She could be pregnant without toll on her body. This is the protective membrane covering over femininity. She linked this to using her feminine body and gestational capacity as a weapon. In this sense, she said, pregnancies can be seen as a revenge against a man who becomes bound to fatherhood whether he wants it or not.

In addition, she had insecurity about sex being injuring or traumatic in some way. This points to the imaginary damage represented by the external vagina appearing like an atrophied small penis. I interpreted that the dream was representing femininity as an injury or deformity. The membrane allegedly is protecting her from penetration, and at the same time, the vagina is an external organ (imaginary phallus) like the penis is.

The dream is a fantasy of imaginary castration as the source of sexual difference. This analysand, although female, had a disdain and contempt for stereotypically feminine and submissive women, which her previous husband wanted her to be. By the same token, she felt insecure in her masculine identifications and sometimes fantasized about desiring to be stereotypically feminine herself.

Another female analysand dreamt that she was using her father's motorcycle. The motorcycle had previously appeared in other dreams, always with her in a position of leadership. In this dream, she used it and lost it because she did not lock it. When she realized that she had lost it, she ran back, but the motorcycle had been stolen. The motorcycle had been broken into pieces, and some pieces had been left behind. A young man appeared who knew the thief, who was part of a gang, and they both wanted to help each other escape from the gang and its scary leader.

In her associations, she said that she belongs to a group she wants to escape from. She also called herself a motorbike woman and said that she always preferred to be a boy. She believed that men are stronger than women when they are alone, but when they are with a woman, they become lacking. Thus, she complained that her husband stayed away from her, and this made her feel lacking. She said that she felt envy of young men and that they have become increasingly aggressive and rebellious, and she linked this to stealing in the dream and how she identified with rebellious young men.

The analysand reported another dream where she dreamt of a female who was a freedom fighter man who eventually got killed. This was a female who became a man to fight against either gender oppression or sexual difference. The responsibility for gender oppression is on society, while the responsibility for sexual difference is on the subject. When the freedom fighter gets killed, it is unclear whether he is a martyr for the cause against gender oppression or if he gets killed as a metaphor for a second death under the Symbolic linked to symbolic castration and sexual difference. In the dream, the second seems to be the case, since the dead man became a living black woman who was slender, tall, graceful, and beautiful. The hero fighter represents the deadly symbolic castration associated with the difference between the sexes that produces either a symbolically castrated man who is heroic and honorable, or a beautiful symbolic woman who acquires graces not available to imaginary femininity or symbolic masculinity.

Analysand believed that 'phallic women' who are sexually seductive and rebellious, and who can dance by themselves without men to the admiration of others, have a boy penis, which would be the equivalent of an imaginary phallus she always wanted to be and have. Another time, she dreamt that she was feeding a baby with her breast, and the nipple turned into a long penis.

In yet another dream, the analysand did not know what a penis was, and the answer came back in the form of a detached penis that all men had to lose in order to understand what a man was. One of the man's pajamas was down to his knees, and his genitals were partially exposed. He did not have a penis and instead had a red sore that she thought he must had been rubbing all the time. She said to the boys: "I don't know what a penis is" and then saw all their penises detached from their bodies and flying in the air. She was embarrassed, and she felt bad for the boys that they had to lose their body parts for her to understand what a penis or a boy/man was. This dream demonstrates how symbolic castration is constitutive of masculinity. In another dream, she was given a motorcycle, and she felt it was very masculine. Her husband told her that he wanted a motorcycle, too, and she told him that only one of them could have it, and she gave it to him.

I interpreted the motorcycle as something powerful between the legs that stands for her identification with masculinity, her father, and the imaginary phallus, and that she wants to steal the 'motorcycle' and at the same time is afraid that it will be taken from her. At the same time, hers and her father's motorcycle is mutilated and broken into pieces. She associated further that I was the one castrating her because I had recently asked for payment and she felt like I was taking her money away from her. She did not want to pay me, in order to keep her money and power. Recently in a family meeting, the extended family recognized and praised her for making the most money in her family, second only to the mother's brother, who is the wealthiest in the family.

Both dreams represent sexual difference, the first with a distorted view of femininity as a form of injury and the second with an identification with masculinity that then confuses femininity with a damaged and rebellious man. In both cases, femininity is articulated as a -1, a lack in the Other, or as the square root of -1 that as an imaginary number does not exist. However, it is not that the male or the father has it and she or the female does not. The father is also castrated in the Imaginary by other aggressive males that in the Imaginary appeared unbarred or not under the Law. Both sexes have a primitive aspiration to be unbarred and symbolically uncastrated men. In the Imaginary, she loses what she does not have other than as a wish and a fantasy. In fact, both sexes have to lose it in order to use it, either as a woman with the help of a man, or as a man with the help of a woman.

But the phallus here does not only refer to sex but also to gender identity as a man or a woman. But what is the difference between a symbolically castrated man and a symbolically castrated woman or how the lack in the Other (Ø) appears in both sexes? One thing is to differentiate between having and not having and another to differentiate between two forms of not having. The symbols for both would be the symbolic phallus, as a missing phallus, or the symbolic phallus for masculinity and the square root of -1 for femininity (Φ and i). The first dream potentially represents masculinity as unbarred or uncastrated, while in the second dream, the father is symbolically castrated in the Imaginary (his 'wheels' are stolen).

In the Imaginary, the mother is seen as dominant and the father as being subordinate to the mother. However, the daughters disobey the mother and obey the father, which might indicate that the father is more subordinate to the Law than to the mother, which makes the daughters obey him despite his lack vis à vis his wife.

In the dream, the father is castrated in the Imaginary by a female or male identified with the fantasy of an unbarred masculinity represented by the motorcycle. Masculinity is identified with a lost motorcycle or with a man who disavows the Law, while woman is identified with a motorcycle that does not exist or that she does not have rather than that is lost. Not-having is constructed as a defect.

Because femininity lacks a signifier, or is a number that does not exist, it is represented in the Imaginary as a deficit or damage. So how does feminine jouissance enter the picture? Well, Ragland said that women don't love or have desire for men and only want to be loved/desired by men, and when they love men, they love them as a mother, since, of course, that is the place where a mother's desire for a child is fundamental. Not that sexual desire is not fundamental for a woman, it is just that it is typically complex, if not problematical. Wanting to be loved is different from a lack of being (desire). Socialized and biological maternal love (doing for others) is not the same as feminine jouissance.

What stopped my analysand from becoming a man desirous of a beautiful woman was having to take care of boys in her dreams or a brother in her real life. In a dream, she had to take care of a teenage boy whom her mother wanted to be happy. The analysand had to make sure the boy did not lose his penis, but his penis dried up and fell off, and she did not want to tell her mother, who kept asking her to take care of the boy.

What is the meaning of a woman loving a man or a child as a mother? Is there a relation between the tender union between mother and child and the fusion of the desire of the mother with the *objet a* cause of her desire that the child signifies? Tenderness is an aspect of the enigma of the life drive, while in the field of the signifier/signification, the desire of the mother becomes determined/signified by the signified of the NoF, otherwise known as the imaginary phallus. Relationships, or object relations, remain vulnerable to the split between tenderness without sex and sex without tenderness. Winnicott (1971) sees no drive in a baby's relationship to the breast, while for Lacan, the *objet a* is both an object of the drive and of desire. Winnicott thinks that only a biological boy has an instinctual relationship to the breast (Freud believed that the libido was masculine). The girl instead only relates to the breast biologically or through maternal identification. Winnicott is probably making a distinction between an anaclitic attachment and a sexual relationship with an imaginary object.

Winnicott (1971) places sexuality on the side of masculinity and Freud's ego drives or life drives on the side of femininity, freezing and reifying thereby gender stereotypes between the sexes (*Machismo* and *Marianismo*, respectively). Men are animals or half-animals, while women follow the virgin Mary, mother of god. For Freud, there may be a distinction between sexual drives and life drives, since the sexual drives also have death drives in them, but Freud does not reduce femininity to the maternal tender element. As we have shown, the fantasy object for a woman also bears a relationship to the *objet a*/phallus. In addition, feminine jouissance is not phallic and cannot be reduced to the maternal orientation either.

When feminine jouissance is realized as something more than a man's phallic enjoyment, or is realized beyond the excitation of being the ideal woman a man desires (being the phallus), then a woman's feminine jouissance lies singularly outside the phallic order. In turn, phallic enjoyment in a man is also realized beyond the surplus or excess preoccupation with virility that denies it.

Feminine jouissance refers to a woman selflessly enjoying phallic jouissance or losing herself in the Other feminine jouissance with a socially permissible metonymic object and signifier that she lacks and that a man appears to have. Since feminine jouissance is under the law and the NoF and at the same time singularly and paradoxically outside the phallic order of the signifier, a woman is able to enjoy phallic jouissance and at the same time enjoy a supplemental feminine jouissance with a man. In the case of femininity, the double loss of not-being the imaginary phallus (for the mother) and not-having the imaginary phallus (that the father appears to have) is transformed into a double form of enjoyment of both phallic and feminine jouissance.

This contrasts when a woman only enjoys phallic jouissance with a man in two different ways. First, as being it, or the imaginary phallus, or an ideal narcissistic object that a man lacks. Second, in the form of the phallic jouissance of a mother woman that sacrifices her own legitimate jouissance, or the good of feminine jouissance, that she has been told is a selfish jouissance, in favor of fulfilling a marriage obligation (presided over by the social Other), or the gender role responsibility of giving a man the phallic jouissance that he wants. Selfishness or narcissism in a woman's sexual jouissance only refers to the wish to be the ideal narcissistic phallic object that a man lacks.

To create an accord between a man and a woman, there must be a relation between feminine jouissance and phallic jouissance, or between $\sqrt{-1}$ and φ (phi = 0.618), rather than man and woman linking up through phallic jouissance, or phi and -phi (presence and absence of the imaginary phallus), which is always related to a third fantasy object (φ) that is found missing within the Other. "This Other jouissance is strictly termed feminine, and on no account does it depend on phallic jouissance" (Lacan, 1971–1972, p. 88). In Seminar XIV, Lacan gives an arithmetical proof of the difference between when a woman functions as an *objet a* or golden number that closes the gap of the absence of the imaginary phallus and when woman functions within femininity proper, represented in the form of the $\sqrt{-1}$. The square root of -1 as the imaginary number represents inexistence or emptiness that also functions within Real and irrational numbers and has a relationship to phallic signifiers. Lacan's proof is shown subsequently (Moncayo and Romanowicz, 2015).

Lacan starts with the Boolean logic of plus and minus and writes the formula as follows:

$$(a - b)\,(a + b)$$

$(a - b)\,(a + b)$ is an important math formula that Lacan utilizes to prove his point that if we use the square root of -1, we get 2, but if we use the golden number in succession of pluses and minuses, we get yet another golden number. He then asks himself what would have happened if we assumed that:

$$a = 1$$
$$b = \sqrt{-1}$$
$$(a-b)(a+b) = a^2 - b^2 = 1^2 - \left(\sqrt{-1}\right)^2 = 1-(-1) = 1+1 = 2$$

> If it is a matter of specifying *a* in two opposite fashions, with plus something and with minus something, and for the result to be 2, it is enough to make it equal to *i*. This is how one usually writes, in an abbreviated fashion, and moreover one much more convenient, this function of the square root of minus one which is described as imaginary.
>
> (Seminar XIV, Lesson 16: Wednesday 12 April 1967, p. 187)

The formula of feminine jouissance in relationship to phallic jouissance is distinguished from the case when man and woman in the sexual act are only related through phallic jouissance.

$$a = 1$$
$$b = o$$

(Here for clarity of calculations, I will represent *objet a* as "o," which is equal to the golden number/phi = 0,618.)

$$(a - b)(a + b) = a^2 - b^2 = 1 - o^2 = o$$

> (1 + o) (1 – o) gives o, on condition that o is equal to this golden number – it is worthwhile repeating it – that I am using to introduce, for you, the function of the little *a*-object. Verify this: when *small a* is equal to the golden number the product of (1 + o) (1 – o) is equal to o (*objet a*).
>
> (idem)

This is a very beautiful mathematical representation of the lack that reproduces the lack. People can plug the hole through phallic jouissance, where in the sexual act, the object does not appear to be missing. However, this is only an illusion, because actually the sexual act replicates the *objet a* and reproduces the lack. Instead, when a relationship between feminine jouissance and phallic jouissance is involved, the sexual act does not lead to more lack for a woman and loss of virility for a man.

It is when a and b are calculated using $\sqrt{-1}$ and φ (phi = 0.618) that the result adds up to 2 according to the math calculations shown previously. This means that feminine *jouissance* must present itself singularly from *outside* the standard phallic frame of reference. The best way to represent feminine jouissance is to 'non-represent' it with the imaginary number that is a number that does not exist or that 'ex-sists.' $\sqrt{-1}$ is a signifier without a signified and where the signified is in the Real of jouissance rather than the signified being another signifier within the Symbolic order.

Finally, sexual differences are not biological (revealed as maternal in a woman and sexual in a man, according to Winnicott), because girl and boy are signifiers within the Other of language and require the intervention of the Other for their differentiated function. When Winnicott associates the female element to Being, if Being is defined as the One's own non-being, then this can be seen as related to Lacan's statement that a woman does not exist. Inexistence is related to the Real and to jouissance and to the lightness of Being rather than to existence in the sense of the signifier and the reality principle.

The Real is not a fabricated sense of a true self behind a false conventional (imaginary and symbolic) self. The Real provides a basis for the jouissance of meaning and for the experience of significance (emotional truth) but cannot be reduced to humanistic categories such as that of meaningful interpersonal relationships or emotional growth. Humanism provides an ideological cover or veneer that does not hold under pressure and leads to lying about and normalizing what actually transpires in relationships where miscommunication is the norm. One cannot represent Being for the Other and fulfill the lack of being in the Other. By the same token, the Other cannot gives us our Being. The subject cannot find the *objet a* or the semblance of Being in the Other.

Neither the Real nor jouissance are solipsistic or narcissistic in the ordinary sense. The Other jouissance requires the Other as a rupture or a tear symbolized by symbolic castration and is eventually realized beyond castration. Once instantiated, the Third jouissance energizes the words of those who speak and structures the exchange value and signification of signifiers without the inconvenient excess of the jouissance of the Other or surplus phallic jouissance.

Maternal desire is not simply a biological form of tenderness associated with nutrition and proteins or a primary identification with the breast/mother, as Winnicott believed, because in human beings, reproduction takes place through the signifiers of desire. In order for a woman to want to have a child, she has to have been differentiated as a woman within Oedipal and family structure. A woman separated from her mother no longer *is* the mother's imaginary phallus/object; for good or bad, this position has been lost. Then, to become a woman, she has to lose the imaginary phallus as a part object in relationship to the father. She loses it both as a part object and as a signifier of the father's phallic jouissance.

As an effect of oedipal structure, a woman wishes to have a child as a substitute for the imaginary phallus that she first was and then lost twice, first by not being the mother's object and second in the sense of what she wanted but never had as a woman due to the prohibition of incest and the symbolic differences between the sexes.

When a woman is pregnant, this double negation is reversed; she experienced the 'father's' imaginary phallus as a metonymic object and phallic jouissance, and the result is a baby whereby she has a part object that now is also part of herself. Her body is ready to produce the biological nutrients for the new life and the hormones that will facilitate desire and tenderness towards the child. Tenderness can be thought as a hormonal effect or as a primary receptivity and sensitivity towards the world that, as a form of discharge or release, directly satisfies the Life drive.

Within Lacanian theory, there are three mothers according to the logic of the Borromean knot. The first mother is the imaginary mother that is driven to want the baby phallus or the object-phallus-baby; the second mother is the symbolic mother whose desire for the NoF as a metaphor and the child as a subject inscribes absence into the child's mind in preparation for the separate identity that will come with the entry into the Symbolic order. The Real mother as *das Ding* is the 'archaic thing' embedded in the object world.

Motherhood, as a sociological gender role that appears in the dream of the analysand mentioned previously, reduces women to an abnegation (altruistic self-sacrifice) that only simulates the phallic function of symbolic castration. In the ideological imaginary, women have to be mothers to serve the patriarchal order or because men supposedly are the ones who offer the sacrifice of their life and work to support women and children. In the dream, the analysand is trying to make sure the boys don't lose their penis, which is the destination that an aspect of her socialized motherhood would lead her to (*Kill Bill*).

A socialized maternal role makes use of biological femininity and imaginary castration but may be devoid not only of genuine tenderness but of the fact that femininity, as a vacuum, an empty container, or a jouissance in the Real, also has a link to knowledge, as in mathematics, for example, that Lacan considered a form of knowledge or knowing in the Real. In other words, feminine jouissance, as a form of the Third, is not only passive. In making an effort to know we are always active. Women do not have to go through masculinity to link up to the Symbolic (there is a woman's way to knowledge), and masculinity does not have to go through feminine jouissance to access the Third jouissance. Different biological males or females may choose to do precisely that, but that is a different story, and the logical relations would still remain the same in any case.

I mentioned that the asymmetry between love and sex is another form of the lack of rapport between the sexes. If a female becomes a man who desires women, there is no sexual rapport with a male; if she becomes the ideal woman, then she is the phallus or object of desire, and she does not desire or lack a man. Who is she then: her devalued self, the ideal woman, a mother, or a man?

This leads to Lacan's declaration that the woman does not exist. Who is she among all these identifications: is she man or woman; alive or dead; normal, abnormal, or eccentric? Obviously, the solution is not for her to have multiple personality disorder and be all of these at the same time. But that 'the' woman does not exist is not sheer inexistence or a form of devaluing negation (I don't have a self). At the level of the Real, feminine sexuality and jouissance is a singularity and a form of generative emptiness available to a femininity that 'ex-sists' outside phallic signification. The phallic function of symbolic castration, and its acceptance or avowal, is the access point to the Real and the Third jouissance of feminine sexuality.

Woman as a trace of jouissance, or a sexed form of emptiness or inexistence, differs from a mother, a man, and the phallic object. From this empty ground beyond the signifier, it becomes possible to distinguish between imaginary phallic simulacrum and symbolic masquerade. Instead of feeling like a fake impostor, or a fantasized ideal object, masquerade becomes the Nietzschean dance of masks, or the stage that the world is, according to Shakespeare. Woman now can function within a phallic symbolic order as a woman rather than only as a female who is a man. Thanks to the phenomenal 'inexistence' of the structure, woman can commune with the Other and the pure form of the signifier (the freshness and aliveness of language, in this case).

The traversal of the fantasy refers to how castration as a signifier of jouissance gives access to the Real of jouissance. The motorcycle for the analysand sustains desire yet defends against castration. Not to be fooled by the fantasy or to be fooled and realize it allows for the possibility of transforming defenses and the modalities of jouissance. The analysand is no longer fooled by her desire to be a man and has to accept symbolic loss and castration either in women or men. Fantasies can be used to sustain desire but have to be divested of their deceptive and defensive aspects.

Lacan's formula for the fantasy ($<>a) shows how the divided subject has lost the object cause of desire and how the subject wants metonymical imaginary objects to close the gap/lack of desire. The subject is the object in the fantasy because the object either divides or completes the subject. In addition, since identification is one of the basic ways of relating to the object, the traversing of the fantasy also entails the deconstruction of identifications and the subsequent subjective destitution or relinquishing of imaginary identifications (woman as either a defective female or castrated man or as the imaginary One that has it all, and man as either an unbarred form of imaginary masculinity or a castrated imaginary man under the Law). If the symptom gives access to the fantasy, the crossing of the fantasy and the traversal of the plane of identification (relinquishing certain identifications) transforms the symptom into a sinthome that can be used for constructive purposes.

References

Freud, S. (1915). A Case of Paranoia Running Counter to the Psycho-Analytic Theory of the Disease. *G.W.*, 10, 242; *S.E.*, 14, 269.

Freud, S. (1916–17). Introductory Lectures on Psychoanalysis. *G.W.*, 11, 386; *S.E.*, 16, 371.

Green, A. (2001). *Life Narcissism, Death Narcissism*. London: Free Association Books.

Lacan, J. (1956–1957). *Le Seminaire. Livre IV. La relation d'object, 1956–57*. Edited by J.-A. Miller. Paris: Seuil, 1994.

Lacan, J. (1966–1967). *The Seminar of Jacques Lacan*. Book XIV. The Logic of Phantasy, Unofficial translation by C. Gallagher from unedited French manuscripts.

Lacan, J. (1971–1972). *. . . or Worse: The Seminar of Jacques Lacan*. Book XIX. Edited by J.-A. Miller. London: Polity Press.

Laplanche, J. and Pontalis, J. B. (1973). *The Language of Psychoanalysis*. London: Norton, p. 318.

Moncayo, R. (2017). *Lalangue, Sinthome, Jouissance, and Nomination: A Reading Companion and Commentary on Lacan's Seminar XXIII on the Sinthome.* London: Karnac.

Ragland, E. (2004). *The Logic of Sexuation: From Aristotle to Lacan.* New York: State University of New York Press.

Winnicott, D. (1971). Creativity and Its Origins. In: *Playing and Reality.* London: Routledge, 1991.

11 Time, and the phases of analysis and Oedipus in analytic treatments writ large

The question of time and the unconscious

Effective treatment is not only a question of waiting until the patient is ready and willing to accept an interpretation and let go of the satisfactions or jouissance (suffering) provided by the symptom, however neurotic. Once it became clear to Freud, and many others after him, that some symptoms are not affected or removed by psychoanalytic interpretations, regardless of the length of the treatment, the attention shifted to the patient's defenses in the here and now instead of waiting for something to happen in the future. Freud and the first generation of analysts provided future analysts with the benefit of years and decades of experience of people in analyses for long periods of time.

To work with the future in the present requires a different approach to time and a distinction of different forms of time in the past, present, and future. People not only need time in analysis, as Freud believed, but need different types or dimensions of time. As stated earlier, Lacan (1966) developed the notion of what he called logical time. What he calls logical time would not seem logical to most people. Lacan's definition of time divides time into two categories: diachronic or chronological time and logical or synchronic time. This is a traditional classification of time: continuous and discontinuous time, or conscious time and the timelessness of the unconscious, or discontinuous synchronic time in the present versus the time of development in the past and future.

Formal linear time can usually be attributed to the function of the father or to a time-tracking, taskmaster boss or obsessive super-ego. This is to be contrasted to the timelessness or circular time of the desire of the mother and of hysteria. Instead of planning and doing in the diachronic linear time of the obsessive, the hysteric wants to let 'being-time' and pure signifiers (*Je* or I) emerge in the here and now according to desire and present conditions and considerations. The caricature of a husband and wife arguing over being late for an event would be a case in point. He is upset over being late, and she says to him: "Relax, we won't be late and if we are, whatever time we arrive will be the right time." Of course, that this would only work for informal engagements. Formal events require a stricter observance of lineal diachronic time such as that enforced by a time-tracking taskmaster.

Timelessness or negation of time in the unconscious should be conceived as a dialectical rather than a formal type of negation. More than without time, the unconscious operates under synchronic time that includes rather than excludes the past and future in the present. In this way, the notion of logical time, or the time of the unconscious, appears related to new notions of time in relativity and quantum theory of physics. Relativity theory requires abandoning the Newtonian idea of a universal time that all clocks measure. Instead, everyone has his/her own personal synchronic time. The standard frame with regard to time would be a Newtonian idea of time applied to all analysands. In contrast, the Lacanian singular length session is an Einsteinian and quantum version of psychoanalytic practice. Standard time runs the same for everyone in every session. Non-standard time runs differently for every session.

The time of the unconscious is non-standard and personal, and therefore it is relative and symbolic, or imaginary time, as it is called in quantum physics. It is not the absence of time but rather a different dimension of time.

> Imaginary time is a relatively simple concept that is rather difficult to visualize or conceptualize. In essence, it is another direction of time moving at right angles to ordinary time. In the image at right (below), the light gray lines (horizontal) lines represent ordinary time flowing from right to left – past to future. The dark gray (vertical) lines depict imaginary time, moving at right angles to ordinary time.
>
> (Corbett, Stafford and Wright [2007]). [The bracketing and the imagc subsequently are mine.]

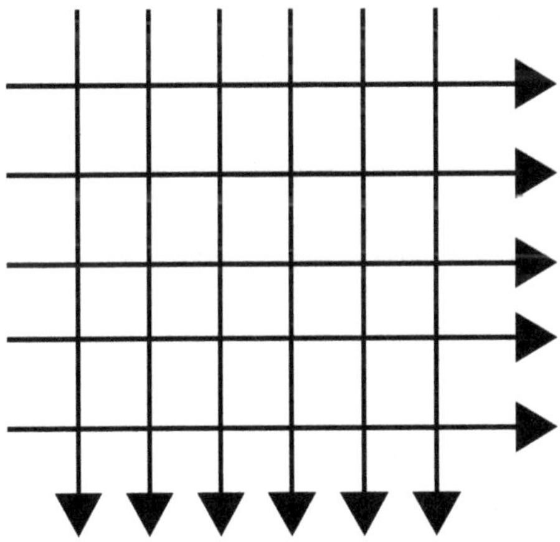

The logic of what I will call symbolic time precisely corresponds to the moment of cutting and concluding the session of analysis. In addition, imaginary, or what I am calling symbolic unconscious, time, "is a way of looking at the time dimension as if it were a dimension of space: you can move forward and backward along imaginary time, just like you can move right and left in space" (idem). Imaginary time, as a dimension of time, is the point of articulation between space and time. Time is not only linear from past to present, but it also goes from future or forward to the past and then to the present. For example, how an analysand looks forward to his/her future career invokes, activates, and carries along all the childhood wishes and conflicts associated with parental identifications.

The question of a different dimension of time is a point of consistency between relativity theory and quantum theory, both of which work with time-space continuity as a unit. Relativity theory works with the general structure of the universe, whereas quantum theory works with the infinitesimally small. In extremely small amounts of matter, time does not appear to be a direct function of movement from one place to another according to the speed of light. Small units of matter, such as sub-atomic particles, function according to non-locality and can travel instantaneously from one place to another faster than the speed of light. Here time stands still as opposed to only slowing down according to the speed of light.

With his notion of logical time, Lacan arrives at a new articulation of these two forms of time. The future is brought to bear on the past in the present. The future ending of treatment is enacted in the ending of each session. In addition, each ending of a session precipitates the working through of the past in the present and between sessions. The ending of a session does not follow a linear sequence, but rather the future end is brought to bear on the present.

With linear notions of time, we think that we recognize or discover something for the first time, then we understand it, and then it is time for concluding or ending a session. When the unconscious opens in analysis, we are looking at the mind as it was in the past. It is the eruption of the past in the present instant. In contrast to space-time in physics, in the mind-time continuum, we don't see the unconscious the way it was then but the way it is now, whereas the reverse is true in the time-space continuum. In the case of the stars, we see them the way they were in the past, but we do not know for a fact how they would appear in the present. The unconscious is over-here not over-there but also appears over-here the way it was in the past.

However, given that we do not have space and the speed of light as mediating factors, there is no way of confirming exactly how the unconscious was in the past. With the unconscious, we only know the past in the present. It is in this sense that Freud said there is no time in the Unconscious. The Unconscious is always in the present time: the present as it was in the past, as how it arises in the present moment, and as it will be in the future. In this sense, no time is the same as synchronic time.

The notion of the unconscious as always manifesting in the present moment reveals an interesting paradox given that the unconscious always seems to divide the subject. Although there is a subject of the unconscious, the subject is not under the conscious control of the ego. Although the unconscious does not fail to present the subject with unconscious truths, it is the ego who is not present or in tune with the reality of the unconscious. The ego lives in the past and the future (or diachronic time), while the unconscious lives in the present moment.

The unconscious appears, opens, or erupts over here, but it also closes within the session. Typically, patients want to continue talking about what they were talking about before the unconscious appeared. The patient does not behave like a lover, a mystic, or a scientist who has been waiting a long time for an event to happen. The patient does not want to know the unconscious subject/object, and therefore the moment of understanding cannot begin or take place. Most people are lovers of ignorance rather than unconscious knowing. This is the case because in analysis, the Unconscious mostly represents a knowing about lack and loss of both the ego and the object. Despite the resistances to unconscious knowing, the analyst directs his/her efforts to maintain the momentum of the opening of the unconscious.

Just like the unconscious appeared in symbolic time, the ending of the session, as a treatment tool, also has to end in symbolic time in order to facilitate the moment of understanding between sessions and not only within sessions. As the appearance of the unconscious refers to the manifestation of the past in the present, the ending of the session refers to the appearance of the future between sessions in the present. Both events are taking place in symbolic time.

The question regarding the effectiveness of the treatment also has to be understood in a non-conventional way in order to work with the unconscious and with what resists rational and conventional intervention. Even if the patient wants to cooperate with the doctor, the unconscious ego and the symptom may not. For this reason, in order to bypass the resistance of the ego or the symptom, the history of psychoanalysis, and medicine in general (placebo), is interwoven with that of hypnosis and suggestion as therapeutic techniques.

A therapeutic intervention takes place on a symbolic net and a mode of jouissance not under the control of the conscious ego of the patient. In most cases, within psychoanalysis, the approach to the symptom is both direct and indirect. It is direct with respect to the identification of the symptom, indirect with respect to its modification. I say in most cases, because there are always exceptions that confirm the norm. In cases of severe and frequent panic attacks, for example, a psychoanalyst, who is also a psychiatrist, may temporarily prescribe anti-anxiety medications, or a psychologist who is also a psychoanalyst may teach the analysand a relaxation exercise.

The Unconscious and the elimination of the symptom are like an experience of Zen enlightenment: if you turn towards it and try to grab it, it eludes you. Enlightenment and the Unconscious cannot be sought, only found. If you want to directly eliminate the symptom, the symptom will resist, but if you accept it as saying something necessary about desire, then the symptom may dissolve of its own accord. If experience is left open, then the Unconscious is right there in the here and now of analytical activity. Both analyst and analysand, sooner or later, should be energetically transformed and revived, or feel psychically enlightened, by the experience and sometimes traumatic encounter with the unconscious signifier. This may not always be pleasant, but it will certainly be experienced as a form of jouissance.

The types of jouissance the analyst experiences will depend on his/her own work and transformation with the different forms of jouissance. The elimination of the symptom is a by-product or a fruit of the manifestation of the unconscious. The objective criterion of effectiveness is subjective and rooted in the subjective experience of the subject. What seemed like an unbearable form of depression or anxiety, all of the sudden, inexplicably entirely disappears (or becomes bearable, like structure in general).

Lacan's interest in the non-standard frame and the direction of the treatment is intrinsically tied to the questions of the effectiveness, duration, and cost of the treatment. Treatments that last forever tend to become predictable. They go over the same material with the same ineffective interpretations. This has become the target of the re-formulations and renewal of Freudian practice in the Lacanian school.

The preliminary pre-treatment phase and the first phase of the treatment

This chapter examines the phases of analysis and links them to the faces of Oedipus to illuminate distinctions between analytic treatments writ large. The breakdown of the therapeutic process into three phases of treatment was initiated by Freud (1913). The word phase can be understood as a developmental sequence, or its meaning could also be understood following the ancient Greek word for appearance. Different aspects of a structure can unfold or appear over time, but the order of appearance may be contingent or arbitrary. In other words, the faces of a structure exist in both continuous or diachronic and discontinuous or synchronic time. The function of retroactivity actually is a way to combine both dimensions of time. What comes before in time determines what comes after (what comes after is built on the basis of what came before), and at the same time, what comes after redefines what came before. Both movements in time are true. What comes before is not built on what comes after: what comes after only redefines what was already there based on the interdependence of the structure. A building is built over time, but it all starts with the architectural and engineering plans that show the building as an entire interdependent structure.

Every event has a beginning and an end, but it also has a purpose or task. The purpose or task is what has to be accomplished during the middle phase in between the starting and ending of something, from the effect of the symptom to the fantasy or trauma and the cause of desire that results in the cure or transformation of the symptom into a post-analytical sinthome. The same can be said about the phases/faces of Oedipal structure. The first phase is the dyadic dual unity between mother and infant, and in the second phase, the father appears in the picture, although the Third and the father already existed as the background and origin of the reproductive sequence. The structure is only developmental for the child, but the child taken together with the parents and the culture represents an interdependent layered structure manifesting at any given point in time.

Taking a detailed clinical and personal history becomes a necessary precondition only for time-limited treatment or treatment in a clinic, including a history of prior treatment. What worked, what did not, and why? What was the focus of prior treatment? What does the patient say about the knowledge gained in previous treatment? It is not ethical to keep charging fees for the same form of treatment that did not work in the past.

Like in any clinical situation, the first interview begins with the question regarding the symptom. Although this is a traditional medical and clinical question, it has a particular psychoanalytic meaning regarding the beginning of the treatment. It creates the analytic space in which the analysand begins to distinguish between a malaise or discontent and the manifestation of a psychoanalytic symptom. In his introduction to the case of Dora, Freud (1905) said that many patients are particularly vague about the description of their symptoms. A symptom must be identified that will be the focus of the treatment, and this symptom must be understood as ego dystonic. The symptom refers to the patient's desire rather than to what others want or have done to them.

Thus, patients with a history of severe trauma are usually not good candidates for analytic treatment, because the question of desire is obscured by the presence of a trauma such as sexual abuse. In these patients, it may be counterproductive and retraumatizing to examine the question of desire. Ultimately, it is essential to reconcile the psychical and environmental dimensions of the trauma. This usually cannot be done in brief treatments or supportive treatments that may be otherwise necessary as a preliminary approach to the trauma.

An exception to this rule would be a case where the analysand has done a significant amount of trauma work but has not reconciled the trauma experience with the questions posed by their own desires and Oedipal structure. I have had patients who came to me because they had already done trauma work but were left unsatisfied because although they had been supported and told they were not to blame for boundary violations or sexual abuse of them as children by adults, the questions of desire had not been addressed. Conversely, some patients and professionals complain that in analysis, years went by and environmental traumas were ignored or not addressed.

We have to remember that aside from environmental traumas, whether sexual or violence related, human sexuality, especially in childhood, is traumatic in and of itself, and there are necessary grief processes that need to take place. The discovery of sexuality and sexual difference in childhood always has traumatic overtones and involves the forbidden aspect of human sexuality. Fantasy life begins in childhood, and therefore memory always has an aspect of fiction. Finally, sometimes fantasies may turn out to be actual events, and at other times, actual events may turn out to be fantasies.

In Lacanian analysis, the symptom will not necessarily be the signifier of the treatment, because in phase II, the symptom will be linked to emerging unconscious fantasies, dreams, and traumas. It is the latter, that will be the thematic and phantasmatic focus of the treatment. With the preliminary sessions and the first phase of analysis, the analysand begins to understand that the knowledge that will help him/her will emerge from them rather than from the professional knowledge of the analyst. The analysand will have to use their own words and language to describe their experience and symptoms. In doing this, the unconscious signifying chain determining the development of symptomatology within language will begin to emerge and manifest in speech and treatment.

By showing interest in what the analysand has to say or knows, whether consciously or unconsciously, the first phase of a transference relationship is also initiated. In contrast to suggestion or the leader/follower relationship of group psychology, the analyst is first in the position of lover rather than beloved. As mentioned earlier in this book, I follow Lacan (1960–1962) in Seminar VIII on the subject of the transference, where he uses the Greek categories of Erastes and Eromenos in order to account for what he calls the metaphor of love as it occurs in psychoanalytic treatment. He speaks of the metaphor of love to account for transformations in the transference during the phases of analysis.

If we speak of metaphor, we are speaking of substitution with respect to the reciprocal substitution that takes place between analyst and analysand in relation to the places of lover and beloved. At the outset of an analysis, the analyst is in two places, the place of Erastes (lover) and the place of what Lacan called the subject supposed to know(ing). These two places of the metaphor of love and the love transference (towards the subject supposed to know) are somewhat discordant.

In the first or beginning phase of analysis, the analysand is in the place of the beloved because he/she is worthy of the analyst's unconditional interest and attention, and the analysand is the object and purpose of the analytical operation. The 'empathic' analyst is the lover wanting to know something about the analysand and willing to hear anything they may want to say. Using the term lover, instead of simply speaking of the empathic function of the analyst, has the advantage of introducing the love dimension of the transference, as well as laying the ground for the introduction of the question of sexuality further on in the treatment.

On the other hand, the analyst is in the position of the subject supposed to know something about the analysand's suffering. Here the analyst appears to be the one in the position of the beloved. Nevertheless, at the beginning of the analysis, the subject supposed to know is not yet a full-blown object of the transference, because the analysand does not yet know what they lack or whether this lack is Real, Imagined, or Symbolic. In addition, the analysand does not know what their unconscious Other knows and desires. The analysand loves the analyst for what they know, but this first takes the form of a conscious therapeutic alliance.

I have also made a distinction between the subject supposed to know, which is how '*sujet suppose savoir*' is usually translated into English, and what I called subject supposed to knowing. The first would be a better rendition of the transference in the first phase of analysis, and the latter would be a better description of the second phase of transference.

In the first phase of analysis, the analyst is a foreground lover and a background beloved (as the subject supposed to know), whereas the reverse is true for the analysand. The beloved analysand offers himself/herself as a canvas on which the analyst may draw some brilliant designs. However, from the beginning, and thanks to the desire of the analyst, as a fruit of the personal analysis of the analyst, the analyst is not seduced into believing in the transference to the subject supposed to know.

The first phase of the treatment also corresponds with the oral and first phase of Oedipal structure in relationship to the mother. By loving the analysand in the sense of expressing an interest and unconditional regard for the free associations of the analysand, the analysand feels as if held by the therapeutic desire of the analyst. This promise and gift of love represents the romantic phase of a love relationship that echoes back to the first phase of Oedipus with the mother.

During the first phase of the treatment, the rule of free association is also given in the form of a paradoxical imperative to speak, but freely. Maternal desire and empathy will be experienced in the form of whatever you say; however insignificant or devalued, it will be accepted in analysis. However, the metaphor of maternal love goes only so far, given that the symbolic function of the father will be the underside of the rule of free association associated with the scansion of time and speech. Interpreting the rule of free association as a manifestation of maternal desire has the value of keeping the analysis of the unconscious central to the psychoanalytic endeavor instead of using good-enough mothering as a basis for redefining psychoanalytic treatment as a form of reparenting, education, socialization, or pastoral counseling.

For Winnicott (1965), the mother–infant relationship was the paradigm of the analytic process. Interpretation in psychoanalysis merely signifies maternal care.

> What matters to the patient is not the accuracy of the interpretation so much as the willingness of the analyst to help, the analyst capacity to identify with the patient and so to believe in what is needed and to meet the need as soon as the need is indicated verbally or in non-verbal or pre-verbal language.
>
> (p. 122)

In this model, the psychoanalytic situation becomes not much more than an extension of infant care and a biological maturational environment conducive to emotional growth. The analyst in fact does become a good-enough mother taking care of the infant's biological needs as if needs were not affected or structurally related to demands and desires that are psychical and oedipal in nature. The good-enough analyst believes in the transparency of biological needs and therefore is keen in responding to and satisfying the demands of the child taken to be natural and legitimate biological needs. By the same token, an analysis ends with an identification with the good breast or good-enough analyst that has reparented the analysand through a personal analysis.

Winnicott, Klein, Bion, and in general the object relations and attachment theorists who privilege the mother and the so-called two-person psychology justified their focus and developmental theories focused on the mother by saying that this new form of psychoanalysis was necessary for more disturbed forms of psychopathology that featured earlier developmental deficits, arrests, and fixations. Neurotics don't need to be reparented, but borderline and psychotic individuals do. We all know, for example, how Marilyn Monroe's analyst invited her to live with his family in order to give her a normal family experience, all to no avail, since she committed suicide shortly after that.

The analyst remains in the internal subjective position of an ideal parent-object that no real human being will ever come to close to matching in the person's life. The analysand may acquire the capacity to be alone but remains dependent on the figure of the analyst/parent. In this, our work is more Freudian than Kleinian, since Freud believed that the cathexis of the internal lost object had to be relinquished in order to find new links and relationships to the Other. Relinquishment in this case means the end of a relationship that also takes place, for example, with the death of a parent, but the parent still lives within the subject as part of the subject himself/herself, not as an idealized internal good object that the subject depends on.

Finally, the relationship to a benign social environment does not only require the desire of the mother and good-enough mothering. An acceptance of symbolic castration, the symbolic function of the f(Other), and entering into a social system of symbolic exchange is also required in order to function within society and inter-subjective relations as sexed beings within a symbolic and cultural environment.

Phase II of the treatment

I will describe this important phase of treatment in terms of the second phase of the transference, the emergence and working through of what Lacan calls the "crossing or traversing of the phantasm," and the intervention of the Other in the second phase of Oedipus. Just like the first phase of Oedipus involved the question of the jouissance of the (m)Other, the second phase of Oedipus involves the appearance of phallic jouissance. The last or third phase of analysis is termination in the sense of the logical end of analysis. In this chapter, we may allude to termination, but it will be relatively ambiguous whether I refer to the discontinuation of treatment or to the logical end and successful termination of treatment. The next chapter will briefly re-examine the phases of analysis, but from the exclusive perspective of the logical end of analysis proper.

With regard to the phases of treatment, the second phase of treatment is related to the moment of understanding in a couple of different ways. During the second phase of treatment, the moment of concluding continues to facilitate the working through of significant material. Once the knowing of the analyst comes to more or less coincide with the unconscious object of desire of the analysand, then the transference, properly speaking, and the second or intermediate phase of analysis has been established. Obviously, this cannot be the end of the story, because otherwise there would be no end or termination phase to the analysis. Analyses that last too long never leave the second phase of treatment, where the analyst is in the position of the beloved.

It is in the second phase of the treatment that the proto or primal fantasies or traumas of the subject will appear in consciousness and in the treatment. The analyst as lover helped to invoke these fantasies, and these same fantasies will come to mediate the relationship to the analyst as a fantasy object.

Symbolic castration represents the symbolic absence of the imaginary phallus for both analysand and analyst. Although the analyst may be perceived as having or being the imaginary phallus, the analysand cannot have this phallus either as an object or as self/object. This is the symbolic meaning of castration within the context of the treatment relationship. Working through this absence is what will facilitate access to phallic jouissance with someone else, not with the analyst.

From the Lacanian perspective on sexual difference and symbolic castration, the third phase of Oedipus is understood in a more complex way than the simple Freudian formulation that the boy has the certified imaginary phallus for when he grows up and identifies with the father, and the girl does not and identifies with the mother but also with the father as a representative of cultural ideals. With regard to the resolution of the Oedipus complex, the question is not so much whether a female will be able to identify with her mother or the female analyst or a male will identify with his father or male analyst. Masculinity, whether in males or females, enters the complex with the sense of having the imaginary phallus but then loses it under symbolic castration vis-à-vis the Other. Masculinity enters the complex by having the imaginary phallus but can only exit or resolve the complex by realizing the only way to securely have it: to lose it and grieve the loss thereof.

Femininity, in females or males, or a woman, whether female or male, enters Oedipal structure by not having the imaginary phallus or the phallus in the Imaginary register. If she comes to terms with this loss, she then may exit Oedipus, realizing that she has the phallus within the symbolic order both as a metaphor/ signifier and in relationship to the masculine other.

An analysand saw herself as a seer into the lack or flaws of others but was blind to her own. It was the defense against lack that generated the tendency to project and induce lack in the other. She thought that others had abandoned her but did not see how she constructed this abandonment destiny (hysteria not schizophrenia). This analysand perceived me as a Carlos Castaneda (1968) type of figure, referring to my qualities as a "seer" or "witch doctor." Her way of saying that I was a worthy Latino was by addressing me by the name of a famous Latino writer. She also flattered me by saying that I was a seer like she was.

During the moment of seeing, the analyst has to see the manifestation of the unconscious, not as a flaw, but as foolish knowing, in the analysand and the analyst. For example, in a narrative statement, the analysand said that her mother did not love her but then said that her mother thought she was the most beautiful of the children. One could say, with Karen Horney, for example, that this is a contradiction the analyst is pointing out to the analysand (her mother does not love her/ her mother loves her) or that this is a manifestation of unconscious knowing that the analysand does not know or does not want to know that she knows. Since she does not want to see (here she is blind) how her mother loves her, or wants to deny it, this knowing is unconsciously held. The analyst sees the unconscious as knowing and not as flaw or defect. Both forms of knowledge are correct but need to be re-interpreted or re-framed. This leads to a therapeutic alliance between the positive idealizing transference to the analyst supposed to know and the unconscious knowing of the analysand.

When the analysand praised me, I did not say "Thank you, that was a nice thing to say about me," assuming that I liked Carlos Castaneda. Instead I said nothing, or perhaps gave a half-smile, but certainly did not proceed to brag or have small social talk about what I know of Carlos Castaneda, or my training and accomplishments, and so on. The small pleasure and imaginary connection that would have come out of this would have been pale in comparison to the criticism it could have generated further on in the treatment. In other words, I did not believe in her transference and instead used her belief in me to point to her own unconscious knowing.

Then as a response to my intervention, instead of feeling that I was taking her mother's side, or the 'Other's' point of view against her, she produced the memory of her sister dressing her as an older beautiful woman whom the mother mistook as a lover of the father. From this, a dream followed that she was supposed to have a child with her father, and so on. Eventually, she felt she had had enough of me and left me rather than the other way, as was usual in her relationships.

This is an example of the analyst giving of what he/she does not have rather than what they have and of occupying the place of the lack or the absent *objet a* of the subject. As I stated earlier, it is the desire of the analyst, or the desire not to be desired as a beloved, or in this case, as a Carlos Castaneda, that functions as the fundamental pivot of the end and aim of psychoanalysis. In his/her symbolic function, the analyst gives the analysand from his own lack of the symbolic phallus rather than the deception of giving an object that does not exist. This analysand wanted her analyst to either be the *objet a* of her fantasy, for me to love her and lack her as my *objet a*, and for me to give her the imaginary phallus that she wanted to receive from her father.

I pointed to emptiness within desire rather than to a desire to be desired as a phallic object by showing the analysand that I accepted the lack within desire, that I was not Carlos Castaneda. My desire remained as a lack without identification with the signifier of the phallus, in this case Carlos Castaneda, or the gaze of the father. The analyst has to keep the lack as it is without identification with the imaginary phallus or with the idealized imaginary father. It is this subjective destitution that helps loosen up, unpack, and reveal the unconscious objects and signifiers at stake in the transference.

Being and not being Carlos Castaneda, or having and not having what he had, is what leads the regression from Carlos Castaneda, as a signifier of the analysand's desire, to her desire for her own father. Now the unconscious knowing of the analysand will replace the knowledge of the analyst. After the transference to the subject supposed to know, the analyst resumes his/her position of lover of the unconscious knowing of the analysand. It is the analysand being in the position of the beloved that will support the analysand in the sometimes-unpleasant task of recognizing unconscious knowing and experiences of lack in privation, frustration, and castration.

The analysand recognized that she was not abandoned by her mother or father and instead found the signifiers of her own unfulfilled desire. These meant that she was loved and desired but that what she wanted was not something that could be given to her. These discoveries or truths of desire do not in any way diminish or conceal the shortcomings or flaws of her parents. They become, however, an accepted aspect of the lack and inconsistencies of the Other.

Had I joined the analysand in her praising of me and proceeded to love her back by pointing out her good qualities and the shortcomings of her parents and supporting her in her grievances against parents and lovers, we would have joined in a narcissistic collusion of mutual imaginary admiration and had a wonderful love fest and romantic first phase of analysis. However, we would have effectively aborted any possibility of real future treatment.

Although the beloved analyst helps heal some of the wounds of the subject, the final removal of the analyst from the position of the beloved, and the demystification and deconstruction of this object into the vicissitudes of a narcissistic phallic object, leads the analysand to the end of analysis via a direct, decisive, and final confrontation with the symbolic rock of castration. In turn, it is from this confrontation that desire can be regenerated and turned towards another, not the analyst, no longer in the hope that the other give the subject something that they don't already have. Once the lack of imaginary castration is symbolized, then both having and not having can be a source of enjoyment and jouissance for the subject and the Other.

I also mentioned that the phases of transference love parallel the phases of love's transference in love relations, but with a few notable exceptions. Seduction represents the first phase of a love relationship. In analysis, seduction, as seen in this case, is the seduction of knowledge or the seduction of the subject supposed to know (the sorcerer or witch doctor). In love relationships, seduction is a promise of love that echoes back to the jouissance of the Other and to the first phase of Oedipus with the mother. This is echoed in the first phase of a treatment when the holding environment holds the promise of a good-enough mother or of the analyst being a better mother than the analysand's mother. The second phase of a romantic love relationship is the sexual and oedipal phase of phallic jouissance, the phase where the fundamental question is to have or not have the imaginary phallus. Romantic love becomes a question of desire, the desire to have and enjoy the imaginary phallus.

In analysis, the movement from love to phallic jouissance is not enacted. Instead, phallic jouissance should be located and deconstructed unto the vicissitudes of the *objet a*, the phallus, and the function of castration. I say should because many treatments do not proceed to this phase and instead stay in the asexual preoedipal or the first phase of Oedipus. In such treatments, if the paternal function is involved, it is usually in the form of suggestion and a reformation of the super ego into better action plans or a more realistic orientation to the patients' goals and objectives.

What, then, is the difference between analysis proper and psychotherapy, or between analyses conducted under different theoretical orientations? In what follows, I will use the phases of analysis and of Oedipal structure to differentiate different forms of analytical treatments. Psychotherapies done by non-analysts fall into a different category of treatment. Supportive therapies done by non-analysts, who have not had a personal analysis, are focused on the therapist being a better good-enough mother/father for the client, and the working alliance stays purely within the Imaginary. An imaginary transference means that there is a fusion between the subject supposed to know and the therapist as beloved and the patient as lover of the therapist. Since there is no awareness or analysis of the transference, the transference as such is not present or considered in these treatments.

In insight psychotherapy done by non-analysts, the treatment also remains within the first phase of treatment and of Oedipus. In these therapies, the therapist remains in the position of the subject supposed to know, but there is a beginning of an analysis of the imaginary transference. Since the therapist has not been analyzed, the therapist remains prone to the desire to be loved and desired by the patient. It is the desire of the analyst that facilitates the analysis of the symbolic dimension of the transference.

In these treatments, the therapist works with the countertransference as projective identification. The unconscious of the analyst is analyzed as if it were the unconscious of the analysand. The concept of projective identification implies that in analysis, the subjective experience of the analyst is determined by the analysand, and the analyst's unconscious has no impact here or is irrelevant.

In contrast to this, from a Lacanian perspective, in such cases, the unconscious of the analyst, as the discourse of the Other, returns to the analyst via the unconscious of the analysand rather than vice versa. In analysis proper, the unconscious of the analysand, or the jewel of their own being, returns to the analysand via the speech of the analyst as the discourse of the Other. Here the Other means the analysand's own unconscious rather than the analyst functioning as a representative of 'objective knowledge.' Alternatively, the countertransference could take therapists, who are not analysts, to their own personal analysis.

As I have already mentioned, there are also analyses that remain within the first phase of the transference and of Oedipal structure as well. This is usually presented as a necessary analysis of preoedipal formations, and although these treatments have clinical value and analytic import, they also may represent overt or thinly disguised disavowals and rejections of both Freudian Oedipal theory and the function of the father and the phallus. Here the analyst works within the transference but only in regard to the maternal transference representing the first phase of Oedipus. Since the function of the third, as the function of the father and of the phallus, is not symbolized, the preoedipal mother differs from Lacan's view of the mother during the first phase of Oedipus.

In the preoedipal view of the mother-child relationship, the inevitable investment of the child with the phallic narcissism of the mother is mistaken for bad-enough mothering. The part played by the father and symbolic castration in generating good-enough mothering or a mother-child-subject relationship is not recognized. In analyses focused on pre-oedipal relationships the questions of the phallus, sexual difference and castration are not addressed in order not to antagonize either the defenses of the analysand or of the culture.

References

Castaneda, C. (1968). *The Teachings of Don Juan: A Yaqui Way of Knowledge.* New York: Pocket Books, 1996.

Corbett, D., Stafford, K. and Wright, P. (2007). http://library.thinkquest.org/27930/time.htm.

Freud, S. (1905). *Dora, An Analysis of a Case of Hysteria.* New York: Touchtone, 1997.

Freud, S. (1913). On Beginning the Treatment (Further Recommendations on the Technique of Psychoanalysis I). *The Standard Edition of the Complete Psychological Works of Sigmund Freud*, 12, 1911–1913.

Lacan, J. (1960–1962). *Transference: The Seminar of Jacques Lacan.* Book VIII. London: Polity Press, 2017.

Lacan, J. (1966). Logical Time and the Assertion of Anticipated Certainty. In: *Ecrits.* Translated by B. Fink. New York: Norton, 2006.

Winnicott, D. (1965). *The Maturational Processes and the Facilitating Environment.* London: Routledge, 2018.

12 The third phase of pure analysis

The aim and end of analysis proper

Introduction

Lacan emphasized that although it is the analyst who ends the session, it is the analysand who ends the treatment. The desire of the analyst differs from ordinary human desire in that for the analysis to succeed, the analyst must not desire to keep the analysand in analysis beyond the logical end of analysis. The analyst does not resist becoming dispensable to the analysand. If the logical end has been reached, the analyst supports the analysand's desire to end the analysis. At the point of termination, there is a loss of jouissance (less is more) for both parties: a subjective destitution for the analysand and a benevolent depersonalization for the analyst.

With human desire, a subject does not want to be left by loved ones unless, of course, they are neurotic and need to fail in relationships because of winning in Oedipus. The successful ending of analysis is like an Oedipal failure, except that it is the son or daughter that rejects the parent rather than the other way around. When ending the treatment with the analyst, the analysand may then have a relationship with their parents and with a lover or beloved. On the other hand, since analysis makes for unity, but not necessarily for normative social relations, an analysis may also result in a realignment and separation from family blood ties.

The desire of the analyst has two main characteristics. First, the desire that the analysand come to sessions and continue speaking and generating unconscious knowing. Second, that the analysand not idealize the analyst and rely on their own unconscious knowing rather than depending on the analyst's professional knowledge. Otherwise, the analysand may not want to end the analysis. The analyst points to the subject's own unconscious because at the logical end of analysis, unconscious knowing will make the analysand independent from the analyst.

Lacan said that analysis is like literature where both the writer and the reader go from the letter to the litter, or from the litter to the letter. A litter represents a creative literary offspring or offshoot and at the same time a disposable yet organic and recyclable waste product. The letters of the unconscious are the signifiers of the alpha objects cause of the subject's desire (the litter). With the litter of letters, the litter, or the objects that letters designate, become objects of desire that have been lost and are in need of symbolization in the experience and life of the subject.

If unsymbolized, the *objet a* becomes a clinker, or an incombustible residue, a non-recyclable toxic product. The installation and symbolization of the analyst as an imaginary phallus or *objet a*, cause of the subject's desire, because of the very nature of the *objet a* as an object of waste meant to be lost, eventually moves the analyst from representing an imaginary object to the place of the *objet a* in the Real. The analytical process moves the analyst from the position of the beloved imaginary object (*a*/phallus) to the position of the absence or emptiness of the *objet a*. The analysis ends when the *objet a* dissipates or evaporates in its approach to the Real of the unconscious. The objective object is first constructed and then destroyed, as Winnicott envisioned.

When the analyst wishes to remain in the place of the imaginary object, cause of the subject's desire, or wishes that the analytical position will result in some gain or benefit for the analyst's own imaginary ego, then the very nature of the object will remove the analyst from this position. In reality, the analytical position, rather than an imaginary or unjust form of power differential or asymmetry, in fact, does nothing for the analyst's own imaginary ego. At the end of analysis, the analyst becomes like fertilizing manure that needs to be flushed, evacuated, and let go. The analyst becomes disposable and dispensable to the analysand. The analyst needs to write himself/herself out of a job, but because he/she can do so, they can actually do an adequate job and make an honorable living.

If the analyst remains in the position of the subject supposed to know or as the *objet a* or phallus of the analysand, the analysand will never want to leave the analyst. Once the transference in analysis has been dissolved, and the analyst becomes an empty other that does not represent the ego ideal for the analysand, the analysand will still have his/her own unconscious, conscious ideals, and love transference to live by.

The objection could be raised that the very fact the analyst does not need to be loved or idealized to feel secure or recognized does not mean he/she is not a master but is precisely what makes him/her a master by not being afraid of being alone or of death. Being towards death "All Alone": this is Hegel's definition of a master, since death is something everyone goes through alone despite how many people may accompany a dying person. This could be all the more a reason to idealize the analyst. However, the emptiness of the symbolic father or analyst is not without lack or limitation.

The master is also a servant. It is not always entirely clear whether the master is a master or a servant. The analyst pays with his person and with the core of his being when he/she lets the analysand see him more as a servant with limitations than as a master, even if the analysand is mistaken in this regard. This is in the service of facilitating the process of termination and separation so that the analysand can '*se-parere*' or give birth to himself/herself.

In addition, the analyst does not fail to not hide his/her failures and forgetting when these actually manifest and to offer interpretations that may put him/her at a disadvantage with respect to his/her own defenses. This is what, in reference to the analyst, Lacan called paying with one's person and with words. It may be that by operating strategically in this way, the analyst remains the master in the end, but if so, then only he/she knows it.

The analyst is alone in the face of the Real and is satisfied with being either a servant or a master to himself and to the other. This is the Other jouissance of the fool, and the idiot who is truly wise and with Oedipus knows that losing can be winning and that winning can also be losing. The child has to be second to the parent and learn to lose the desired parent to the forbidding parent so that they may win in life and marriage or relationships. At the same time, in treatment, succeeding is succeeding and failing is failing. Sometimes analysands will say that you did not help them, and you did. Other times, they will tell you that you did help them, and you did not. To be wise is to quietly and calmly know the difference.

The aim and the end

The question regarding the end of analysis implies something beyond the final moment of a process. In fact, the way the final phases of analysis are conceived influences the direction of psychoanalytic treatment from the very beginning.

In Spanish and English, the same word is used to describe an aim or objective (fin/end) and the end of something (fin/end). Thus, it is the aim or objective concerned which allows for the definition and/or the termination of an activity. For this reason, in this chapter, both of these themes will cross-fertilize and interact with one another: the aim of analysis and the termination of analysis. Depending on how the aim is defined, the aim and the end may be similar or different.

For example, if the aim of analysis is to build the identity of the ego and the therapeutic alliance, then, given this premise, it is not surprising that psychoanalysis would end with the identification with the analyst. In the case of the object-relations school, if the aim of analysis is the development of secure attachment (Bowlby), good-enough mothering (Winnicott), or the acquisition of the alpha function (Bion), then it is not surprising that analysis would end with the identification with the good object (the Kleinian analyst).

In contrast to these perspectives, within Lacanian psychoanalysis, the aim of the analysis of identifications is the end of the identification with the analyst.

> Any conception of analysis that is articulated – innocently or not, God only knows – to defining the end of the analysis as identification with the analyst, by that very fact makes an admission of its limits. Any analysis that one teaches as having to be terminated by identification with the analyst reveals, by the same token; that its true motive force is elided. There is a beyond to this identification defined by the relation and the distance of the objet petit a to the idealizing capital I of identification. . . . This crossing of the plane of identification is possible.
>
> (Lacan, 1964, Sem. XI, p. 272)

> Anyone who has lived through the analytic experience with me to the end of the training analysis knows that what I am saying is true.
>
> (p. 273)

> For the fundamental mainspring of the analytic operation is the maintenance of the distance between the I – identification – and the a (idem).
>
> It is in as much as the analyst's desire, which remains an x, tends in a direction that is the exact opposite of identification, that the crossing of the plane of identification is possible, through the mediation of the separation of the subject in experience.
>
> (p. 274)

The aim of the desire of the analyst is to eventually work himself/herself out of a job by becoming dispensable rather than indispensable. When the analysand no longer identifies with the analyst, the analyst becomes dispensable and the analysis has reached its logical conclusion. Lacan argues that at the end of a Lacanian analysis, the analysand identifies with the sinthome rather than with the analyst.

Psychoanalysis goes around the circle of identification twice. "The termination of analysis occurs when one has gone around a circle twice; namely, to re-discover that which holds one captive" () (Lacan, Seminar XXV, Session 4: Wednesday 10, January 1978). Identifications have to be first recognized and deconstructed and then relinquished or taken away. This process is part and parcel of the path by which the desire of the subject is recognized and differentiated from the desire of the Other or from the desire to be recognized by the Other. When identifications (with the analyst and other significant figures) are abandoned, the subject finds his or her identity in the larger symbolic structure and the wondrous emptiness of unbeing (désêtre of the subject and the Real according to Lacan, 1966–1967).

> When he puts himself there [in the position of psychoanalyst], after having himself taken the psychoanalytic path, he already knows where he will be led to then as psychoanalyst by the path to be re-travelled: the désêtre of the subject supposed to know by being nothing but the support of this object called the object a.
>
> (Lacan, Seminar XV, Session of 1/17/1968, VI 100)

Terminable, interminable

Given Lacan's call for a creative return that retroactively re-founds the meaning of Freud's work, I will begin by examining Freud's approach to the subject. It is important to remember that Freud's discussions with Ferenczi regarding Ferenczi's "active technique" played the role of a precipitating event in motivating Freud to write *Analysis Terminable and Interminable* (1937). In the history of psychoanalysis, the question of introducing technical modifications is often linked to attempts to abbreviate the process of the cure. The criteria used to determine the termination of analysis becomes a question of the utmost importance.

The meaning of Freud's title establishes the guidelines of a clinical program. Freud does not propose an option or alternative, but, quite the contrary, he emphasizes that an analysis is both terminable and interminable, a veritable paradox, therefore. And this does not apply to some analysands and not to others but to each and every one of them. On the other hand, an analysis has to have an end, because otherwise it would be interminable. And if regular sessions end, how can analyses be interminable?

Freud remarked that when he began his psychoanalytic practice, he did not know what to do in order to have his analysands conform to what he termed an analytic or therapeutic pact. Conversely, once Freud had fine-tuned the analytic situation, he did not know what to do in order to terminate the analysis.

> In the early years of my psycho-analytic practice I used to have the greatest difficulty in prevailing on my patients to continue their analysis. This difficulty has long since been shifted, and I now have to take the greatest pains to induce them to give it up.
>
> (1913, p. 130)

In analysis terminable/interminable, Freud proposes two criteria by which to determine whether a treatment can be ended and considered successful: if the symptoms have been resolved and whether enough unconscious material has been evoked and resolved in the treatment and the transference relationship so as not to have concerns about possible relapses in the future. The latter point is important, because only if the treatment has had a therapeutic effect on the symptoms could one consider the treatment as having produced robust and long-lasting effects. Otherwise, the symptoms could have temporarily resolved for reasons unrelated to the treatment. In this case, the analysand could remain prone to relapses in the future.

However, Freud stops short of claiming that a treatment could have future preventive power. Although the treatment produced the remission of the symptoms, the analyst or psychoanalysis cannot predict accidental or environmental factors that could have an adverse or regressive effect on an analysand's condition in the future. Psychoanalysis has an effect on symbolic causality but not on chance or causality in the Real in the form of a gap (Tyche, according to Lacan [1964]). Causality in the form of a gap refers to the Real unconscious modeled after a cut and topology more than a signifying structure. The Real of jouissance intersected by the signifier manifests within a signifying chain or within the gaps of the signifying chain but is not caused or conditioned by Symbolic causal series.

According to Freud, the resolution of the symptoms is directly related to two factors: either the strength of ego defenses or the weakness of the drives. The reverse is true for the persistence of the illness or the failure of the treatment: they are due to the weakness of ego defenses or the strength of the drives. What is ambiguous in Freud's description is the meaning of the strength or weakness of defenses. By the weakness of defense, Freud means not only the absence of necessary defenses but also the predominance of unconscious defenses.

Paradoxically, unconscious defenses weaken the ego, although unconscious defenses are supposed to emanate from an unconscious part of the ego. Based on the same premise, one could make the opposite argument: the ego is so strong because it has roots in both conscious and unconscious processes, and it is this strength that is responsible for the development of symptomatology. Freud was a believer in conscious and rational forms of repression or of "mastery" of the drives. He only rejects unconscious forms of repression as being counter to healing and the therapeutic aims of psychoanalysis.

In this, Freud is a traditionalist, and his writings are co-extensive to the more general process of secularization of religious principles characteristic of modernity. Freud pictures the ego and the drives in equivalent terms to the distinction between good and evil. However, we also know from his theory that ego defenses can also be problematic and that not much happens in life without the drives. In addition, the repressed amounts to more than simply the drive as a kind of evil inclination that needs to be tamed by morality and reason.

Freud's theory is more nuanced and less moralistic and dualistic when he speaks of the repressed in terms of repressed conflicts, traumas, or developmental fixations. In this context, he emphasizes the principle of undoing rather than redoing ego-repression and how the repressed needs to emerge and be resolved and worked through in the course of the treatment. The more the unconscious played a central role in the treatment, the more likely the resolution of the symptoms will be. However, in my work, the unconscious encompasses both the Ucs. of the repressed and the Ucs. of the repressive.

When symptoms are not resolved, then this is due to the intensity of the symptom or to the jouissance of the symptom (pain/pleasure linked to it). The jouissance of the symptom in Lacan is equivalent to the intensity of the drive in Freud's work. Freud attributes the failure of the treatment to either the jouissance or the strength of the drive or to the failure of defenses. The first is what leads Lacan to develop the notion of the sinthome tied to the jouissance or drive dimension of the symptom. For Lacan, since the drive cannot be extinguished, the symptom continues after analysis in the form of the sinthome. However, the sinthome also has an aspect of defense built into it. The sinthome allows for jouissance but also contains it by re-knotting the three dimensions of experience (RSI).

Before proceeding on to the analysis of the question of ego defenses, an important point must be made in relationship to the question of the stubbornness or the insistence and repetition of the symptom. This point is usually made to invalidate psychoanalysis as a form of effective treatment. The case of the Wolf man is often cited as an example of a fraudulent or false claim on the part of Freud. It is claimed that Freud claimed that he had cured the Wolf man of his symptoms, when in fact his symptoms persisted throughout his life. However, Freud was clear on the process by which and how the Wolf man returned to treatment, with him and others, and had a way of accounting for the successes and failures of the treatment. The Wolf man spent over 70 years in analysis, and this example is used to discredit psychoanalysis as a form of medical or psychological treatment.

What is often overlooked is that there are plenty examples of failed treatments in other psychiatric treatment modalities. Experienced clinicians know that medications are never as effective as reported in empirical or controlled statistical studies. Symptoms of depression and anxiety persist despite years of anti-anxiety or antidepressant medications, not to mention the case of antipsychotic medications. Medications are less expensive but not necessarily more effective than psychoanalysis. The same can be said of behavioral treatments. If one focuses attention on the patient and the symptom, by writing down the symptom as it manifests on a daily basis, for example, or seeing the patient several times a week for the purpose of suppressing the symptoms via various kinds of behaviors that strengthen defenses (exercise, entertainment, relaxation, etc.), then this intervention will indeed have an effect on the symptom, but the question is for how long will the modifications last, or how robust will they be? It is kind of unbelievable that behaviorists think that symptoms can be reliably eliminated for good without any consideration given to the patient's history, family, relationships, sexual life, or passions.

The analysis of ego defenses: obstacle or treatment?

According to Freud, when the ego is "crippled," regular ego defenses cannot defend against anxiety, explosiveness, addiction, or depression, just to name a few examples. Freud attributes the intensity and the pathogenic nucleus of these symptoms to the quantitative factor of the drives. But the question that follows from this assumption is whether the buildup of healthy defenses reinforces unconscious defenses or allows for them to be undone and modified. Freud answers this question when he says that the better is the enemy of the good. If, by building healthy defenses, the analysand feels good, he/she will not want to do the painful work of undoing unconscious defenses. It is ego strength, not weakness, that is an obstacle to the cure.

When considering the obstacles to effective treatment, Freud asks what obstacles there are to build stronger defenses rather than what the obstacles are to undoing repression or to revealing/disclosing the truths about the subject's desire. He considers that he had already done the latter with limited success in the early period of psychoanalysis. Lacan (1955), for his part, wants to go back to the early Freud but does not address the legitimate reasons that Freud gave for his later focus and theorizing on ego defenses.

When focusing on the defensive process rather than the repressed content, Freud is more interested in strengthening ego defenses than in finding a new way of working with or undoing unconscious defenses and resistances. Of the initial group of early analysts, Reich (1933) was the one follower of Freud who focused on ego defenses to undo rather than strengthen them (the technique of character analysis). Lacan's answer to Freud's interest in (strengthening) ego defenses was to shift the analysis of resistance to the analyst. I shall return to this further on.

Freud writes as if generosity and kind-heartedness, for example, were qualities associated with the alleged harmony of the ego, whereas miserliness and hostility are quantities of the id. In the developed character, the strength of the ego prevails over the strength of the id. This refers to the question of identification involved in the formation of the ego ideal. According to Freud (1900/1923), the ideal qualities of generosity and kindness are formed by identification with what is opposite to the tendencies and quantities of miserliness and hostility that have been abandoned. A child identifies with the generosity and kindness he/she is shown by his parents. However, such generosity and kindness may have been there all along, since Freud grants that at the beginning, the ego and the id evolve out of a single matrix. The actions of parents strengthen certain traits and weaken others.

The ego and the id are never completely synthesized nor separated (not one/not two). The ego is never pure and undefiled, and the id is not only impure and defiled. Often there is more honesty in the id and in desire than in the presumptions of the ego, tainted as they are with narcissistic forms of self-love and self-righteousness. The ego lives by the fantasy of being the master of his/her own house. It is this fantasy of becoming someone important, of replacing or vindicating the father, which represents an attempt to close or suture the gap in the ego. It is this attempt that leads to a division rather than a unity of the subject. The ego lacks the object that would make him/her a master. The true master is not a master, or is the emptiness above the crown of power, political, administrative, or otherwise.

But to get to the emptiness beyond the crown of power, the subject has to work through the quantitative factors that were associated with the imaginary projects of the ego: anxiety, loss, lack, grief, and anger. Although these quantitative factors divide the ego, they contain useful and pure qualities needed to produce a psychical state that does not spontaneously occur within the ego, or at least is usually found obstructed within the imaginary dimensions of the ego. It is the combination/amalgamation between the quantitative id factors and the qualitative factors associated with the ego that, taken together, lead the subject towards the emptiness of both ego and object.

I link the qualitative factors in the ego to what I call "It" (das Ding or the 'no-thing'), as the emptiness of the subject of the Real that comes into being at the place where the subject disappears from the statement. The subject comes into the scene as the Being of non-being. The Being of non-being, as the lack in the Other, gives access to symbolic understanding and new permutations/realizations of the symbolic structure. As Lacan pointed out, after Lao Tse, within the Symbolic, the subject knows without knowing that it knows. This unknown knowing of the subject or of a non-ego differs from the unconscious part of the ego of the defenses.

Freud was optimistic that better, shorter, and less expensive treatments can be achieved by giving more help and strengthening the ego. However, better therapy that will strengthen the ego is the therapy that suppresses/represses the symptom, or masters the drive, in the style of common sense and behavioral interventions. Ego psychology goes hand in hand with behaviorism or cognitive therapy. Freud intends to replace pathogenic unconscious repression with current, flexible, rational, and healthy defenses.

But can better repressions be developed without conjuring up the repressed? Does treatment fail because better defenses cannot be built due to the weakness of the ego or because repression has not been undone? Ego defenses do not allow pain and want displeasure over in the shortest amount of time. So how is it, then, that a stronger ego is good for treatment? Would a stronger ego tolerate more pain, or would it want the pain over in the shortest amount of time? This is another contradiction. In fact, it is the ego that needs to be let go and replaced by a different organizing principle.

It is the symbolic order and the subject that can allow for the signification of desire, for its manifestation and clarification, and at the same time for symbolization that places desire squarely within the dimension of the Law. One could object that this is a square desire and argue in favor of the romantic and postmodern notion of drives and desires that are independent of any law. However, this leads to postmodern chaos, catastrophe, early deaths, and suicides, if not perversion. The borderline and narcissistic conditions are ample evidence that such notions lead to problems with impulse control, unbridled individualism, and the illusions of a sexuality not determined by the regularities of social or natural laws.

How can the ego be the part of the analysand that the analyst can ally with in order to further the cause of the treatment if the ego is one of the biggest obstacles to the cure? Related to this is whether the ego works under the pleasure principle or the reality principle and how the pleasure principle is defined: as the organizing principle of the drives or of the ego? The notion of the therapeutic alliance, for example, relies on the link between the ego and the reality principle, not between the ego and the pleasure principle.

Freud defined the reality principle as the temporary tolerance and acceptance of displeasure in order to achieve a more lasting, stable, long-term satisfaction. But this definition contradicts the definition of the ego as being intolerant of displeasure. The desire to avoid pain interferes with the possibility of more long-term solutions to mental problems. The ego has to be willing to put up with some temporary pain in order to be released from suffering. The ego is an obstacle to this objective.

The ego of the defenses is also the ego of narcissism because the pain involved in making the unconscious conscious necessarily involves the recognition that the ego is not the master of the psyche. It is a mistake to think of the ego as the dominant mental agency. This is what Lacan (1969) called the master's discourse that interferes with the discourse of the analyst and the aims of psychoanalytic treatment. The undoing of the defenses requires the recognition that the subject does not know a lot about himself/herself and that some of the historical fictions/memories/narratives may be incorrect or at least fantasized and that the symbolic Other, and the discipline of the signifier is also required to restore continuity to experience.

The challenge for psychoanalytic treatment is how to achieve the twin goals of helping the analysand accept suffering as part of the analytical process and at the same time maintain a positive transference in the analytical relationship. There are some built-in gratifications in the transference that make this tolerable or possible. The analyst does not provide recognition or support for narcissistic identifications, and the empathy with ego defenses needs to be short lived. But what takes their place? The answer lies in the dynamics of transference love, another aspect of the practice of analysis that Lacan illuminated. I will return to this in a section up ahead.

Another requirement of this therapeutic task is not only the suspension of ego defenses, or the tolerance of a narcissistic injury, but also the deconstruction of the super-ego. By this, I mean that whatever the analyst does, it should not be intended as a form of punishment, since this is what the illness is thriving and depending on.

Freud established equivalence between the ego and a text, when in fact the better comparison may have been between the unconscious and a text. Lacan (1957a, 1957b, p. 163) calls the unconscious "the discourse of the Other." It is this discourse that is "riddled" with holes, allusions, avoidances, distortions, and so on. In the interpretation of dreams, Freud (1900) used the example of a censored public text to explain the workings of the dream censor in the production of a dream. However, in *Analysis Terminable and Interminable*, Freud only thinks of censorship in terms of either the ego or the pleasure principle.

In addition, both Freud and Lacan ignore the fact that Freud early on used the pleasure principle to explain the sexual drive and the tendency towards wish fulfillment. It is this double aspect of the pleasure principle that is related to the unconscious as a discourse. The unconscious and the pleasure principle not only represent and organize drives but also the unconscious tendency towards symbolization and censorship.

For Freud, pathogenic defenses weaken the ego or produce what he calls an ego modification that affects and interferes with the course of treatment. Pathogenic defenses cripple the ego or healthy ego defenses and function. This formulation would work if it were not for the fact that pathogenic defenses are also fixated at the level of the ego or, more strongly, emanate from the unconscious ego, according to the Freud of the Ego and the Id. It is a case of the ego crippling the ego. So, again, do we want to strengthen or weaken the ego to further the cause and success of psychoanalytic treatment? One possible answer that Freud gives is that we want to weaken the unconscious ego and strengthen the conscious ego. This would also work if it were not for the fact that the conscious ego is also an obstacle to the treatment. The ego says: "I'm fine, I am not so bad after all, I am feeling better now, and I would rather not talk about that."

The analysis of the formations of the repressive unconscious

Symptoms persist due to the jouissance at play, that is to say, the pleasure involved in even the most horrible forms of psychical pain. A person wants to both cling to the pleasure in the symptom and avoid the pain in the same, a kind of impossible (Real) state of affairs. It is the avoidance of unpleasure that constitutes one of the main motives behind defenses. On the other hand, it is the seeking of pain that constitutes the second opposite motive for preserving the symptom. The ego wants to suffer for two reasons: to cling to pleasure or jouissance and satisfy the need for punishment or pain. The latter represent two aspects of jouissance and of the super ego: the demand to enjoy and the equal demand to suffer, two aspects of passion or pathos (suffering).

One of the key manifestations of ego defenses is denial or defensive rather than creative negation. The ego says, "I rather or I don't want to talk about that, and if you insist, I can make life very unpleasant for you." The patient routinely avoids talking about certain subjects (topics and people), to the point where the analyst finally gives up asking and begins to collude with the patient's defenses. This leads to stagnation and interrupted or partially successful/unsuccessful treatments. This example underscores the convergence of the aim with the end. If a treatment is going nowhere, the treatment may end without having reached its logical end point. In this sense, termination refers to a phase in treatment that comes after a significant amount of unconscious material has been evoked and worked through. If a treatment ends without having passed the beginning or middle phases of treatment, then this is not an end in either sense of end as aim or conclusion. The end simply means the stopping of the sessions.

It is always unclear in Freud's texts, as in life, whether the problem/obstacle is the strength or the weakness of ego defenses. Sometimes Freud writes as if the treatment would have been more successful if the ego defenses were stronger and the ego was able to successfully suppress a symptom, the jouissance and impetus of the drive, or the Oedipus complex. In this, Freud's approach to treatment is quite similar to common sense and to behavioral treatments that depend on various successful defenses against symptoms. Sometimes Freud also writes as if pathological defenses/repressions in childhood had altered the ego's ability to use healthy defenses. Unconscious repression stemming from childhood alters the ability of the ego to use conscious or rational defenses against the symptom/drive. At other times, Freud refers to the need to alter the ego defenses in the treatment. Here he attributes unconscious repression to the ego rather than identifying the ego with health, rationality, and consciousness or self-awareness.

In my opinion, this is what led Lacan to reject the analysis of ego resistances altogether and to identify the latter with an unsuccessful attempt at repression and social conformity, equivalent to behaviorism and adaptation to the environment. In "Variants of the Standard Treatment," Lacan (1955) critiques the analysis of resistances insofar as it relates to the school of ego psychology and the analysis of the ego. He believes that this variant of the treatment ignores the analysis of the formations of the unconscious that truly represents the right treatment for the symptoms. What I have called the multiform criterion, or the non-standard frame, refers to the variants of the standard treatment. The non-standard frame responds to a logical or mathematical (metaphorical) framework more than stemming from Lacan's idiosyncrasies or psychopathology, as some have wanted to claim. The non-standard frame is a subfield or a different model of the frame rather than simply the absence of a frame. I don't consider the variable-length session a short session, since the short session is a variant of the former. Finally, the variable-length session takes place against a background of a unit of chronometrical time (the analytic hour within which analysands are scheduled).

Lacan emphasizes that the analysis of resistance is always within speech and that defenses are taking place within the discourse. Lacan contrasts the analysis of speech and discourse, from the view that attributes to the ego the sense function that determines the understanding and meaning of words. For Lacan, the truth-value of words is found in unconscious desire and not at the level of the ego.

However, Freud's ambiguity with regard to the ego and to defenses may continue to be a source of exploration and of new discoveries that may advance the course and future of clinical psychoanalysis. In this regard, Lacan may have thrown out the baby with the bath water. I agree with Lacan that the problem is the strength and not the weakness of the ego and that the imaginary ego needs to be deconstructed and let go in the process of analytic treatment. However, I believe that, precisely for this very same reason, the analysis of defenses remains a crucial aspect of analytic treatment and of an analytic understanding of suffering (psychopathology).

A clinical example can help to illustrate this point. In the example provided by a new case of a supervisee of mine, the analysand told him that he had sex with a different man every day since his last session. The supervisee did not know what to do with the material and feared correctly that a transference interpretation would increase the defenses against the analysis. At the same time, the analyst candidate did not want to say something that would make the analysand feel judged by the analyst.

I suggested that he needed to ask the analysand simply to speak about what he thought or felt about what he told the analyst. The subjunctive mode within the statement is what is called an '*irrealis* mood' that allows the speaker to have their own responses to what he/she said and in particular to be able to disagree with himself/herself. Such responses are sayings that reveal the subject of the enunciation and the unconscious rather than producing the closure associated with the dogmatic ego of the statement.

In this instance, the analysand may tell the analyst that he feared or was angered by the possibility that the analyst could judge him for his 'acting out.' In response, the analyst could help the analysand explore how the analysand himself felt about his actions. In turn, the analysand could become conscious of how he has some judgments about his actions and how he projects his own judgments unto the Other (for the analysand, the Other represents a social authority). Via the projection, and the inversion of demand, his own desire for the Law becomes the desire of the Law or of the Other.

This example helps illustrate how desire is acted out, or repressed by 'expression,' and, in turn, what is overtly repressed is the repressive activity of the analysand's own conscience and unconscious censor. The analysand may also be provoking the analyst to make a transference interpretation so that the analysand could tell the analyst all about his sexual fantasies with the analyst. Here possible unconscious fantasies with a father figure are being acted out rather than repressed or are being repressed by acting instead of remembering. In this example, what needs to be addressed first is the repressive rather than the repressed unconscious. But is there a difference between unconscious judgments and the workings of the unconscious censor, or between the repressed super ego and the repressive unconscious?

As Freud himself acutely observed, all the dream work censor does is use the same processes involved in language and judgment to confuse the relations among the terms. The terms don't change, but their location does (an interruptive dislocation pattern, therefore). Self is replaced by other, love by hate, and inclusion by exclusion, just to name a few. In addition, the structure of judgment, unconscious censorship, and the symbolic order of language are all coextensive to one another, with only one exception.

The exception involves the drive or the affective component of judgment or censorship that justifies carving out a separate category for the super-ego. The repressed and unconscious repressive super ego is the same as the repressive unconscious, with the exception that the super ego appears to be personally angry with the subject, much like a sadistic angry parent. The super ego is the personal and drive dimension of unconscious judgment. Personal here refers to lived experience, but, paradoxically, personal also refers to the impersonal death drive working through the laws of the Code.

The difference between the analysis of the repressive unconscious and Reich's technique of character analysis is that despite the common objective of deconstructing ego defenses, Lacan does not believe that desire can exist without the Law. In contrast to this, Reich believed it was possible to reach an unrepressed desire buried under social prohibitions and defenses. For Lacan, the prohibition of desire generates desire at the same time.

Lacan often emphasized how desire is intrinsically intertwined and entangled with the function of the Law. The Law for Lacan functions unconsciously and unconsciously produces the effects of repression. The Law not only conceals but also reveals and produces desire. We want what we can't have and don't want what we have or can have. The formations of the unconscious, or mental formations, are compromise formations between unconscious desire and unconscious defenses.

When an analysand omits or refuses to speak or symbolize something, not only does he/she refuse a particular wish, thought, or emotion, he/she also refuses to recognize a narcissistic injury resulting from the loss of an object: a loss that is central to the constitution of the subject. Lacan associates this misrecognition with denial or negation (*verneinung*) as an unconscious function of the ego (ideal-ego/ego-ideal).

Now for Freud, denial, as a defense, and as a form of negation, was not unconscious. Unconscious repression utilizes denial, and denial is a form of the negative, but in denial, the repressed is intellectually accepted and unconsciously negated at the same time. The ego can recognize his/her division and the existence of repression but deny that it applies to the ego at a particular circumstance. In denial, negation is not unconscious, since it requires a deliberate action/decision, a judgment or choice by the subject. The ego says: "I am fine, I am not lacking anything, have not lost anything or anybody, I am not 'less than,' and I don't want anything that I can't have."

When the ego says, "I am fine, I am in control," although these statements are conscious affirmations that deny their opposites, the fact that they are denying their opposites is preconscious, while the fact that the ego is protecting a narcissistic injury resulting from the castration complex is entirely unconscious.

The alteration of defenses in treatment depends on the ability/capacity to alter pleasant and unpleasant feelings and to accept or seek what is or is not true within experience or within the subject or the object. The analysis of resistances is not an ego analysis per se, because the actual question is to analyze the repressive unconscious, or unconscious repression, and not only the repressed and the return of the repressed. The analysis of resistances or of defenses is not only a question of undoing rather than strengthening ego defenses, because the so-called ego defenses may be unconscious linguistic formations rather than ego processes.

In his paper on negation, Freud (1925) describes a defensive reflex and repression under the pleasure principle as preliminary forms of judgment. The pleasure principle, or what he calls the original pleasure ego, attributes a good or bad quality to something and "wants to introject into itself everything that is good and to eject from itself everything that is bad" (p. 237). The decisions of the pleasure ego under the influence of the pleasure principle thus play the decisive role in operations determined by instinctual factors such as swallowing and spitting that are also motor operations that establish the first distinctions between inside and outside.

However, the decisions of the pleasure principle or of the pleasure ego can also be understood as the laws of the unconscious. And in this regard, the laws of the unconscious and the pleasure principle are equivocal: they serve both the purposes of wishful thinking or pleasure and object seeking and the defensive moves of pain/anxiety avoidance and of unconscious displacement and distortion. Seeking pleasure is the other side of avoiding pain, as well as vice versa.

This is the archaic aspect of the unconscious that organizes the primitive relationship to the mother and the partial object (breast). However, early on, and via the paternal metaphor, the unconscious becomes embedded with the structure of desire, the name of the father, and the structure of language. "Repression may without doubt, be correctly described as the intermediate stage between a defensive reflex and a condemning judgment" (1905b, p. 175).

The process of affirmation and negation at work in language seems to be intrinsically related to the acquisition of language via symbolic parent-child relationships: 0/A, Gugu/dada, daddy/mommy, yes/no, and so on. It is the parent as Other that affirms or denies, grants or stops certain actions of the child, which are then found duplicated in the child's own judgment vis à vis themselves as well as others. The identification with the opposite, as a union of opposites, is internal to the process identification. Objects are abandoned or negated/repressed through the process of identification at the root of the formation of the ego ideal.

> I have asserted above that dreams have no means of expressing the relation of a contradiction, a contrary or a 'no.' I shall now proceed to give a first denial of this assertion. One class of cases which can be comprised under the heading of 'contraries' are, as we have seen, simply represented by identification-cases, that is, in which the idea of an exchange or substitution can be brought into connection with the contrast.
>
> (1900, p. 318)

Separation is achieved via identification with a parent, and the identification is the affirmation of a contrary wish or desire to that which is being negated/repressed via the identification with the Law. The castration of the mother/child dyad leads the boy to identify with the father as the holder of the imaginary phallic attribute. At the same time, this identification places the boy in a rivalrous position with the father vis à vis the mother's attention. The boy is no longer the mother's *objet a* but now wants to have what the father has that the mother wants. To exit Oedipus, the boy has to lose the imaginary phallus in order to use the phallus under the auspices of symbolic castration. As Freud said, the loss of the imaginary part-object is compensated with an identification. It is the loss of the mother, as well as the loss of the father's imaginary phallus, that constitutes the fuel for the formation of the ego ideal. The loss of the imaginary phallus, and the love of the father, also places the boy at risk of taking a feminine position vis à vis the father.

The boy accepts symbolic castration and the loss of the imaginary phallus and represses his eroticism towards his mother, as well as the hostility and homoeroticism towards the father, by identifying with the NoF. If the mother rejects or contests the NoF as a structure, or the father's symbolic function, then it is the hostility and/or the homoeroticism towards the father and the Law that will prevail.

The case of the girl is not symmetrical. She enters oedipal structure through the castration complex. Both the boy and the girl enter the second phase of Oedipus through separation from the mother, but in this separation, the girl realizes that she does not have what the mother wants from the father. If she accepts not being the mother's *objet a*, and not having what the father has, then she will want the phallus and a baby from a man but within the context of symbolic castration. In addition, this position will also give her access to the cultural symbolic order. The girl has also identified with the ideals of the symbolic mother and father. Finally, what the girl has repressed through the identification is the eroticism towards the father.

Since Freud says that oedipal structure is always composed of varying combinations of the positive and negative aspects of the myth, recessively, the boy may acquire a passive position towards the father, and the girl may also acquire an active position vis à vis the mother. Thus, through a symbolic identification, the girl represses dominant and recessive forms of eroticism towards both parents. In so-called positive oedipal structure, the dominant desire towards the parent of the opposite sex, and the recessive homoerotic desire towards the parent of the same sex, will both be repressed via an identification.

In a negative oedipal structure, the reverse will be the case. The dominant homoerotic desire towards the parent of the same sex, and the recessive heterosexuality towards the parent of the opposite sex, will both be repressed. The repression of the recessive tendency is stronger given that the dominant erotic bond to an oedipal parent has to be preserved in the form of a general sexual orientation that eventually will yield the fruits associated with biological maturity.

This formulation, which incorporates both Freudian and Lacanian views on the Oedipus myth and the castration complex, is somewhat at variance with the usual Lacanian interpretation of the castration complex as simply representing the separation from the mother and the loss of being the end all and be all fantasy object of the mother. From then on, the demand for the phallus is addressed to the father, and it is the father's response that differentiates between the sexes. However, the girl will also lose the imaginary phallus that the father has, as a part object, and this comes, as it were, as a second moment of the castration complex for the girl. The boy, in turn, after losing the *objet a* that they were for the mother, will think that he has what the father has, only to have to lose it in order to exit Oedipus and be able to use the fantasy of the imaginary phallus as an adult man with other women.

Freud also distinguishes between repression and negation by saying that negation is the way that censored thoughts can make their way into consciousness. Negation facilitates the undoing of repression by allowing a thought into consciousness and denying it at the same time. But the act of conscious negation is a repetition of the similar unconscious act that led to repression. The affirmation and negation that take place in judgment at the front end of consciousness are similar in form to the affirmation and negation that take place in language and in the dream-work in the unconscious back end of the mind. The latter represent the interplay of the primary forces of being and non-being, life and death, from which the conscious intellectual functions of judgment originate.

Dream distortion and dream displacement, for example, are due to the agency of unconscious censorship. Dream censorship is an integral part of dream representation, the same way that negation is an integral part of linguistic representation. In a psychoanalytic conception of symbol, a symbol represents something that has been repressed. In language, negation works differently: there is a substratum of negation or erasure of the relationship to the object at the same time that the object is represented. The object is not repressed.

The object elephant, for example, is represented in absentia by the signifier elephant but is also partially represented or misrepresented as a difference in relationship to other words. But within letters, there are primitive relationships to objects that the letters no longer refer to. These objects have been erased or repressed. For example, certain letters initially bore an iconic resemblance to a particular animal. The spirit of the animal passes onto the letter and comes to animate the energetic sparks contained within the letters. The relationship to the animal has been replaced by the question of the Real or what exists or does not exist in reality independently of images and language.

In dreams, this process is reversed, instead of words replacing images and objects, it is images that negate dream thoughts and words. The same happens with conscious perception of visual reality. The world is perceived as existing out there and 'as if' names were contained within the essence of things. How naming and language condition perception remains ostensibly unconscious.

The unconscious can represent either the repressive or repressed force, and the same is true for consciousness: consciousness can be repressive or repressed. Freud gave contradictory accounts of how the unconscious represented repressed desires and consciousness represented the power of ethical repression or conscience. In the same way, he said that there was no negation in the unconscious but then had to explain how repression took place unconsciously. He gave accounts of how the super-ego, as the unconscious repressive force within the ego, could itself be repressed by the ego and at the same time distinguished a form of unconscious that was not repressed. This latter form of unconscious approximates his view of the preconscious as being unconscious in a descriptive sense (Freud, 1915).

Since there are three psychical systems and three registers, the unconscious will oppose the rules of consciousness and use images to represent such rules by their opposites. At the same time, words and the rules of the Pcs.Cs. system will suppress and forget the meaning of images. This is the conflict between the Symbolic and the Imaginary.

The inside/outside movements between images and words, between desire, the drive and the law, between conscious and unconscious experience, between the repressed and the repressive, parallel the unconscious structure of language. The act or the decisions of speech involve the same choices and judgments of affirmation and negation that reveal or conceal the truths about thought, words, and desire.

Language reproduces the symbolic functions of Culture, the Law, and the paternal metaphor. The prohibition of incest, the rules of kinship, of grammar and logic, are all interrelated. Although in one sense, the dream-work can be identified with the primary process of energy in dreams (free flow of energy-immediate satisfaction-unlimited condensation and displacement) characteristic of the repressed unconscious, in another sense, condensation and displacement, as the laws that regulate the dream-work in the unconscious, are the laws of the unconscious censor or of the repressive unconscious.

The repressive unconscious is another name for the laws of the signifier or of the word, of the Other, the symbolic father, the phallic function of symbolic castration, and the locus of the Code, as Lacan called it following the linguistics of Jakobson. A Code is a system of constraint and possibility or inhibition and facilitation that exists within language, the psyche, the brain, and the family. In addition, the laws of the Code, or of the Other, are not necessarily within the subject but rather are a Third Dimension between sender and receiver, dream thoughts and dream images, thoughts and words, self and other.

Lacan considers the signifier ruled by the pleasure principle, because he considers the pleasure principle the principle of defense and repression and not what stimulates the sexual drive as a craving for pleasure/pain or for jouissance. Instead he associates jouissance with the death drive. Jouissance is linked to both pleasure and suffering, and suffering is linked to both the craving for pleasure and the repression of desire.

The Law is a transitive experience, since the subject is both the subject and the object of repression. The decision to say or not to say something is co-extensive or parallels the process of symbolization and of affirmation and negation in the unconscious.

In *The Ego and the Id* (1923) Freud wrote that "the faculties of self-criticism and conscience – mental activities, that is, that rank as extremely high ones – are unconscious and unconsciously produce effects of the greatest importance" (p. 26). Yet in other texts, Freud writes that unconscious repression is only a preliminary form or stage of judgment. The question at stake here is not only whether unconscious repression involves the faculties of self-criticism and conscience but also Freud's conception of conscious and unconscious repression. I have pointed out that Freud regarded conscious repression as necessary and positive or rational and unconscious repression as irrational and negative. It is unclear in his quote whether he regards an unconscious conscience as something rational or irrational akin to his concept of a malevolent super ego.

Freud derives his belief that 'in unconscious thinking no process that resembles judgment occurs' from the fact that in dreams, a term can be transformed into or be represented by its opposite. A similar word can be used to express antithetical meanings. Freud does not consider Hegel's concept of 'sublation' or 'Aufheben' whereby something is eliminated only insofar as it has come to situate itself in a unity with its opposite. Freud does not consider the operation of negation in sublation and therefore claims that there is no negation in the unconscious. The determinate being of an element in the dream image is the unity in which its opposite has been preserved/negated.

In other texts, Freud (1905a) seems to be acutely aware of this process when he writes:

> Contrary thoughts are always closely connected with each other and are often paired off in such a way that the one thought is excessively intensely conscious while its counterpart is repressed in the unconscious. This relation between the two thoughts is an effect of the process of repression. For repression is often achieved by means of an excessive reinforcement of the thought contrary to the one that is to be repressed.
>
> (p. 200)

The transformation of a dream-thought into its opposite in the dream-content is precisely a way of repressing that presupposes the activity of negation. The element in the dream-content is affirmed at the same time that the censored dream thought is negated. Moreover, the function of affirming or negating applied to a pair of opposites is extrinsic to the opposition itself. The attribution of a quality or value (positive/affirmative versus negative) will depend upon the meaning given to the terms by a wider associative context or assemblage. 'Old' could be strength or weakness/lack and represent either having or not having something. The same could be said of the signifier 'young.' Whatever signifier comes to signify lack will be negated and its opposite affirmed. With human beings, the pleasure principle is modified by cultural and linguistic modifications that will reduplicate the duality found within the pleasure principle. Both desire and defenses will be unconsciously signified within language and visual perception.

Finally, although the analyses of unconscious defenses, narcissistic injuries, and formations of desire are crucial for the treatment and elimination of symptoms and for improving the social, sexual, and productive function of the subject, the structure and division of the subject and of the psyche will not end or disappear with the ending of the treatment. This is the interminable aspect of analysis.

Narcissistic injury and resistance

Lacan associates the misrecognition of the division of the ego with denial or negation (verneinung) as an unconscious function of the ego. The ideal-ego and the ego-ideal in their own ways both attempt to cover over or conceal the basic division of the subject. The ideal ego covers the division by using body images, while the ego ideal does it using ideas and words. Although division and splitting are common to all subjects, they nonetheless produce a narcissistic injury since tertiary ego-ideal narcissism is often represented by an ideal of unity, completeness, and even perfection. From this perspective, narcissistic injuries and defenses are not exclusively or intrinsically linked to so-called pre-oedipal phases of development. In addition, early injuries to the ideal ego are not necessarily due to lack of maternal empathy or mirroring behavior, as is commonly believed.

The specular image, as a body image and as the ideal ego, incorporates and resolves the intensities of the life and death drives that were linked to the absence and presence of the breast. The body image replaces the presence of the object and compensates for its absence.

At the same time, life and death drives continue to be revealed and manifest through the ideal ego as a new mental formation or "matheme." The absence of the *objet a* will appear in a blank spot, defect, flaw, or something missing within the body image. If the absence does not appear, then this leads to a grandiose self-image, linked to an idealized good breast and to the mother's imaginary phallus. The absence of the absence also leads to developmental arrest because the self does not move in the direction of the Other. The absence of the object within the image stabilizes the body image and prevents it from becoming a grandiose image. In the papers published by the International Psychoanalytic Association, the differences between the ideal ego, the ego ideal, and the grandiose self are often confused and are all explained in terms of fusion states with the mother (Lichtenberg, 1975; Hanly, 1984).

In addition, fusion with the mother, leading to a grandiose self, is also confused with neglect, deprivation of "emotional sustenance," or the lack of maternal desire for the child. The lack of maternal desire is also confused with the mother's conditioned desire for a fantasized object. All of these factors are seen as determining either a form of depressive ego weakness or a defensive grandiose or false self.

The absence of a specular image, as an ideal ego, fixates the ego at the level of the partial object and renders it subject to the jouissance of the Other and to persecutory psychotic anxieties, as well as primitive forms of fusion with the partial object. There is no self or subject at this point. This condition can be produced either by privation of maternal desire or by the foreclosure of the name of the father. Either too much or too little amounts to the same result in this regard.

The denial of the division of the ego takes two forms: one related to the ideal ego, the other to the ego ideal. The first includes the denial of any bodily or physical limitations or flaws. The denial can also take the form of narcissistic overestimations of the body in all its glory. An example of this would be the case of an analysand who dreamt that she was a superwoman. Her associations included a sense of the great dexterity of her body and a memory of her father recognizing her as the "birth of perfection."

The second denial of the division of the subject is linked to the ego ideal. Here the subject finds its unity via identification with ideas, ideals, and relationships that seem to complete the subject. An example of this is an analysand who considered her relationship idyllic and a source of great happiness and yet had a repeated dream where she was with different men and feared that her partner would find out and risk losing the relationship. She denied that she had any ambivalence about her partner and feared exploring the possibility that she might be too dependent or fused with the partner. Any exploration of ambivalence immediately translated into a fear that the analysis could cause an end to the relationship.

In general, the division of the subject appears when the other does not recognize or misrecognizes the identifications of the ego either with bodily or specular images or with the mass or aggregate of ideas that constitute the ego ideal. It is important for the analyst not to be fooled by the strength or unity of the ideal ego or ego ideal. At the same time, the analyst needs to be empathic with defenses in a purely strategic sense. The judo-style flow with ego defenses, while preserving the awareness of their defensive purposes, enables the analyst and the analysand to work with and through the divisions of the subject. The apparent support of ego defenses is purely strategic for purposes of their eventual dissolution and transformation into the symbolic functioning of the subject.

Symbolic castration

In *Analysis Terminable and Interminable*, Freud also points out how the joint efforts of the analyst and analysand to recognize and work through resistance run aground upon the rock of symbolic castration.

Although castration is prefigured in the loss of the breast, the hole in the image of the ideal ego, and the loss of feces, strictly speaking, the fear of castration is what triggers the development of the super-ego and the ego ideal. For example, an analysand of mine reported feeling guilty that he had not taken his shoes off before getting on the couch, despite the fact that there was a piece of fabric under the analysand's shoes and that I had never asked him to take his shoes off. I interpreted his experience as a good example of guilt rather than remorse over a bad deed, since he was creating a restriction where there was none.

In response to my interpretation, he recalled that as a five-year-old, he was left by his parents sitting on a bench outside the supermarket. When they came out, they found him sitting on the bench and masturbating rubbing his penis over his pants. His parents had a hysterical reaction towards a five-year-old that perhaps they should not have left sitting alone in public by himself in the first place. He remembers them shaming him over how he could humiliate them in public like that. He was mortified and to this day he has a significant amount of shame over his sexuality. This is a good example of unconscious fear of punishment and the role that castration anxiety has in the development of the super ego and ego ideal.

I say ego ideal because the analysand had identified with several parental ideals towards which the analysand had a significant amount of ambivalence.

Retroactively, castration can also determine the meaning of the loss of the breast and the lack in the body image. An example of the first, and of identification with the partial object of the drive and desire, would be the sense of loss and dispossession that small breasts can trigger in women and the castration anxiety that the small breasts of a lover can trigger in some men.

The example of people who go to medical doctors requesting the removal of a hand or arm would be a glaring example of castration producing a retroactive effect on the body image. The super-ego retroactively affects the image of the body as described in the Bible: "If your hand causes you to sin, cut if off" (Gospel according to Mark 9:38–48). It is interesting to note how although the pre-modern cruel super ego has disappeared from the ideals of the culture, its unconscious effects re-emerge via developments of new forms of psychopathology. In traditional biblical culture, there was a direct correlation between cultural ideals and the pathologies of the primitive super ego. In postmodernity, traditional ideals or super ego formations that have been suppressed in the culture return from repression via new forms of psychopathology.

According to Lacan, Freud discovered the existence of a true complex when he came across what has been called the problem of castration. It is well known that by using that term, the founder of psychoanalysis attempted to account for a threat that in fact is never fulfilled. Symbolic castration as a developmental complex has nothing to do with emasculation or an effective bodily loss. But then why is castration so decisive and marking, to the point that Freud calls it the living rock which signals the unsurpassable limit of any analysis?

Castration is effective by virtue of being a symbolic condition. Symbolic here refers to a theory, or to what Freud calls the sexual theories of childhood. Freud says childhood theory, not fantasy, fiction, or lie. Freud presupposes that childhood sexual theories regarding the difference between the sexes are an invariable step in the constitution of the subject. Symbolic castration does not arise from the inside as a phase or an ontogenetic stage of development but rather comes from the *field of the Other*. The mother is perceived as lacking something that she wants from the father, and the same is true for the father. The mother lacks/desires the imaginary phallus that is attributed to the father, while the father lacks the *objet a* (of love and drive) the mother is perceived as being.

The Other is revealed as both complete and incomplete. The complete or imaginary aspect of the (f)Other is the one that threatens castration or, in other words, the one that generates the lack or loss that refers to the anecdote of the castration threat. The Other will take something away from or reveal a lack in the subject. On the other hand, the (m)Other herself is perceived as incomplete, inconsistent, or having something missing, which refers to the anecdote of femininity as the absence or lack of the phallus.

Given this, what does the Freudian limit of castration imply? According to Freud's understanding, the analysis of masculinity does not go beyond a point the passing through of which would signify a giving in, a submission into passivity before the father. Said conflict would be equivalent to the castration complex provoking all the consequent duels, challenges, combats, rebellions, and ingratitude which usually are expressed as stagnation and a worsening of the analysand's condition. Correspondently, the analysis of the female collides with the demand for the phallus and its status as a missing phallus or a lack makes for varied dissatisfactions and complaints, if not for plain depressions.

Symbolic castration is beyond Oedipus

According to Lacan, castration is a genuine complex. Based on Freud's writings on femininity, Lacan argues that castration is the logical premise that then and only then as a defensive consequence generates what before Lacan had been called the Oedipus complex. From a Lacanian perspective, Oedipus becomes a myth and no longer a complex. Moreover, in Seminar #VIII, "On Identification," Lacan (1960–1961) states that Oedipus is a dream of Freud and should be interpreted as such. What is implied? Oedipus is repressive before it is repressed. The Oedipus story and the rivalries and passion concerned conceal the truth that desire is established as a function of the law and prohibition – the incest prohibition being the paradigmatic example of all prohibition. As written in the Gospel of Paul:

> The sinful passions aroused by the law were at work in our bodies. . . . I would not have known what sin was except through the law. For I would not have known what coveting really was if the law had not said, do not covet.
>
> (Romans 7:7)

In the case of Paul, the Law is rejected for causing the very problems that it is invoked to cure (Lacan, 1957–1958, Sem. V, p. 470). On the other hand, the rejection of the Law also causes the elimination of desire and therefore raises the severity of the Law to a level previously unprecedented within the Jewish religion (for example, the absence of a celibacy ideal for the priesthood within Judaism). Castration and the prohibition flowing from it compel one to desire. In addition, the partiality of desire imposes a limitation that the subject finds difficult to accept. The resistance to desire appears to follow from a neurotic conflict between the law and desire, but, in fact, it is a desire not to desire because the law of castration itself causes desire. In this sense, the very posing of a conflict between the law and desire may be seen as defensive in and of itself. I shall return to this later on.

Can one go beyond symbolic castration?

The answer is yes. Lacan, with legitimate ambition, proposes to go beyond castration. This new aim is associated with a central tenet of Lacanian clinical practice: the question of the resistance of the analyst already explored in Chapter 9.

The resistance of the analyst is resistance to listening, to intervening (the horror of the act, as Lacan calls it), and, especially, it is resistance to set aside the wish to function as the analysand's wished-for ego ideal instead of getting past imaginary castration by accepting the lack as it is. The analyst functions not with his/her ego ideal or his/her formal professional identity but with what Lacan calls the "desire of the analyst." The desire of the analyst is neither the countertransference nor the vocational desire to work as an analyst.

The desire of the analyst is a lack that is not a deficit and that functions as an organizing principle of the analytic process. The analyst's desire facilitates the manifestation of the unconscious in the analysand's speech, a speech act that together with the act of interpretation results in a restructuring or a retying of the Borromean knot or psychic structure. Desire as lack, or lack as pure desire, is the Third that structures the direction of the analytical dyad (group of two). Pure desire should also rule a psychoanalytic organization instead of the dual imaginary unity that prevails in groups structured around the adoption or rejection of the inexistent imaginary phallus of a leader. The lack within the desire of the analyst, together with free association, are the foundational rock of psychoanalysis that every analyst has to pass through and beyond.

In addition, the desire of the analyst is also characterized by the intention of directing the desire of the analysand first towards the analyst but then turning it toward others. After having gone through the process of being various types of imaginary *objet a*, the analyst ends in the place of the *objet a* as an absence, or All-alone in the Real, which is the same as pure desire. The desire of the analyst is something like a second-degree desire which differs from the common and "human all too human" (Nietzsche, 1878/1996) "desire of being desired." What is at stake here is that the analyst, on the basis of his or her desire, succeeds in overcoming the resistance to work in favor of becoming dispensable to the analysand and working through the mourning thereof.

The beginning and middle phases of pure analysis proper

The end of analysis is played out and prepared from the beginning in accordance with the aim of the analyst. If the aim of analysis is not resisted, then analysis will be regulated by the desire that defines the analytical position and the psychical state of the analyst. As I said previously, at the end of analysis, the aim changes from the analysis of identifications and the identification with the analyst to the identification with the sinthome.

Lacan (1974/75) says that the neurotic "believes in his symptom" (Seminar XXII RSI). The neurotic understands that the symptom is trying to say something not yet understood. The symptom is an enigma, therefore. Put differently: she knows that there is something she does not know and is certain that if that "knowing" were to be known, the cure would follow. The analyst therefore is localized in Lacan's terms as the subject supposed to knowing (the S.s.S. position) what the analysand ignores. It is the unconscious knowing of the analysand that is being attributed to the analyst. The analyst needs to move from the position of the subject supposed to a knowledge about the imaginary *objet a* to the suspension of certainties and *connaissance* (knowledge).

Contrary to what would be expected, the neurotic is not looking for the person and virtues of the analyst (the good object) but for that "knowing" which he/she ignores. Knowledge of any kind results in a transference relationship to the Other. As soon as a subject is being attributed to knowing, the basis for the transference has been established. Therefore, the transference is defined by "unknown-knowing" and not by conscious knowledge or by feelings or affective states. Affects are subordinate to knowing according to the following characterization: I love whom I presuppose to be a subject of knowing; I hate whom I withdraw this supposition from (Seminar XX, Encore).

To assume the analytical position, the analyst must first 1) ignore or not be attached to what he/she knows in order to apprehend the singularity of a new analysand and 2) with respect to what he ignores, intend to understand it. This double game reveals one of the richest paradoxes of analysis: although the analysand supposes the analyst knows many things about him or her, in truth the analyst ignores everything about it.

Unknown knowing is situated within the analysand. Granted that without the analyst, the unveiling of the unknown becomes impossible. Such is then the *via di levare* (by way of extracting or taking away) which Freud (1905c) talked about: namely to be like a sculptor who chips away the stone in order to make the appearance of the sculpture possible by following the lines of the material itself rather than the designs of the artist.

But the analysand (and suggestive/behavioral treatments) is searching for the *via di porre* (way of superimposition or putting on). The analysand offers and gives herself as a canvas upon which the analyst may draw or offer some brilliant designs. The analysis installs the analyst in both the S.s.S. position and that of the ego ideal. Just as in love, one loves in the other that which one lacks in oneself in order to reach one's own ideal. The other of love is who allows the subject to deny the lack. I am referring to a narcissistic type of bond or union that reveals what is deceiving about romantic and sexual love. In truth, ordinary dual love is to want to be loved. And if I am loved by an ego ideal, then I am an ideal ego. This follows from what Freud said regarding the childhood desire to be one's own ideal. This is an aspect of the relationship between the ideal ego and the ego ideal.

Thus, when Kohut (Kohut and Wolf, 1978; Baker, 1981) notes that some narcissistic analysands did not experience him as a separate object or even a separate body, he is only discovering a narcissistic characteristic of love or Eros itself. The object or the other is expected to be an extension of the subject precisely because such other has been situated in the place of the ego ideal or ideal ego. The ideal ego or the alter ego, as they refer to object love, can be conceived as a mental image of this or that body.

Thus, this other body, which is an extension of the subject's body, is what allows the imaginary ego to complete what it thinks (albeit unconsciously) it lacks in the body. In the love of the object, the other as object is what the subject desires in order to conceal his/her own incompleteness of being. To put it differently: the desire and love of the object as it relates to sexuality cannot escape what has been called a narcissistic type of bond or union. This would not be a characteristic of "selfobject needs" only found in narcissistic character disorders.

In addition, we are referring here to a fundamental lack of being which in Freud's theory is intrinsically interwoven with sexuality, the castration complex, and the symbolic function of the phallus. In this case, a concern with loss or rejection, for example, has more to do with the inevitably lost metonymic object of desire (which becomes symbolized as a loss at the level of the subject) than with whatever symbolic object-love historical parents in the family had or did not have to give or not give.

But the most decisive point has not yet been made. A neurotic is a specialist in the art of becoming the object of the demand of the Other. Of course, that without being willing to pay the price for it or recognizing that this demand of the other is unconsciously emanating from the neurosis itself. Therefore, the defining formula of the neurotic is that he/she situates the demand of the other uppermost. And what does he/she think the Other wants from him/her? That he/she be just like the Other to the point of nullification. From this follows the decisive character of the identification that the analysand comes to look for in the analysis. And if one falls into the trap of neurosis by offering to give what one has that the other seems to be lacking, one is – despite all good intentions – only aimlessly swimming in the depth of the neurosis without further recourse. In summary, the identification with the analyst that many believe to be a formula for the final phase of analysis implies nothing but the stagnation in one of the stages of the process. In this scenario, the analysis becomes interminable.

Ego identification with the analyst has more to do with the neurosis itself than with what Greenson (1978) called a realistic object relationship characterized by the empathic alliance with an analyst achieved during the initial stages of an analysis. Greenson states that humanness consists of giving insight and understanding in an empathic and serious fashion. But as shown with Lacan, this knowing and understanding is a basis for the transference.

From another perspective, empathy and the alliance with the analysand run the danger of becoming an imaginary reinforcement of the defensive ego which analysis is supposed to deconstruct. The suffering of the analysand is commonly connected to secondary or false presenting problems which often function as some of the repressive substitute ideas which keep repressed and unconscious contents away from consciousness. In this context, the demand made upon the analyst is to be empathic and understanding of the analysand's problems as presented by the analysand and his or her ego defenses.

In addition, the patient initially wants to speak about what she or he wants to talk about; an empathic analyst should respect the patient's agenda or the defensive selection of material. Thus, it should be remembered that the alleged alliance is being established with the ego of the defenses themselves. Finally, if the demand of the analysand is actually about being loved and recognized, the task of the analyst does not end with an offering of the image of the analyst as an auxiliary ego and an explanation of where the parents of the analysand failed.

Therefore, if the demand of the analysand directs the transference towards identification with the ideal, the desire of the analyst should attempt to break up such a situation. The analyst has to cultivate a state beyond the crown of power and authority represented by the ego ideal. In his/her own analysis, the analyst has to have reached a state beyond the ego ideal in order not to wish to be such for the analysand. Transference love represents the analysand's resistance aimed at erecting an ego ideal or a complete Other in the figure of the analyst. This transference resistance defends against the lack in the subject as well as in the Other.

When the analyst does not remain in the place of the ideal and does not respond to the demand of the analysand, then in that void, the analysand's fundamental fantasies will become apparent. The analysand not only wants for the analyst to tell him/her what to do or not do, a demand of a demand, but also demands that the analyst give him or her the signifier of the phallus as well as the object of love and of the drive. Finally, the analysand also wants to become and give the analyst the object that the analyst desires, lacks, and needs. The analysand wants the analyst to demand this object from him/her.

It follows from the previous that the analyst's position/state and desire is that of the silence or equanimity of the Buddha, of the stoic who does not respond (ataraxia),[1] and/or who responds in surprising or unexpected manners to the many ways in which the analysand unconsciously sets up the analytical situation so as to widen the reach of his/her demand. By proceeding in this way, the analyst does not set himself/herself up as an ego ideal for the analysand in order to occupy the place of what Lacan denominates the *objet a*. By not representing an ideal parent, or the 'subject supposed to know,' the I(O) of the ego ideal is transformed into the signifier of a lack in the Other (S(∅) that in turn is interpreted in the light of the formula for the fantasy ($◊a). The analyst lacks the object that the subject wants/lacks. The analyst is not the ego ideal or the imaginary *objet a* that could complete the subject and make him/her their own ideal thereby.

Thus, it is possible to understand that the conflict with which the analysand entangles the analyst by means of the transference neurosis and the Freudian limits that point to symbolic castration and its accompanying rivalries, arguments, dissatisfactions, ingratitudes, and so on do not yet constitute true limits. The conflict still continues a theme and a plot which allow for the concealment of a void or emptiness that Lacan (December 10, 1959) calls the pain of existence (the reality of emptiness as an absence). In this respect, the imaginary fixation to the wish to murder the father or mother serves the purpose of avoiding contact with the abyss of the Real as emptiness. Emptiness is not to be '*a*-voided' but rather accepted and realized as true being or unbeing (désêtre) rather than as absence (relative nothingness).

The experience of the pain of existence does not lead to nihilism or skeptical doubt. On the contrary, the circular experience of emptiness, of perfection and imperfection, finitude and infinity, wholeness and incompleteness or 'holeness' leads toward the One, energizing the possible word or unary trace of all who speak. It becomes possible, then, to set aside the pretension that one has been allocated the worst in the distribution of the jouissance of life. When mutating the subjective position, one abandons the myth of guilt and interdiction by accepting the impossibility of the jouissance of the Other. The latter jouissance implies the fantasy that the Other enjoys something inaccessible to the subject. For example: the mother in the Oedipal myth.

To sum up: what is especially or actually implied in forbidden jouissance (which otherwise may be possible if the prohibition is transgressed) is the confrontation with the fact that the jouissance of the Other and the imaginary phallus as such do not exist. But as mentioned in previous chapters, when one form of jouissance is eliminated, another form of jouissance is attained. During development, symbolic castration of the jouissance of the Other, or of the mother-child fusion, leads to the manifestation of phallic jouissance, while the symbolic castration of the imaginary phallus leads to the Third Other jouissance. The Third is realized as 'non-existing' or inexistence in the sense not of nothingness but of what 'ex-sists' in the Real outside language.

To terminate: the interminable

When, how, and why do analyses end? Let us return once again to our starting point in order to take this time another converging road. The analysand transforms into what at the end of analysis? Lacan gives a strange response to this question. The analysand transforms into an analyst. But does this mean then that, after all, the analysand did in fact identify with the ideal? Not if the analysis was able to go beyond identity or identification via the deconstruction of the analysands' ego-ideal and the analysand's wish to mimic and identify with the analyst. Although the analyst's practice of listening to the ways of the Unconscious produces a similar subjective position/state in the analysand, the analysand has to discover this truth in his or her own psychical structure rather than by identification with the analyst.

The possibility that the analysand may be able to listen in a singular way to himself/herself serves as a guarantee that the analysis may in fact be interminable. Therefore, if there is self-analysis, such only begins when an analysis with the Other has ended. All in all, analysis succeeds in producing an adverted subject able to re-cognize desire without confounding or hiding it behind the demand of the Other. The subject then may disregard the Name-of-the-Father precisely because he/she knows how to use it. In Lacan's later work, the self-analysis that continues after the end of the personal analysis and the use and disregard of the NoF are both linked to the sinthome, and to the Borromean knot of four.

Note

1 A calm or imperturbable mind. Equanimity or *im*passivity (as a benevolent alternative to absolute indifference) in the sense of inner mastery or freedom from being controlled by disturbing emotions or an inconvenient form of *jouissance*.

References

Baker, H. and Baker, M. (1987). Heinz Kohut's Self Psychology: An Overview. *American Journal of Psychiatry*, 144, 1.

Bion, W. R. (1970). *Attention and Interpretation*. London: Tavistock Publications.

Ferenczi, S. (1928). The Elasticity of Psycho-Analytic Technique. In: *The Evolution of Psychoanalytic Technique*. Edited by M. S. Bergmann and F. R. Hartman. New York: Basic Books.

Freud, S. (1900). *The Interpretation of Dreams: The Standard Edition of the Complete Psychological Works of Sigmund Freud*. London: The Hogarth Press and the Institute of Psychoanalysis, pp. 4–5.

Freud, S. (1905a). Fragment of an Analysis of a Case of Hysteria. In: *The Freud Reader*. Edited by P. Gay. New York: Norton and Norton.

Freud, S. (1905b). Jokes and Their Relation to the Unconscious. *SE*, 8.

Freud, S. (1905c). On Psychotherapy. *SE*, 7, 260–261.

Freud, S. (1912). Recommendations to Physicians Practising Psychoanalysis. *SE*, 12, 111–120.

Freud. S. (1913). On Beginning the Treatment. *S.E.*, 12.

Freud, S. (1915). *The Metapsychology: The Standard Edition of the Complete Psychological Works of Sigmund Freud* (Volume 14). London: The Hogarth Press and the Institute of Psychoanalysis, p. 109.

Freud, S. (1921). Group Psychology and the Analysis of the Ego. *SE*, 18, 67–143.

Freud, S. (1923). The Ego and the Id. *SE*, 19, 3–66.

Freud, S. (1925). On Negation. *SE*, 19, 235–239.

Freud, S. (1937). Analysis Terminable and Interminable. *S.E.*, 23, 209.

Freud, S. (1960). *Group Psychology and the Analysis of the Ego*. New York: Bantam Books.

Freud, S. (1973). *Three Case Histories*. New York: Collier Books.

Greenson, R. R. (1978). The Working Alliance and the Transference Neurosis. In: *Explorations in Psychoanalysis* (pp. 199–224). New York: International Universities Press.

Hanly, C. (1984). Ego Ideal and Ideal Ego. *International Journal of Psychoanalysis*, 65, 253–261.

Kohut, H. and Wolf, E. (1978). The Disorders of the Self and Their Treatment: An Outline. *International Journal of Psychoanalysis*, 59, 413–425.

Lacan, J. (1955). *Escritos 1. Variantes de la cura tipo*. Mexico: Siglo XXI, 1985.

Lacan, J. (1957a). El seminario sobre la carta robada. In: *Escritos 2*. Mexico: Siglo XXI, 1975. The Seminar on 'The Purloined Letter.' In: *Écrits*. Translated by J. Mehlman. Yale French Studies 48, 1973, pp. 39–72.

Lacan, J. (1957b). The Instance of the Letter in the Unconscious. In: *Ecrits*. Translated by B. Fink. New York: Norton.

Lacan, J. (1957–1958). *Formations of the Unconscious: The Seminar*. Book V. Edited by J. A. Miller and Translated by R. Grigg. London: Polity Press, 2017.

Lacan, J. (1959). *El Deseo y su Interpretacion*. Buenos Aires: Nueva Vision.

Lacan, J. (1959–1960). *Seminar 7: The Ethics of Psychoanalysis*. Translated by D. Porter. New York: W. W. Norton, 1992.

Lacan, J. (1964). *The Four Fundamental Concepts of Psychoanalysis: The Seminar of Jacques Lacan*. Book XI. Translated by A. Sheridan. New York: W.W. Norton, 1977.

Lacan, J. (1966–1967). *The Seminar of Jacques Lacan XIV: The Logic of Fantasy*. London: Karnac.

Lacan, J. (1967). *Proposition of 9 October 1967 on the Psychoanalyst of the School*. https://lacancircle.com.au/wp-content/uploads/2017/11/Proposition_of_9_October.pdf. Accessed July 7, 2020.

Lacan, J. (1967–1968). *The Seminar of Jacques Lacan*. Book XV: The Psychoanalytic Act. Translated by C. Gallagher. www.lacaninireland.com/web/published-works/seminars. Accessed November 17, 2019.

Lacan, J. (1969). *The Seminar of Jacques Lacan: Book XVII: The Other Side of Psychoanalysis* (Bk. 17). New York: Norton and Norton, 2007.

Lacan, J. (1972). *On Feminine Sexuality: The Limits of Love and Knowledge: Encore: The Seminar of Jacques Lacan*. Book XX. New York: Norton and Norton, 1998.

Lacan, J. (1974/75). *R.S.I.* Translated into Spanish by R. E. Rodríguez Ponte, 1999. Unpublished.

Lacan, J. (1978). *Momento de Concluir.* XXV. Unpublished.

Lichtenberg, J. (1975). The Development of the Sense of Self. *Journal of the American Psychoanalytic Association*, 23, 453–484.

Nietzsche, F. W. (1878). *Human, All Too Human: A Book for Free Spirits.* Translated by R. J. Hollingdale. Cambridge: Cambridge University Press, 1996.

Reich, W. (1933). On the Technique of Character-Analysis. In: *Essential Papers on Character Neurosis and Treatment.* New York: New York University Press, 1989.

13 Clinical psychoanalysis in the public clinic and the question of trauma

The nature–nurture dialectic and the complemental series

Freud (1934) conceived of psychiatric disorders as falling into a continuum of causal series. The series begin with what he called the sexual constitution and which now outside psychoanalysis would be called the biological and genetic factor leading to developmental disturbances. The second series is composed by events experienced. At one end of the series (or the continuum) stand those people who would have developed a disorder regardless of the most benevolent of life experiences. Here Freud stood in stark contrast to the exaggerated environmentalism that prevailed in the rest of psychology during the first half of the twentieth century and was continued by behaviorism and the interpersonal schools of psychoanalysis. At the other end of the series stand cases that would have escaped a psychiatric disorder if they had not endured the burden of traumatic environmental experiences. In the intermediate cases, both factors are combined to varying degrees. Thus, at the turn of the century, Freud already propounded the present interactionist paradigm between nature and culture.

More recently, congenital or genetic factors involved in the production of psychopathology are associated with biochemical vulnerabilities of the brain and not as dispositions related to sexual or aggressive drives. The different disorders involve failures in the release or uptake of different neurotransmitters, which either facilitate or inhibit the transmission of nervous impulses. For Freud, impulse was equivalent to drive, whether it be sexual or aggressive, and was closely related to the love/hate and pleasure/pain emotional core of the psyche/brain. Although, on the one hand, contemporary neurobiology does not make the same assumption, on the other hand, temperament is in fact currently being defined by behavioral researchers as "constitutionally based individual differences in reactivity and self-regulation" (Rothbart and Ahadi, 1994, p. 55).

Temperament is considered the inherited personality traits which develop early in life and which manifest in the form of emotional reactivity and emotional self-regulation. Intense aggressiveness or negative affect and excessive demand and desire for attention and gratification characterize a "difficult" (neurotic, we would say) temperament. To make things worse, or to bring entropy to the mix, in the course of development and life, and perhaps through character, increased complexity is realized in the temperament that changes over time from self-regulation to reactivity and from reactivity to self-regulation.

The notion of reactivity coincides to a significant degree with the notion of drive as an inherited potential for impulsivity and aggressivity which is prior to or at least not reducible to the objects and targets provided by the environment. High reactivity refers to the intensity of emotional and physiological arousal and excitation (either due to desire or aggression) and low reactivity to the ability to tolerate frustration and for emotional self-regulation.

Relative degrees can be attributed to either the quantum of arousal and stimulation or the strength of inhibitory and self-regulation processes. Thus, a child's high reactivity could be attributed to either the strength of impulse and drive or the weakness of the inhibiting function. The reverse is true for low reactivity: strength in self-regulation could be attributed to either the weakness of impulse or the strength of the inhibiting function.

In addition, low reactivity, self-regulation, and the capacity to inhibit the transmission of nervous impulses can be considered the conceptual equivalents of the psychoanalytic notion of defense. The same way that Freud thought of the drive as a limit concept between the genetic/biological and the more symbolic and environmentally based notion of desire, inhibition can also be conceived as a bridge or limit term which can be understood either as cultural/symbolic phenomena (defenses and symbolic laws/rules) or as a biological executive function of the frontal cortex associated with the neural and chemical capacity to inhibit the transmission of impulses. The latter also speaks to there being a constitutional and biological base for the brain related functions of inhibition and defense. In this regard, Freud thought that the super ego, as the representative of social rules within the mind, could be transmitted via heredity and not only through the environment.

Constitutionally based differences in levels of impulsivity and irritability are expressions of genetic aspects of the sexual and aggressive drive which predict future ability to control or act out various desires and impulses (hysteria). On the other hand, high repressiveness and inhibition are associated with a shy or inhibited temperament, low levels of aggression and impulsivity, and a propensity towards anxiety and neurotic disorders (obsessional neurosis).

Finally, contemporary neurobiology also recognizes the ability of life events to affect, alter, and modify brain processes. Loss experiences, for example, could very well lead to changes in the action potentials for the transmission of impulses. Therefore, genetic dispositions cannot be totally identified with brain or biological processes, given that brain processes can respond to both congenital and environmental conditions.

In fact, one could argue that language is in effect a symbolic net that wires, sprays, and imprints its structure unto neuronal chains within the brain. Language functions as a code superimposed on the semiotic structure of the brain that regulates the facilitation and inhibition and the on/off position of impulses. Genes may also function differently in different environments. A genetic predisposition may or may not manifest itself, depending on the nature of the environmental and cultural-symbolic conditions.

Childhood and later traumas, the function of fantasy and of recovered and pseudo or screen memories

After having distinguished the first two ends of the complementary series, Freud (1934) proceeds to also emphasize that "a complemental relationship exists between the intensity and pathogenic importance of the infantile and of the later experiences" (p. 373). In other words, the environmental series needs to be further subdivided into childhood and later experiences. In the case of later conflicts and traumas, childhood experiences exert their influence by the effect of regression alone. In other words, a feedback loop exists between the two. Later experiences are given additional intensity by childhood experiences, and childhood experiences are retroactively interpreted in the light of later experiences.

Childhood experiences, in addition to genetic predispositions, would explain why a trauma could trigger a disorder in one person but not in another. Moreover, the importance of the parental environment (and Oedipal structure) has also been confirmed by contemporary research within the field of developmental psychology. If a child, for example, has come out of the early family experience in childhood with antisocial character traits, this is much more likely to influence his or her choice of peers during adolescence than the likelihood of the latter having a structural and enduring impact on character structure.

For Freud, childhood had a double significance. First, the congenitally determined drives are shown here for the first time, and second, external influences and accidental events can awaken other drives than those preestablished by heredity. Accidental experiences in childhood are capable of inducing fixations and changing the object, aim, intensity, and source of impulses. During critical periods of development, accidental events can have lasting and structural effects, which would not be the case once developmental milestones have been established.

Moreover, from a Freudian perspective, in order to arrive at an accurate and comprehensive depiction of the complemental series at work in the production of psychiatric disorders, the experiential end of the complementary series, whether in childhood or later on in life, needs to be further subdivided into material reality and psychical reality. With the notion of psychical reality, we arrive at what I will call a tripartite model of causality for mental disorders which includes the congenital and the biological, the psychical and social-environmental dimensions. The psychical is differentiated from the purely psychological dimension, because the latter refers to behavior and/or conscious and preconscious cognitions, while the former also includes unconscious processes.

The psychical dimension can be considered a properly psychoanalytic dimension established by Freud after the development of the early trauma theory of psychiatric disorders. It is interesting to note that current practice within the mental health field, as seen within the scope of practice of counselors, social workers, and psychologists, can be said to have regressed to Freud's early trauma model of unconscious function and psychiatric causality. In addition, due to ideological and market pressures, psychiatrists have also abandoned the psychoanalytic field in favor of a return to the properly medical and biological field.

Freud's transition from the early trauma model to his theory of the unconscious and the Oedipus complex is much more subtle, objective, and complex than we have more recently been led to believe by those who have embraced Masson's (1984) controversial account of the reasons behind Freud's abandonment of the trauma and seduction theory. Masson argued that, in disregard of the well-being and sanity of his patients, Freud abandoned the trauma theory in order to protect the wealthy and socially influential parents of his patients from charges of sexual abuse. As many have already argued, this accusation becomes preposterous when one considers that Freud would have not discovered the Oedipus complex, or the function of unconscious fantasy, had he not gone beyond the early trauma theory.

Although it is true that a type I error could occur if a clinician takes an actual trauma for a fantasy, it is equally true that a clinician can make a type II error by taking a fantasy for an actual trauma. Sometimes a client may report a fantasy when it is actually a trauma, and sometimes a client may report a trauma that in reality is a fantasy. Both types of errors could be equally misleading and damaging. But if clinicians ignore the psychical reality of fantasies alongside the material reality of traumas, they become liable to make type II errors and therefore lead their clients to believe that they have been abused when there is no actual basis for such a conclusion. In this, I think that psychoanalysts, by considering both material and psychical realities, are potentially better off than those clinicians who only hold onto material reality to the exclusion of psychical reality.

In Freud's introductory lectures, one can find a candid and current account of the intricate relationship between material and psychical reality, trauma and fantasy, and between recovered and 'pseudomemories.' From a psychoanalytic perspective, pseudomemories or 'screen memories' are not trumped-up charges or willful false statements but rather stories or beliefs that have been acquired to defend against unconscious fantasies.

In either case, pseudomemories constitute a psychical reality for the subject. With the conceptual tools provided by a framework that contains a notion of psychical reality alongside that of factual or material reality, the clinician is able to escape falling into the trap of either/or propositions with regard to true or correct or false and incorrect memories. By and large, current-day clinicians (Enns et al., 1998) who work with adults who may have experienced childhood abuse, and who establish professional standards for the psychology profession, have working knowledge of how memories can be both repressed or forgotten and recovered (although often underemphasizing the psychoanalytic origin of these concepts) but disregard the relationship among pseudo or incorrect memories, the function of defense, and what Freud called psychical reality and unconscious fantasy life.

Moreover, it is important to note that fantasy and trauma share the experiential but not the environmental end of the series. Although fantasy can contain fragments of environmental experience, it remains non-identical with it. In addition, fantasy and trauma function within a dialectical relationship. Just as fantasy and sexuality in general, whether imagined or actual, can be traumatic, so can trauma contain fantasized elements. Fantasy may continue to elaborate and reshape events occurred. Referring to unconscious fantasy, Freud writes that there is still a surprising, astonishing, and bewildering factor at work in the production and development of symptomatology. These adjectives describe his reluctant and undesired realization that infancy scenes are not always found to be true. Freud's (1934) ideas on this matter are worth quoting in full:

> You will see that this discovery is more likely than any other to discredit either the analysis which leads to such results, or the patient, upon whose testimony the analysis and comprehension of the neuroses as a whole is built up. . . . If the infantile experiences brought up to light by the analysis were in every case real we should have the feeling that we are on firm ground; if they were invariably falsified and found to be inventions and fantasies of the patients we should have to forsake this insecure foothold and save ourselves some other way.
>
> But it is neither one thing or the other; for what we find is that the childhood experiences reconstructed or recollected in analysis are on some occasions undeniably false, while others are just as certainly quite true, and that in most case truth and falsehood are mixed up. So, the symptoms are thus at one minute reproductions of experiences which actually took place and which one can credit with an influence on the fixation of the libido; and at the next a reproduction of fantasies of the patient's to which, of course, it is difficult to ascribe an etiological significance.
>
> (p. 376)

Given the current relevance of Freud's remarks, they can be regarded as Freud's own foreshadowing of the resistance and discredit that the theorizing of unconscious fantasy could bring upon psychoanalysis and Freud himself, not only in the immediate future but also 100 years later. The discredit under consideration would bear upon psychoanalysis not only because of the resistance of incorporating something of fantasy or fiction into a scientific endeavor but also because of the implied discredit that a fantasy element could bring to the client's testimony and statement.

The previous quote also shows how Freud's discovery runs contrary to his expectations and inclinations. Moreover, he recommends that reality and fantasy are to be treated alike and that the clinician initially should make no effort to distinguish them. Fantasies are also real and are an integral part of childhood experience. And as an aspect of psychical reality, fantasies are the second and perhaps the determining factor for the production of symptomatology. However, Freud also disproves those critics who still at this point may think that he disregards actual trauma and environmental experience:

> Do not suppose, however, that sexual misuse of children by the nearest male relatives is entirely derived from the world of fantasy; most analysts will have treated cases in which such occurrences actually took place and could be established beyond doubt.
>
> (p. 379)

Finally, Freud believed that "constitutional predispositions are undoubtedly the after-effects of the experiences of earlier ancestry" (idem). In other words, the relative strength of both desire and its inhibition/prohibition, and the ensuing ethical and incest-related conflicts experienced and enacted during a lifetime, are transmitted from one generation to the next both at a genetic level and a symbolic, familial, and environmental level. Both the genetic inscription and the symbolic narratives and significations take place and are transmitted structurally and beyond consciousness as a doing or activity that escapes the subject.

The objection could be raised along self-psychology lines that I am anachronistically overestimating the importance of the traditional conflict between law and desire given that in the contemporary, permissive, and post-patriarchal society, repression is no longer a problem. Instead, problems with lack of object constancy, maternal empathy, and impulse control have become the etiologically significant factor behind the prototypical malaise of contemporary society: the borderline personality disorder. Actually, both the phenomenological and epistemological dimensions constitute mirror images of the same condition. Both the borderline condition and the self-psychology or object relations paradigm reflect the absence and disavowal of the symbolic and developmental function of the father.

Advanced technological societies have gone from the traditional overcontrol of desire leading to neurotic conditions to a generational problem with identity and impulse control. Society has gone from the brutal, authoritarian, imaginary father to the absence of the necessary symbolic paternal function. Society may have solved the problem of neurosis but in the process has created new problems and conditions.

Finally, the symbolic function of law and prohibition at stake in character formation does not refer so much to questions of relative ethical values but to the anthropological structure of the incest prohibition. Current awareness of childhood sexual abuse or epidemic violations of the incest prohibition only serve to confirm its legitimate and necessary function. It is the prohibition of incest that lies at the core and foundation of the Oedipus complex and most fantasy formation.

Case examples will help illustrate the heuristic value, relevance, and operational importance of the concepts in question. The examples selected are based on two first interviews done by the author. First interviews were chosen to emphasize the diagnostic and assessment dimension of the series.

Example #1

The first is a case of a woman psychiatrically diagnosed with bipolar disorder and a history of manic episodes. In contemporary psychiatry, bipolar disorder is regarded as having a clear if not exclusive genetic and biological component, as already discussed in the first chapter of this book. There was no prior history of bipolar disorder in the client's family. During childhood, her parents separated when she was six, and she remained with her father. Client reported not liking her mother very much then and that she therefore was not that affected by her loss. However, she was bothered by the appearance of a stepmother on the scene whom she described as cold and strict. Thus, this traumatic experience would be placed at the environmental end of the complemental series.

With respect to childhood environment and moving towards the psychical dimension of the continuum, it is common knowledge that children may often blame themselves for their parents' divorce or for being unloved by a parent. Children may think that the parent left because they were bad or did something wrong. This, of course, assumes that the absence of the mother was experienced as a loss, although she denied this. In fact, client said that at the time, she did not experience it as a loss but rather as a relief. Client also denied that mother was physically or sexually abusive. In addition, it is commonplace that people suffering from major depression have had significant losses in early childhood. The loss is compounded and aggravated by guilt and self-blame, which we know have a major part to play in the production of pathological grief.

In this client's case, not only did her mother leave when she was six, but the fact that mother left her could be construed as indicating a failure in good-enough mothering to begin with. "What kind of mother would leave behind a six-year-old?" However, such an assumption may be also difficult to determine, because, for example, the father may have not allowed the mother to leave with the child. In addition, the problem with considering good-enough mothering as such a central etiological factor is that, short of massive neglect and abandonment and the total disappearance of the mother from the child's life, there is no standard by which to measure how much is good enough. In addition, there is a necessary loss linked to separation and the incest prohibition, which could always be confused with deprivation or a failure in good-enough mothering.

From a Freudian perspective, the psychical proper would refer to the oedipal dimensions of the phenomena in question. For the client, for example, the theory would predict that the mother's absence was experienced as an oedipal victory. This victory would be consistent with the victorious feelings associated with a manic condition. In addition, denial is a defense commonly observed with manic disorder. In the client's case, she denied the accusations emanating from her conscience in several ways. Not only did she deny the loss and the self-blame that many children experience but also that she ever was second place or in a subordinate place vis à vis her mother with regard to her father's affections. In addition, a further denial could be that she ever had hostile feelings towards her mother. Of course, that the hostility would return full force via manic symptomatology. Psychoanalytically speaking, mania has been defined by Green, and following Freud and Caligula, as the victory dance over the body of the dead enemy (Green, 1973). The dead enemy stands in for the oedipal rival.

Strictly speaking, a rape she suffered at age 18 and which precipitated the manic episode represents the third series of the etiological continuum. Thus, the environmental series can also function as the precipitant factor for a mental disorder. At this point, and without further knowledge of the client, one could only speculate as to why she had a manic reaction to the rape trauma. But the tripartite model outlined in pages previously would argue that this question could only become intelligible by establishing structural relations between the manic symptoms and all of the other traumatic and psychical factors at work within the continuum, including the biological series.

Example #2

The second example is that of a patient suffering from major depression with psychotic features. The current stressor was that of her adored father having had a stroke while vacationing, being in a coma, and her not having the money to go see him.

She divorced nine months ago and is furious that she didn't do anything better with her life other than being a housewife. Client said this in such an intense, self-loathing way that it alerted the clinician to search beyond the social dimension of the statement. Not surprisingly, the intensity of self-loathing ties in with the self-loathing that's typical of depression. In addition, given that traumas make it difficult to recognize fantasies and desires, the latter are often expressed in the form of guilt and shame.

The clinician focused on the self-loathing and wondered what she could be punishing herself for beyond the already stated. She then disclosed that she had a lover for 17 years while she was married. He was her husband's brother-in-law. She said she was forced at gunpoint to be this man's lover for all that time. She was asked whether she had reported him. She said no because she feared for her life. He had never made actual threats, but she was afraid because he owned a gun and made references to it in their conversations. He didn't have a history of criminality or previous violent behavior.

Then she said that once she had a chance encounter with his daughter, and the daughter was so furious at her for "having an affair while her father was married" that she threatened to kill client. Client immediately went to the police and reported her. Clinician pointed out that in this case, the man's daughter did actually make a threat, and she was very quick to go to the police. The clinician wondered whether there were some needs of hers that were being met in this relationship. The interviewer was surprised when she quickly changed her demeanor and said yes. There were economic needs involved, because the husband didn't have enough money. This story has all the psychical reality of drama and tragedy: the hate, the forbidden passions, the betrayals, all of which could be missed if one simply takes the material reality of the traumatic series at face value. Lacan has called the unconscious the discourse of the Other, which in this case would signify the potential interdependent net of meaning which could be woven if you asked all the significant others involved (lover, his wife and daughter, client's husband, etc.) to speak about their versions of the events at hand.

Further on in the treatment, I was able to ascertain further elements of this dramatic story. The client came to acknowledge that the first year of her relationship with her lover had been voluntary on her part. She had been compelled to accept his advances, because she had tried to warn both his wife and her husband about the developing situation, but neither had believed her. His wife told her that she was too much of an "ugly Indian" for her husband to take notice of her. Angry and insulted, the client set out to prove to this woman that she was "woman enough" and capable of taking her husband. As far as her husband was concerned, it later turned out that she felt rejected by him and that he was either gay or bisexual and therefore did not feel jealous and may have even welcomed her affair. The risk of this kind of probing increasing her self-loathing must be weighed against the possibility that by being able to talk about the complexity of the actual situation, and how her need and desire are also at play, this would help alleviate her burden of guilt without implying that she is at fault ethically or legally.

Descriptive psychiatry organizes diagnoses according to different clusters of symptoms or a series of body-mind signs-signifiers. In anxiety and mood disorders, for example, the two major signs are affects: depression and anxiety. As affects, depression and anxiety fall on the side of bodily, semiotic, and biological phenomena, but as effects of signifiers linked to the Symbolic order, affects generate a lack, or its absence, that is then experienced as signal anxiety. But from a psychoanalytic/cognitive point of view, the affective or the bodily component is secondary to the psychical or cognitive component. Psychoanalysis and cognitive psychology explain affective states according to certain ideas, representations, and signifiers. These cognitions are preconscious or unconscious in a descriptive sense, as Freud would say. They are things that are accessible to consciousness or things that the person reports to the clinician as having to do with their anxiety or depression.

From a strictly psychoanalytic perspective, these preconscious cognitions are substitutes or substitutive representations for unconscious signifiers that represent either fantasies or traumatic experiences or both. Within linguistics, signifiers are units of signification such as phonemes, words, or sentences. In the case of neurotic conditions, the substitute signifier is a phobic object (i.e. dog), an obsessive idea (i.e. God), a somatic symptom (vomiting), or a depressive negative self-statement (I am bad). In the case of character disorders, character traits constitute substitutive signifiers. Just as within the biological series, neural impulses are transmitted from neuron to neuron via neurotransmitters and their receptors, within language, as an organizer of social and environmental experience, signification circulates from one word to the next via language rules such as syntax, grammar, and/or the rhetorical figures of metaphor and metonymy.

Thus, given that ideas or cognitions are organized by language, it can be argued that symptoms are constructed via the intercession of both neurotransmitters and the rules and figures of language. Symptoms are signs of the body and signifiers/metaphors of the mind, which mutually determine each other. Sometimes the body plays the part of the horse (cause) and the mind that of the cart (effect), and sometimes the mind is the horse and the body or brain the cart. In this interaction, the qualitative aspect of affect is determined by cognition, signification, and the words of the Other. The quantitative or intensive aspect of affect that defines it as pleasant, unpleasant, or neutral is a type of jouissance that refers to the subject, the Real, and the drive, but the subject commonly misrecognizes and confuses the quantitative and qualitative aspect of affects. The subject is blind to how affect is not only the effect of the words and actions of the Other but is also an interpretant of the drives and desires of the subject.

Thus, an affective state is both a bodily experience of jouissance as well as a thought or metaphoric signification. Metaphor, as a unit of meaning or signification, is something of the mind or a mental construction. Mind, thinking, and subjectivity are all organized and structured within language. From a phenomenological standpoint, affect is a feeling and not a thought, and yet, although an affect as jouissance can only secondarily be described in words, an affect, as a bodily experience of anxiety or depression, is dually determined by the signifier and jouissance. For example, affect was transformed from aggressiveness to depression as a result of the signifiers that were linked to aggression in the first place.

In the case of panic disorder, for example, clients often declare their ignorance, stating, "I don't know why I am anxious," hoping that the clinician may know something about it. Psychoanalytically speaking, ignorance is an effect of repression. Repression acts on the ideas that could give meaning to the affective experience of anxiety. With some help from the clinician, the client may come up with some preconscious ideas linked to the experience of anxiety. These preconscious ideas may have nothing to do with sexuality and, therefore, the clinician has a choice as to which therapeutic paradigm to use. Because what is preconscious is what is most accessible to the client, a cognitive behaviorist could legitimately say, "I don't see how this disorder could be associated with sexuality." But when the clinician knows how to listen for key signifiers appearing within speech acts and symbolic actions, and the client is able to move through the different links within a signifying chain, the client may indeed arrive at the question of sexuality. From this perspective, the psychiatric diagnosis only becomes intelligible within the field of the unconscious.

The clinical mental health field, and the field of a clinical interview, is confined to acts and facts of speech and language. Whether a psychiatrist, psychologist, social worker, or marriage/family/child counselor, the clinician is confined to acts and facts of language. It is within the field of language that a diagnosis and then a therapeutic relationship can be established. Lacan (1953) gave so much importance to the analysis of language because he realized that the beginning of any psychiatric endeavor most commonly takes place within language. Even if the client uses body language, its interpretation is still taking place within language. On the other hand, language and metaphor are in fact in interaction with and can evoke dimensions of experience that may lie outside or beyond language.

Typically, language has a dual function: to reveal and conceal, to express and suppress meaning. As we speak, a process of selection, of inclusion and exclusion, takes place. Thus, for example, the evocative power of metaphor, as a linguistic expression, lies not only in what is said but also in what is not said. Speech also has ways to reveal what is not said. This way, the field of language may contain a varying mixture of truth and fiction or imagination. A statement is both a half-truth and a half-fiction. The half-truth refers to the saying, while the imaginary construction refers to what is said, in the light of what is not said or what is unconscious. This double structure of meaning also coincides with a division within subjectivity itself. This is what Lacan (1958) has called the divided subject ($).

When utilizing social language, the ego says, I think, I speak, and by this, any person refers to a level of intentionality that he views as his own; it refers to an intentionality that fits in with his self-image (Fink, 1997, p. 24). This is why Lacan made a conceptual distinction between the enunciating ego of the statement and the subject of the enunciation and between meaning and signification. Meaning is imaginary because "it is tied up with our self-image, with the image we have of who and what we are" (idem). Instead, Lacan conceives the subject of the unconscious as an effect of the operation of the signifier. The classical Freudian slips, the parapraxis, the double meanings, the polyvocal significations, in short, all of the formations of the unconscious, are effects of the language-like symbolic structure of the unconscious. All of these psychic formations have the effect of betraying what the conscious ego intends or means to say within an interview. The unconscious and the signifier speak through the subject. Finally, significance as distinct from signification and meaning points to the Real of jouissance rather than the signifier.

The clinical consequence of the divided subject is that usually a person is not straightforward or transparent with respect to their desire. People are often confused about what they want and if what they want is what they want or what others want from them. This dilemma is also at work in the interview situation from the very beginning. The Other to whom the statement is addressed guides the selection process at work in the statement. In choosing words, the interviewee is also considering what the interviewer may or may not expect from them in that situation. On the side of the interviewer, this means that he/she is receiving their own message coming back from the interviewee. The interviewer is hearing what they want and expect to hear.

Thus, because language has a metaphoric structure, the speaker is always saying something other than what they are saying. This paradox and predicament were expressed in the proposition of the pre-Socratic philosopher Epimenides the Cretense, who said, "All Cretenses are liars." Being himself a resident of Crete, if Epimenides is telling the truth, he is lying, and if he is lying, he is telling the truth. So, it can't be that all people are liars and yet, wittingly or unwittingly, consciously or unconsciously, everybody lies, because speech, intrinsically and structurally, contains half-truths and half-fictions. As I have indicated elsewhere (Moncayo, 2018), paradox, in analysis, functions at a different logical level than true and false in a court of law. In the latter case, the truth is, while the false is not. In the former, every truth in language is a half-fiction, and every fiction has a point of truth.

Finally, the latter has a direct bearing on the whole question of fantasy and reality, pseudomemories, and recovered memories. Speech and memory always contain an element of fiction, and pseudomemories or fantasies always contain a reality and traumatic component. This recognition is also related to the professional consensus within psychology regarding memory containing a varying mixture of the accurate and inaccurate (Knapp and VandeCreek, 2000). Professionals, in clinical or court settings, and who only consider material reality, tend to think that people or children never lie or distort their statements. In contrast to this, within analytical discourse, a child analyst, for example, makes good use of paradox and equivocation to do justice to both sides of the controversy and the complexity of human experience.

Practically speaking, beyond taking client's statements at face value and jumping to conclusions about causality, listening and hearing (*J'ouis-sense*) may be the only tool of investigation that the clinician has. In psychoanalysis, listening to the patient's speech is privileged over inferences of causality or classification of the symptom. In listening, the clinician is listening to both what the client is saying and what they are not saying, for the content of what is being expressed, and what and how something of their desire is being suppressed or distorted. The clinician listens for those places of intersection and meeting between conscious and unconscious discourse, material and psychical realities. If initially clinicians only think about diagnostic classification or causality, they may arrive at a fixed and artificial, if not downright false, relationship between etiology or causality and symptomatology.

The initial diagnosis is always provisional because the diagnosis may only be confirmed once the treatment is well underway. This latter point may be especially true when diagnosing character or subjective structure. In the case of depression or anxiety, for example, a description of symptoms during a clinical interview would only tell the clinician whether these symptoms or affects are the predominant phenomenological or biological symptom. But whether this depression lies within the context of the dynamics of desire and the Oedipal configuration of a hysterical or obsessional structure will not become clear until further on. In an interview, psychical structure manifests in terms of the clients' process: the act of speaking and the relationship to the interviewer more than the content of their utterances. As Dor (1997) has stated, "the specificity of a subject's structure is characterized first and foremost by a predetermined profile of his/her desire" (p. 14). For example, the type of relationship a client has to their own desire will begin to appear through the words and distortions that the person uses when talking about what brought them to treatment.

The singular non-standard frame

The singular frame is also very important for the practice of analysis within a public or institutional setting. If only the post-Freudian classical frame is considered psychoanalysis, then psychoanalysis risks becoming irrelevant for large portions of the public mental health field. This is precisely what happened in the United States to a large degree. Psychoanalysis was stereotyped and dismissed as a private practice model used with white affluent or European American analysands. It was also considered too long, costly, and ineffective in the long run. Psychoanalysis or psychodynamic psychotherapy eventually failed in community mental health in the United States, after two decades of psychodynamic psychotherapy (Kennedy's bold new plan for mental health) being the prevailing model used to deliver psychotherapy to the poor, the marginal, and the underserved.

The efficient reason for this failure was the standard frame. First, there was a 50 percent no-show rate for appointments in public clinics, but this was not the main problem. The biggest problem was the scheduling and acceptance of more disturbed patients that needed to be moved from acute services and back into the community, and the community mental health clinics were all full and with long waiting lists, while half the time, clinicians were waiting for clients to show up to their appointments. This was untenable, because more acute cases were going without services, while clinicians had time available due to no-shows. A psychoanalytic model here needed to quickly switch to an applied mode in the service of the community. Since this did not happen, the families of the mentally disordered went to the legislature to complain that their severely disturbed family members were not receiving needed services. Changes and new directives were quickly implemented that changed the way that community mental health services operated.

The 50 percent no-show rate to psychotherapy appointments within public mental health settings happened within the context of the standard frame or the holding environment that prescribes a regular appointment every week or every other week. "Tuesday at 2 is your time, and your responsibility is to show up on time, and mine is to be here to see you on time." This is the idea of the psychotherapy contract, the standard frame, and the holding environment all in one.

In contrast to this, I proposed that within public mental health, the symbolic function proper is at work in the singularity of each session. The patient is in treatment, but each session is different, and the time and day may change. At the end of the session, the patient has to express a desire for another session. The therapist is willing to let go of the patient, a desire that is regulated by the desire of the analyst, which in turn causes the treatment to be regulated by the desire of the patient to attend to appointments. The session could stay on the same day, same time next week, but this needs to be confirmed at the end of each session and not taken for granted.

The singular session (not a one-session treatment) and frame work better for advanced access to public mental health treatment. The clinician has available hours within which many different patients could be seen. Most patients do not have fixed times, and many more analysands can be accommodated according to their need, demand, and readiness for services. The no-show or the inactive treatment need not be seen as no treatment but rather as a different modality of treatment, similar to the work in between sessions and in between treatment episodes. Being in the caseload of a clinic, or having an open case, functions as belonging to a symbolic register within which clients are still receiving treatment by virtue of being part of a symbolic circle of names. While one patient is in the inactive modality of treatment, in between treatment episodes, or even in between sessions and cancelled sessions, other patients can be seen whose demand and desire for treatment make them more readily available to benefit from an analytic intervention.

Trauma, psychical causality, and the complementary series

The strategy within transference is even more important in cases coming with a history of moderate to severe trauma. This is another example where the tendency towards environmentalism and ego psychological object relations within psychoanalysis converges with a psychodynamic and/or social work perspective that makes trauma the exclusive focus of psychopathology and psychotherapeutic treatment. Although it is true that in public mental health there is a greater prevalence of trauma, due to the socioeconomic and cultural characteristics of the populations served, it is also true that within the trauma model perspective, the notion of psychical causality and unconscious fantasy is in danger of extinction. Trauma only appears to be free of psychical causality and operate solely on the basis of chance factors. As discussed in the introduction, Aristotle argued that there are five forms of reason and two forms of chance or accidental forms of causality: automaton and Tyche. Only Tyche is true chance; automaton appears to be accidental, but it is still determined by psychical causality.

Psychiatry tends to fold over what is a three- or four-dimensional structure into a dualistic behavior-brain, or genetic-social dichotomy. The psychical series and the concept of a structural unconscious tend to eventually disappear from this perspective. As argued in Chapter 1, what is needed is a model that can hold three or four dimensions of causality firmly in place. The problem with DSM, in this respect, is that it collapses the notion of the psyche or psychical causality into a surface definition of personality disorders.

Although it is true that every instance of post-traumatic stress includes a history of trauma, not every trauma leads to post-traumatic stress. This explains the hidden causality of the psychical dimension of the unconscious. What is required for the development of PTSD is the interaction of the trauma with unconscious fantasy and with structural phases of development. In addition, the fact that sexual abuse is the prototypical form of abuse and that statistically sexual abuse occurs most often within the family and within the parent-child relationship (the father–daughter relationship, though not exclusively, since there are plenty examples of mother–son incest) should have alerted clinicians to the presence of psychical causality and to the inevitability of the prohibition of incest as the foundation of the Oedipus myth (in the positive meaning of the term 'myth').

What prevents clinicians and professionals from realizing the nature of psychical causality lies in the misrecognition of the protofantasy of seduction and the origin of sexual desire in the desire of the Other. In addition, clinicians, and the social order in general, tend to collapse the legal, moral, and psychical dimensions of trauma.

Jeffrey Masson (1984) contributed to the confusion and dichotomy between trauma and fantasy by regressing to Ferenczi's (1932) emphasis on trauma and holding onto the seduction hypothesis long after Freud had converted the seduction hypothesis into the seduction protofantasy. This is even though in some respects, Ferenczi's analytical practice seemed to scan the analysand's speech in ways that Lacanians do in order to allow fresh associations to emerge.

The seduction hypothesis fits well with the view that wants to deny the existence of childhood sexuality, the prohibition of incest, and the Oedipus myth. Ferenzci's view regarding the confusion of tongues refers to how perverse parents may abuse their children's oedipal fantasies. However, this view has migrated to a contemporary humanistic view that children are innocent and free of sexuality, and if any sexuality is to be found in children, it is because of the perversion of the adults around them. Children's innocence may be true, but it exists in a non-dual state with the polymorphous perversion of childhood that Lacan has differentiated from perversion proper. In addition, the protofantasy of seduction is consistent with the fact that sexuality comes from the outside, from the desires/fantasies and care-giving behavior of the parents. This, however, does not mean that all parents sexually abuse their children.

The repression of the protofantasy of seduction, at theoretical and subjective levels, can lead to the paranoid view that sexual abuse is widespread and takes place in the majority of households ruled by a patriarchal order. When the inevitable reality of sexual *fantasy* between parents and children is repressed, this leads to the paranoia that if anything like that exists, it must mean then that there was actual sexual abuse in the family. Beginning therapists, as well as those influenced by a kind of activist and partial political mentality, are particularly prone to this kind of distorted perspective. The fact that children may sexually arouse parents, or vice versa, is not sufficient proof that they abused their children but rather of the cultural necessity of the prohibition of incest. Both the arousal/desire of the parent and its prohibition, taken together, give rise to a culturally produced sexuality in children.

This is an important point because within certain psychoanalytic circles in the United States, for example, there is the belief that the only alternative to an environmental trauma hypothesis is to rely on a dated concept of a biological drive. Such a view does not consider how unconscious fantasy, sexuality, and psychical causality are constructed within an unconscious symbolic cultural universe that Lacan called the discourse of the Other. The question of the universality of the prohibition of incest in anthropology was settled long ago by Levi Strauss' structuralist response to the functionalist perspective of Malinowski (1927). Levi-Strauss (1949) pointed to the fact that the examples of cultural exceptions to the prohibition of incest were in fact the exceptions that confirm the rule. If the sexual relationship to the parent is not forbidden, there is always a primary family tie or relationship that is forbidden in every culture. In other historical cases, incest has only been allowed for an elite group but forbidden for everyone else. In fact, the current enforcement of mandatory reporting of child sexual abuse is a historical manifestation of an otherwise ahistorical and structural prohibition of incest that makes a historical social structure possible.

That a child may have wanted to seduce a parent because of the child's Oedipal wishes, or that they felt seduced by a parent for the same reasons, does not make them legally or ethically responsible for a violation of the incest boundary. On the other hand, when therapists focus exclusively on the symptom of trauma and empathize with the symptom and the patient by telling them that it is not their fault and that their parents violated their otherwise pure childhood innocence, this by itself does not seem to relieve the patient of their PTSD symptomatology. I have treated many clients who already had this form of treatment and were dissatisfied with the results. What they wanted was for someone to listen to their unconscious feelings of guilt due to their Oedipal desires.

On the other hand, it is also true that analysts that focus on the psychical to the exclusion of the environmental traumatic series also suffer from the same kind of one-dimensional myopia. To exclude one or another form of causality from the genetic/psychical/environmental series leads to different kinds of clinical errors (type I and type II errors). With his concept of the complementary causal series for the production of symptomatology, Freud had already provided a solution for the seduction hypothesis/seduction protofantasy dichotomy/dilemma. The latter is part of the psychical series, the former part of the environmental/accidental series.

What is needed is a dialectical perspective that can simultaneously hold the view of sexuality as traumatic and of sexual trauma as Oedipal in nature. This reality is also coextensive to the relationship between truth and fiction, material reality and psychical reality, and historical memory and screen memory. These pairs are always found in various degrees of combination, and the work of the clinician/analyst is to recognize their relative contributions to the mental life of the subject. I would dare to say that it is only psychoanalysts who are equipped to make this assessment and diagnoses. Although psychological researchers have debunked the notion of repressed memories of trauma (Freud had abandoned the one-dimensional trauma theory long ago) and have experimentally shown that children can distort memory with their own fears and wishes, they don't have the theoretical framework to put the pieces back together into a coherent structure.

With respect to the therapeutic relationship, the presence of a history of trauma complicates the question of the symptom, the therapeutic alliance, and the phases of the transference. It is very difficult to focus on questions of desire, sexual difference, and sexuality with a patient with a history of severe sexual trauma. It is also difficult to redefine the symptom involved in a repetition of the trauma without risking blaming the victim of the trauma. These clients tend to either be very inhibited with respect to sexuality or engage in a fair amount of sexual acting out and have difficulty controlling their impulses. In either case, there is a resistance to symbolize and articulate questions of unconscious sexuality.

When there is sexual acting out or a repetition of abuse, but as perpetrator rather than victim, the perverse abuser has succeeded in transmitting to the victim the basic ingredients of a perverse structure. In these cases, and if the patient stays in treatment, either the focus on the trauma, or the focus on the Oedipal ramifications of the trauma and its manifestation in the transference relationship, has to wait for later phases of the treatment. This waiting does not come without a price given that in the meantime, unconscious guilt continues to generate a significant amount of anxiety for the patient. I have already stated that self-blame does not only come from the trauma but from the unconscious fantasies associated with it. The golden mean between generating excess anxiety by a premature focus on trauma, and not alleviating excess anxiety by not doing so, has to be decided on a case-by-case basis and not in standard fashion.

References

Dor, J. (1997). *The Clinical Lacan.* NJ: Jason Aronson.

Enns, et al. (1998). Working with Adult Clients Who May Have Experienced Childhood Abuse: Recommendations for Assessment and Practice. *Professional Psychology: Research and Practice*, 29 (3), 245–256.

Ferenczi, S. (1932). Confusion of the Tongues Between the Adults and the Child: (The Language of Tenderness and of Passion). *International Journal of Psycho-Analysis*, 30 (4), 225–230, 1949.
Fink, B. (1997). *A Clinical Introduction to Lacanian Psychoanalysis.* Cambridge: Harvard University Press.
Freud, S. (1934). *A General Introduction to Psychoanalysis.* New York: Washington Square Press, 1963.
Goldfried, M. R. and Wolfe, B. E. (1996). Psychotherapy Practice and Research: Repairing a Strained Alliance. *American Psychologist*, 51, 1007–1016.
Green, A. (1973). *La Concepción Psicoanalítica del Afecto.* Buenos Aires: Siglo Veintiuno Editores, 1975.
Jones, E. E. (1993). Introduction to Special Section: Single-Case Research in Psychotherapy. *Journal of Consulting and Clinical Psychology*, 61, 371–372.
Knapp, S. and VandeCreek, L. (2000). Professional Psychology: Research and Practice. 31 (4), 365–371.
Lacan, J. (1953). The Function and Field of Speech and Language in Psychoanalysis. In: *Ecrits: A Selection.* Translated by A. Sheridan (pp. 30–113). London: Tavistock, 1977.
Lacan, J. (1958). The Signification of the Phallus. In: *Ecrits: A Selection.* Translated by A. Sheridan (pp. 281–291). London: Tavistock, 1977.
Levi-Strauss, C. (1949). *The Elementary Structures of Kinship.* Boston: Beacon Press, 1969.
Malinowski, B. (1927). *Sex and Repression in Savage Society.* London: Routledge, 2001.
Masson, J. (1984). *The Assault on Truth: Freud's Suppression of the Seduction Theory.* New York: Farrar, Strauss & Giroux.
Moncayo, R. (1998). Cultural Diversity and the Cultural and Epistemological Structure of Psychoanalysis. *Psychoanalytic Psychology*, 15 (2).
Moncayo, R. and Harari, R. (1997). Principles of Lacanian Clinical Practice. Anamorphosis. *Journal of the Lacanian School of Psychoanalysis*, 1, 13–28.
Moncayo, R. and Romanowicz, M. (2015). *The Real Jouissance of Uncountable Numbers: The Philosophy of Science within Lacanian Psychoanalysis.*
Moncayo, R. (2018). *Knowing, Not-Knowing, and Jouissance. Levels, Symbols, and Jouisssance.* London: Palgrave Macmillan.
Rothbart and Ahadi. (1994). Temperament and the Development of Personality. *Journal of Abnormal Psychology*, 103, 55–66.

Appendix I

Energy, jouissance, and affect versus signifiers and representations

In this appendix, I want to say a few words about the controversy within and outside psychoanalysis regarding the relative importance for psychoanalytic practice of bodily affect, jouissance, and energy versus the focus on mental representation, language, and the signifier. Many have argued that Lacan's theory neglects Freud's theory of affect and gives too much importance to an over-intellectualized theory of linguistic representation. This is not the place for a careful analysis of Freud's theory of affect in its relations to a Lacanian theory of affect, emotion, or jouissance or to address the body-mind question. The point of this appendix is to examine Lacan's later thinking on how jouissance marks the symbolic body and incorporates itself there.

Lacan's capable early students, such as Green and Laplanche, that later turned against him, were used by the IPA against Lacan and as a wedge against Lacanian psychoanalysis. This, of course, does not mean that Lacan is always correct about everything, although his views are always worth considering in some detail. I agree with many who argue that Lacan's later work was in fact a response to many of his fellow intellectuals and critics (Green [1973] and Laplanche among analysts, Deleuze and Derrida among philosophers, Barthes and Jacobson among semiologists and linguists, Levi-Strauss in anthropology, etc.).

Lacan (1977–1978) has a unique way of thinking that language is the symbolic body of thought. The signifier is the representative, or the body, of thought and mentation. This is a different formulation than Freud's, who wrote that the body is represented in the mind by representations and signifiers. Instead Lacan says that the signifier is the body of thought rather than the thought of the body, as Freud believed. The question here is how jouissance contributes to thought rather than how the mind represents the body. The body within thought or representation, rather than thinking, represents a biological body or organism.

Thought, or thinking with the body, is part of the body or brain, rather than separate from the body, and thinking as part of the body is wrapped around the symbolic body of the signifier. The symbolic body can refer to how different types of 'bodies' are represented within the culture. The thought of the body instead refers to the Real of the physical body of the subject. This formulation also implies that there can be thought, without language or code, as a form of non-thought or jouissance.

In a previous work (Moncayo, 2018, p. 13), I spoke of the 'Umwelt' as a subjectively perceived environment, a three-dimensional bubble or membrane, an unconscious symbolic image of the body. In Seminar XXIII, Lacan refers to the body as a sack or a bubble (Moncayo, 2017, p. 39). The sack, and the bubble or membrane, are examples of the Imaginary as structured by the Symbolic. Like translucid images, a bubble and a membrane are subtle, low-density forms of matter, yet their form and consistency are held together by ciphers (structural elements) that regulate the surface tension and pressure of formless states of matter. Visual images are also like bubbles inside of which we place perceptual concepts. This new topological concept of the body and of the ego arose in Lacan's later work to replace the earlier optical schema for the bodily ego.

The symbolic body of signifiers is like a sack, a topological cross-cap, or a bubble as a three-dimensional body image. Lacan differentiated between the specular image and the body as a cross-cap. The cross-cap was necessary to differentiate the *objet a* and the body. The *objet a* is the first form of thought as the representative of the experience of satisfaction in relation to a part of the Other's body. In fact, thought begins in how a part of the mother's body is introduced into the subject's body as a cross-cap. The *objet a* is inserted inside the previously two-dimensional surface of the ideal ego, establishing thereby the subject as a topological cross-cap or projective plane.

The signifier and *objet a* circulate within the projective plane (cross cap), accessing both the object and concept inside the bubble, as well as the thing itself outside both the image and the concept of the thing. The Umwelt, or membrane/bubble, surrounds the subject and separates and differentiates the subject from the larger environment that every other Umwelt is also subjectively perceiving. An ordinary form to describe it is the three feet of personal space that surrounds every subject, or the colloquial expressions: "Keeping someone at arms length" or "close to one's heart." The larger world of objects in the biological environment, as seen from the perspective of a speaking-being, is the-thing-in-itself, or '*la chose*' and the '*a-chose,*' as Lacan calls them. The signifier or image on the screen separates the self-internality of the concept from the self-externality of the thing. The thing falls outside the net of language and is found instead through mathematics or the matheme, the poetics of lalangue, and the experience of jouissance (pleasant/unpleasant pathos).

> It was all the same Greek philosophers who tried to give body to the idea. An idea has a body: it is the word that represents it. And the word has a quite curious property, which is that it makes the thing (*qu'il fait la chose*). I would like to equivocate and to write that as: '*qu'il fêle achose*', it is not a bad way of equivocating.
>
> (Lacan, Seminar XXV, Session I: Wednesday 15 November 1977, p. 2)

Here Lacan speaks of the thing (*chose*) or the *a-chose* (the 'no-thing') rather than the body. It is the word that makes and splits the thing and incorporates it in the process. When the word splits 'the thing,' *das Ding* is incorporated into the signifier. Representation does not merely represent but rather defines or makes the thing and splits it in the process. What does this split mean? The thing is split between the Real and the Symbolic. When the word embodies the thing, or the object, just like when the signifier represents the subject, the Real thing or the *a-chose* or 'no-thing' falls outside or in between signifiers (the subject-qua-'no-thing'). It is the in-between or the outside of jouissance that incorporates itself and structures the relations among signifiers. At the same time, while represented in the Symbolic, 'the Thing' is split up between S_1 and S_2, becoming imaginary in the process, or an image set in or stuffed with an unconscious linguistic signifying structure (like algorithms for virtual images).

Within human beings, there is an absolute difference that makes all the difference: the thing is split into the S_1–S_2 relative relation, while the pure signifier (S_1 without the closure of S_2) points to the Real, or what is unmarked within the thing and within jouissance, and outside the Symbolic. The split of the thing refers to the (conflicted or binary) relations between the Imaginary and the Symbolic, concretely or empirically represented by the image and word of a thing that, once marked, is known as an objective object. The thing instead refers to the Real.

In the split of the thing into S_1–S_2, visual images appear to be independent from language, but in human beings, visual images are objects that are used within a functional, image-processing, symbolic alphabet. The letters of a symbolic alphabet energize the visual representation of the world. The Imaginary attempts to rebel and break loose from the Symbolic, as seen in the examples of animism and the uncanny. In the latter, the figures of the Imagination (through the projective plane) become the (intimate and 'extimate' at once) '*thinginess*' (using Lacan's use of the feminine suffix described subsequently to describe a thing), mana, or animistic version of the world that temporarily replaces, thereby, the letters of the symbolic alphabet that energize the visual representation of the world.

A third alternative is when the Real resolves the conflict between the Symbolic and the Imaginary at a different level or in a different configuration of the topological knot of three. The new knot of three is made when the consistency of the knot is kept in place by the duplication of the Real into the second Real that is the sinthome. The pure signifier (S_1 without the closure of S_2) of absolute difference points to the Real, or what is unmarked within the thing, within jouissance, and outside the Symbolic.

Lacan (1970) says that the signifier is the body or bone of thought and that the bones of the body are also incorporated into the signifier. A Freudian symbolic body, or an aggregate of representations, represents a biological body or organism, and a Lacanian biological body is incorporated into the symbolic body of the signifier. The signifier refers to the killing of the thing or the primal father, while ancestral bones are incorporated into the signifier.

> I return first to the body of the symbolic that must be understood as not at all metaphorical.
>
> (Radiophonie, p. 4)

The first body makes the second from incorporating itself there.

(idem, p. 5)

The dead body keeps what gave the living its character: body.

(idem)

The signifier as an incorporeal and dead ancestral body conveying a second symbolic death marks the biological body and is not only metaphorical in this sense. Lacan argues that the Symbolic is made up of the bones of the body (Hegel said the spirit is a bone. Besides, one could write with and on bones) as the remaining irreducible Real elements that order the elements of the symbolic body (the Symbolic is made with how bones are incorporated into the signifier) and vice versa: the elements of the incorporeal symbolic body mark the bones of the body in such a way that from the fossil record, for example, paleontologists can extract cultural elements from the numbers and letters written on the bones.

The latter is much easier to understand than the first: How is it that bones are incorporated into the Symbolic? Is this a metaphor of how the spirit and mind of ancestors continue to live within traditional symbolic forms? Well, Lacan just told us that the Symbolic is not only metaphoric. What is the relation between bones and signifiers, aside from both being structural elements? Bones and signifiers represent the replicator relation of the homomorphic principle, of different structural elements manifesting at different levels that constitute the same/similar structure of matter in steps: biological life, language, and mathematics. But in this sense, we would be speaking about parallel meaning but not about the Symbolic being literally made up of the bones of dead ancestors. How is it that the marrow of the bones of the ancestors' body and being is transmitted into the marrow and being of future successors? How do letters animate the marrow, and how does the marrow animate the letter in the body–mind relationship?

The latter would be a delusion if it were not taken as a metaphor, and yet Lacan said not to take it as a metaphor. Since we do not know what the materiality of the concept of metaphor is made of, why not say it is made of bones? If you say a metaphor is made of neural circuits, this would not explain the materiality of the signifier itself, although, of course, the brain, and the frontal cortex in particular, is a necessary condition for language.

The Real of the bone and of the relic, and the *objet a*, as a semblance of jouissance, are associated with what Lacan called the littoral of "*litterality*" in "*Lituraterre*." Literature is made of earthly waste (litter) elements of jouissance that are as valuable as offspring. Literature, or the letter, is the meeting place between letters made of varying combinations of earth and water, as the place of intersection between the two. Earth is the ground of the signifier and water is its jouissance. Sticking to the letter, or writing with the bones, does not mean concreteness without metaphoric abstraction in this case but rather how the body of jouissance contains Real links that energize the abstraction of the letter from within (jouissance is the heart of the signifier) or lodges itself there, as Lacan said. Thought, as a reflection of light, is the luminosity and jouissance that incorporates itself into the letters and Name that signify the body of a Real subject.

The *objet a*, as a semblance of being, is the bone or jouissance of thought, or the unsayable inscribed into the signifier as an affect, at the same time that an affect is the effect of the signifier in a subject. This entire formulation could be a delusion, and we could be much safer sticking to the concept of the bone as a metaphor and attributing the rest to Lacan's later dementia or pseudodementia. But perhaps this is not the case, and Lacan may have been pointing at something real.

Cultural symbolic elements enumerate and represent the jouissance that structures their relations, rather than making jouissance become something bodily, organic, or biological once again. Jouissance-value structures the relations between exchange value and use value. Lacan believed that the symbolic and cultural body in the form of instruments of jouissance (he gives the examples of jewelry and weapons, etc.) is the place where the biological body is incorporated in culture and the only way that jouissance can be known, ciphered, and deciphered in culture.

Throughout his work, Lacan spoke of jouissance and the Real in various ways: as lalangue, mathematics, and various types of jouissance, including '*J'ouis-Sense*' (to hear significance and jouissance in speech), feminine jouissance, and the jouissance of the mystic as forms of the Third jouissance. A writing *on* the body refers to numbers and letters and their impact on bodily jouissance, but a writing *with* the body also refers to the impact of bodily jouissance unto the structure of thought and symbolic exchange.

Lacan (1970) said that energy is "nothing but the numerical value of a constant" (p. 18), implying that energy does not exist other than as a number. So, what is the difference between it does not exist period and it "ex-sists," or it exists outside the signifier but within experience? In Seminar XX, Lacan (1972–1973) says that feminine jouissance and the jouissance of the mystic are something that the subject experiences but knows nothing of. Jouissance can be experienced and transformed in relationship to the deciphering of Sense, but jouissance is something Real and not a mere fiction produced by hermeneutic deciphering within the Symbolic and the Imaginary.

Experience here refers not only to what we already know but rather to what we know nothing of, but we may experience in the Real of jouissance. I would like to clarify that when I call Freud's Pcpt.Cs. system a membrane, a blank screen, or a sheet of paper that also doubles up as a form of awareness that does not retain impressions derived from the senses, I am not referring to Locke's (1632–1704/1996) white paper or tabula rasa. Sensory impressions are always inscribed, coded, or represented by the other two systems standing behind and providing structure for new sensory impressions. The empirical aspect of sense information refers to the fact that the first system is not saturated and remains blank. This way new impressions and information can enter the psychical system despite contradicting prior history, prior experience, and instinctual and cultural knowledge embedded in signifying systems.

Lacan's paradox or equivocation refers to a particular form of jouissance: phallic jouissance and surplus jouissance within phallic jouissance. Is it an experience or a cipher? Is jouissance only a cipher, or is jouissance outside the signifier? Phallic jouissance is linked to the signifier, signification, and the erogenous zones, while the first and the Third jouissance are outside. The first is outside but not within the signifier, as represented by the example of psychosis and the early dual unity of mother and child. The Third jouissance is outside but after the signifier. The second phallic jouissance is mental and mediated by the signifier and marks the biological body, as Lacan says.

The first (jouissance of the Other) and Third (Other jouissance) stem from the Imaginary and Real bodies, respectively. The signifier has a greater impact on phallic jouissance than on the other two forms of jouissance. Phallic jouissance disrupts the jouissance of the Other, because the first is before the establishment of the NoF in a particular child. The Third is a product of the second and also goes beyond the second or the NoF and lodges itself inside the signifier (making and marking its "body") in the form of lalangue or *J'ouis-Sense*. Both are experienced in the body, but the first is inconvenient, while the Third is not.

Affect, the *objet a*, jouissance, and contemporary society

In the section on the Furrows of the Aletosphere of Seminar XVII, Lacan (1969–1970) says that there is only one affect. This one and only affect is the effect of the object in the subject as a speech effect, or an effect of discourse. In the one affect, the subject is affected and 'effected' by discourse as an object. Discourse produces the *objet a* as an affect in the subject. This nameless or unpronounceable affect is the *objet a* as the lack of being. Affect is the effect that the *objet a* has on the subject insofar as the object is a missing object or the index of a loss and a void. Grief would be the corresponding "world" affect or mood for the normalizing losses that take place in human development.

Every loss is a void, but not every void is an absence, because the void can also represent a plenitude, plane, or dimension (the Real). The latter would be a different form of enigmatic and benevolent affect or jouissance. On the normal side of grief, the lack of being or the being of non-being passes unto serenity, while on the side of the vacuum plenum, plenitude passes unto elation and bliss. Manic depression is the pathological version of both: when the loss is denied, lack turns into depression or a concave false hole without an object, or, conversely, into an exploding and luminous convex hole that dislocates and pulverizes the subject (mania).

A noun can be a name for something, for example, a party, to which you can add another noun as a suffix in order to turn a particular quality or aspect of the party into its main characteristic. In this case, for example, a party could be designated or called a *partouse*. Lacan uses this form of a feminine suffix that ordinarily can be used to turn words into slang or informal language to think about the relationship between the *objet a* and affect. Another related form would be the use of the diminutive in speech, as a form of endearing language, to reveal affect in speech and sound.

The use of the diminutive to reveal love or affection is what Lacan uses as a paradigm to think how the *objet a* is extended into objects of capitalist consumption.

The diminutive points to something very small or infinitesimal, almost immeasurable, or impossible to calculate. Such objects or social goods of consumption require a certain amount of sacrifice or loss to be produced, as is also the case with children. In the diminutive, there is tenderness in the voice and in the use of the suffix and the noun in language, and Lacan believes this is the place where the fabrications of science are located. The *objet a* is an object of desire and of the drive. Desire is the unnamable between signifiers, while jouissance is the outside speech located within the speech that surrounds the object.

But with regard to what moves around the object, the truth of jouissance is not unveiled. The object is the Imaginary, speech is the Symbolic, and jouissance is the Real. Affect is the effect experienced, while feeling is what language calls what language produces in the personal experience of the subject. Jouissance, in turn, is the Real effect, unnamable otherwise, of the *objet a* (in the Real). The *objet a*, as the object of the drive, mediates the relationship to visual environmental objects. Visual objects produce various effects on the subject, but the magnitude of the effect is mediated by the extent to which an environmental image has been charged or invested with a quality or aspect of the *objet a*.

The *objet a* is what makes a subject a sucker (*ventouse*) for a consumer good. The *objet a* as an energy wave is what energizes, vitalizes, and animates an object. The subject is spirited by the wind of the *objet a* or the *objet a* as a wind (spirit) or form of the breath (soul). However, when the wind of an energy wave is disclosed in the form of a concrete object, without remainder, then the inevitable result may be anxiety. We are drawn to the *lathouse* or *objet a* quality of an object of the drive, and at the same time, when the *objet a* appears in the form of a concrete object, it can quickly turn into anxiety. The *lathouse* is a hidden truth impossible to demonstrate.

At special times relative to the existence of an object, the agalmic aspect, or *objet a* quality of the object, can be revealed in an aorist verb form. The aorist verb form refers to the unmarked aspect of a verb that can be used to reveal or designate the unmarked or traceless aspect of an action, such as a bird flying through air, or a fish swimming in water. The aorist verb form can be used to evoke or signify, but not theorize, savoir rather than *connaissance* (knowing rather than knowledge), since the latter requires logical entailment, arguments and discrimination, and conclusions. The aorist verb form reveals savoir but does not explicate knowledge or *connaissance*. The aorist form is what gives any repeated action the quality of something unique, singular, creative, and new, rather than simply being a repetitive action. The aorist verb form is how Tyche, or Aristotle's true form of chance and fortune, manifests within language. The aorist tense of a verb refers to a continued, inclusive, or undivided activity that is taking place in a present that contains its own past and future (even then, or in future and past presents).

Goods are a category of environmental objects that are of particular significance to the subject in terms of the satisfaction of needs and desires. The availability of objects is itself mediated by the number of demands. The more demands, the more availability of the object. Goods are particularly in demand when they represent a quality of the *objet a*. In this sense, we can say that *objet a* mediates demand and production. In the demand for the *objet a*, there is always one more subject and one more object (1 + a).

> The o-object is what is grasped in the app.al/apparel of love. Love is supported by the narcissistic coatings of the o-object that give an object it's mystical element, it's "*Je ne sais quois*", the indefinable quality that makes an object something distinctive or attractive.
>
> (Lacan Seminar XV, Session of February 28, 1969, XI 3)

For Lacan, the *objet a* is a jouissance-effect. Sound and light waves are forms of jouissance that point to the *a*-thing or *l'achose*, or the lack of essence of the essence, that represents the lightness and insubstantiality of things. Insubstantial here means the presence of energy and vibration but the absence of matter. Sound and light waves are so-called fabrications of science. Lacan does not want to follow theology and call quanta, or light and sound waves, the noosphere. Instead he proposes the term aletosphere. The aletosphere is like a cloud of information hanging out in space or another planet (a reference to Plato's topos Uranus or world of ideas), although it can also be accessed from any planet.

The neologism *aletosphere* is related to *lathouse* and *aletheia.* Truth, or *aletheia* in Greek, can only be half disclosed or unconcealed as the true. The other half remains concealed or undisclosed. *Lathouse* is the neologism obtained using the feminine and diminutive suffix out of the Greek word for truth. From *letheia* to *lathouse. Objet a* is the truth-value, jouissance-value in this case, of the object for the subject. Jouissance represents the transference effect of a sound or light wave as an *objet a.* The *objet a* is a wave of jouissance, or of true affect. An affect may be suppressed not only because of associated representations but because the affect, as a form of jouissance, and as a wave, also contains an aspect of *lethe* or forgetting in Greek.

> As far as the feminine unsubstance is concerned, I would go as far "Parousia." And these tiny objects little *a* that you will encounter when you leave, there on the footpath at the corner of every street, behind every window, in this abundance of these objects designed to the cause of your desire, insofar as it is now science that governs it – think of them as *lathouses.*
>
> (Lacan, 1969–1970, p. 162)

Lacan uses the concept of *lathouse* to designate the globalized consumer phase of capitalism and civilization, marked by the use of computer and internet-based information or techne to impact overall economic exchange. This globalized world, which presents itself as 'transparent' and 'measurable,' is far from being what it claims, since *objet a*, injected into the objects of consumption, are not visible to the naked eye, and require psychoanalysis to be seen. The loss of the capacity to experience something outside techne is a quality increasingly present in the technological world. Media entertainment is the new form of archaic animism. Media entertainment, as a new form of animism that masquerades as technological development, has, metaphorically speaking, replaced the benevolent magnetic waves of jouissance that wrap or curl around the pure aorist or symbolic experience of the world.

In the final analysis, I am not so sure if the differences between the early form of protestant capitalism and the later form of capitalism, known as the consumer society, or even between socialism and capitalism, are still relevant nowadays. These differences have been replaced by the difference between crony and democratic capitalism or the social management of private capital beyond a reasonable level of excess + 1. Either private individuals can determine how to publicly use the surplus to benefit society, or the state can do the same under the supervision of private industry as the generator of wealth. Under social capitalism, the super ego says: "Work hard, save, and buy or exchange the goods you and your loved ones want, or need." The super ego in the case of crony capitalism say, "Don't save, don't be satisfied with what you have (at the cost of debt and the environment), and don't think about tomorrow (live in the immediate false consumption of the present moment)."

For ethical capitalism, the good is not in the goods, or in capital, but in the work process itself. Human goods are not the payment or reward for human effort and exertion but rather its fruit, side benefit, or added bonus: its jouissance value. A value is added and given for the jouissance that the subject already has (+1). The added Other jouissance, evoked in universal undivided activity (*Il'ya de l'Un*, after all), is a species-doing, a going-on-being (a *m'etre* or *maître*/master), that escapes or exceeds the subject. Because an excedent of jouissance 'ex-sists,' meaning that productivity and capitalization continue to be organized in the Other, whether you know it or not, productive subjects can drain small pieces of jouissance from the larger 'homo economicus' that escapes us.

The Other-jouissance, linked to undivided human activity, is where the aim of the activity is included in the activity itself rather than in the profit motive or a financial surplus value outside work activity. The surplus value instead lies within the experience of jouissance linked to a productive activity. One can observe this even in blue-collar workers who want their jobs back in the carbon or oil industry despite the environmental risks and physical exploitation involved. They don't want to learn new skills for new and healthier industries for themselves or others, because they are used to the expected jouissance associated with their work.

Surplus jouissance is what leads to expanding productivity rather than the profit motive. The surplus jouissance value of productive activity is an alternative to the revolutionary political passion that does not last more than a generation or two, as shown in the Russian and Latin American socialist revolutions. The Chinese case is different, since *Wu-wei* (non-action) is an integral aspect of Chinese civilization that leads the culture to expanding productivity based on the unity of the *lathouse* or *aletheia* that is sought (jouissance as a no-thing or a non-doing) and the work that does not fail from being thoroughly accomplished.

The same convenient Other jouissance that propels the process of discovery in science fuels the productive process and militates against the exploitation of fellow human beings, unless so-called nihilistic revolutionaries proudly and in ignorance insist on so-called pure forms of violence that justify perpetrating sadism and cruelty upon others. The violence of the sun cannot be used as a justification for political violence, since the livable zone of the solar system in which we live is not random or accidental and is organized by a golden mathematical structure. The violence of the sun is one of the terms for which the habitable zone, the magnetic field surrounding the planet, and our living and breathing atmosphere is the Other.

References

Green, A. (1973). *La Concepción Psicoanalítica del Afecto*. Buenos Aires: Siglo Veintiuno Editores, 1975.

Lacan, J. (1969–1970). *The Other Side of Psychoanalysis*. New York: Norton, 2007.

Lacan, J. (1970). *Radiophonie*. Scilicet 2/3. Translated by J. W. Stone. Paris: Seuil, pp. 55–99.

Lacan, J. (1972–1973). *Encore. The Seminar of Jacques Lacan*. Book XX. London: Norton.

Lacan, J. (1974). *Television*. Edited by J. Copjec. New York: London, 1990.

Lacan, J. (1977–1978). *The Seminar of Jacques Lacan*. Book XXV: The Moment to Conclude. Translated by C. Gallagher. www.lacaninireland.com/web/published-works/seminars. Accessed December 17, 2019.

Locke, J. (1689/1996). *An Essay Concerning Human Understanding*. Indiana: Hackett Publishing.

Moncayo, R. (2017). *Lalangue, Sinthome, Jouissance, and Nomination: A Reading Companion and Commentary on Lacan's Seminar XXIII*. London: Karnac.

Moncayo, R. (2018). *Knowing, Not-Knowing, and Jouissance: Levels, Symbols, and Codes of Experience in Psychoanalysis*. London: Palgrave McMillan.

Appendix II

Two half-sides of truth: *Aléthes* and *Léthes*, truth and forgetting

In his work, Heidegger (1943) tries out different approaches to the question of truth. *Aletheia* or *aléthes*, for example, refers to two things: both *aléthes* and *léthes*, truth and concealing or forgetting, as well as the difference between truth proper and the true at the level of representation and the signifier. "In every entry of being into its habitation in words, there's a margin of forgetting, a *lethe* complementary to every *aletheia*" (Lacan, 1953–54, p. 192).

The true signifier forgets the silent Truth of jouissance, and yet *Léthes* is the heart of *aletheia*. The privative *a* in *a-letheia* negates *lethes*. Truth is both the unconcealed (the social agreement regarding a proposition) and presupposes concealment, hiddenness, or the outside social agreements and representations. The true negates forgetting, or the fictional side of truth negates the secret that truth in the Real of jouissance signifies. "We are used to the Real, the truth we repress" (Lacan, 1966; Ecrits, p. 169). "It is with the appearance of language that the dimension of truth emerges" (Lacan, 1966; Ecrits, p. 172). Truth presupposes a concealed or repressed outside representation, while the true or false emerges at the level of representation and speech. Deception and lies are not the opposite of truth, because they are inscribed in the text of truth. The truth 'outside' the Symbolic is not only the repressed but what lies outside representation altogether.

Heidegger (1961/2008) clarifies that unconcealment, in the sense of the clearing, is not the same as truth, as representation, I would add. He refers to unconcealment as a quiet meditative form of thinking, a place of stillness. This is what I have called non-thinking as a form of thinking. Can thinking even raise the question of non-thinking so long as it thinks philosophically? Philosophy or science don't know what thought is, and Lacan tells us, in a Zen moment, that thought is a form of jouissance. This is thinking at the end of Greek philosophy with an Eastern and topological twist of the knot. This is why I propose in this appendix that there are two truths, and two versions of the two: *aléthes* and *léthes*, truth and concealing or forgetting, as well as the difference between truth proper, and the true at the level of representation and the signifier. I also link 'J'ouis-Sense' to *alétheia*, or the clearing aspect of truth, or the non-thinking aspect of thought.

The true that is said through mistakes and half-true/half-false statements circumscribes Truth as what remains outside the equivocations of the signifier. "Or again we could say that there are two truths: one that is the opposite of falsehood, and another that bears up both the true and the false indifferently" (Miller, 1974, p. XX). Truth is equanimous with respect to the dialectic of the true and false within speech, or how the true often requires mistakes or the false to be said first. Truth is similar to the Real because it is impossible to articulate the whole truth or the Real as a plenum. But precisely due to this impossibility, truth aspires to the Real. *Aletheia* is both untruth and fiction, as well as truth. The true (not truth) is both true and a form of untruth or fiction. When 'being-there' (Dasein) falls or is thrown into the world, it misinterprets, but senselessness or emptiness, as falling and impermanence, means more than this.

In the conformity or correspondence between representation and reality, the place of truth shifts from the original unhiddenness of Being to the correct statement of a human being. The unhiddenness of Being is revealed in the statement rather than in what remains outside of the statement, yet the latter equally grounds the statement.

Aletheia, or unconcealment, in the sense of the opening of presence, was originally only experienced as the correctness of representations and statements. However, for Heidegger, in addition to the truth of propositional judgments, there exists a more essential form of truth that lies largely not in a judgment but in the human '*ek-sistence*' (Lacanians write 'ex-sistence') itself, insofar as it reveals what remains outside existence. The agreement of judgment with the real thing presupposes that reality has already been drawn from concealedness in a more fundamental way. To draw real things from concealedness to unconcealedness (*aletheia*) requires a certain 'light.' This light is Dasein's ek-sistence itself, its being-in-the-world from which originally all meaning draws its light. The being-in-the-world of ek-sistence is the light or jouissance in which a phenomenon is revealed.

Meaning is the light of representation, or of the word as a revelation of the hidden light of jouissance revealed within speech. The illuminating or illustrative and heuristic aspect of the word is its ability to draw a form of jouissance that is experienced as meaning, as a form of enchantment or invocation. Every being stands in the light, and at the same time, the light of Being or of the Real withdraws from the light of representation. The light of Being is not revealed in the light of representation or explanation. Episteme obfuscates the light of Being, and yet with all correct linguistic representations or statements, we get nowhere without the Real. In every form of lowercase being, the word stands for Being, and at the same time, uppercase Being or the subject of the Real remains something more than the signifier.

Being withdraws from the cleared ground of representation into the groundless ground of the One's own non-being (Lacan, 1971–1972). Clearing is actually the groundlessness in which the ground is revealed, the space in which the earth floats. Refusal or negation is not just another repressed or concealed signifier, what limits dissemination, or what every other signifier or the Other could also be (i.e. it is this particular signifier or thing, not that). For example, I am this particular signifier rather than another signifier. The singularity of the Real of jouissance at the heart of the signifier is something else. The Real of jouissance represents a refusal of the correspondence between the Symbolic and the Real.

The Real is an absolute difference, something outside signification and not only another repressed signifier; the Real unconscious, not only the repressed unconscious. A true hole lies concealed or hidden by the signifier, while a false hole only appears like a gap or nothing, but, in truth, the concealed or hidden is another signifier. Yet the lack of correspondence between the Real and the Symbolic is precisely what organizes the Symbolic (what is outside organizes what is inside). What organizes the Symbolic is both a repressed signifier of lack and the lack of a signifier to represent the Real, a false and a true hole, respectively.

When an entity places itself before another, when we take the one for the other, when a being appears but presents itself as other than it is, this concealment is dissembling. Here we have an indication of the possibility of error, deception, and/or lack of oversight. Dissemination is a dissembling of truth.

Unconcealedness as clearing involves denying that truth can be rendered through unconcealing in the mode of representation. The clearing of Being is more than representation or language. Representing or speaking is not truth but the true in the mode of lying: I am not lying about lying. Speaking is lying or the truth in the form of a true untruth (relative truth not falseness), and truth proper withdraws or falls into the Real and stands on emptiness or is a bringing forth from emptiness, elation, or jouissance. This is the happening of the conflict between unconcealedness and concealment (not concealing but rather unrevealing the secret mystery). Truth is a happening or a conflict between secret mysteries and fictional representations of truth.

Beings stand on the basis of language, while capital Being is set in the background as what remains outside the signifier yet grounds it at the same time. The One's own non-being is the intimacy of the opposition between language and the Real of jouissance for which the opposition between the Imaginary and the Symbolic is only a semblance. The Imaginary and the Symbolic are external to one another: images conceal signifiers and signifiers disassemble images, while the Real of jouissance is the bodily outside that organizes the heart of the signifier. As I said in Chapter 6: "Strife, misunderstanding, or equivocation, as the conflict of opinions and identifications, is not a rift, as a mere division or hate ripped open, but rather the intimacy with which opponents belong to each other" (p. 208).

By thinking of the world and the word as a specific structured openness, the opposition between openness and concealment is not eradicated. The undetermined openness, in which decisions are made, does not make these decisions less significant. The openness is not some kind of controlling power or deity but rather "what" generates a relationship with things and the 'no-thing.' What will occur in an event before the "happening" in it is altogether undetermined. In this indeterminateness and immediacy of Being also lies what remains unmastered in the sense of the concealed.

In an event, it is truth, and not merely something true, that is at work. Truth differs from something true. The true refers to determined or conditioned forms of being within the signifying structure. Being as the unconditioned presentness of beings, or the emptiness of form as ek-sistence, remains concealed or outside representation (the One's own non-being).

The common understanding/misunderstanding of the metaphysics of presence refers to the idea or the presence of the signified as another signifier functioning as meaning. The idea is another signifier, while thought, as the unsayable of jouissance at work within the signifier, is the body of thought. Presence or 'presentness' of emptiness refers to the body of thought, or to thinking with the body, as distinct from cognition or thinking. Thinking grounded in non-thinking or thinking with the body. Thinking with the body is not metaphysics or includes rather than excludes the body. Thinking with the body of jouissance drops both body and cognition and elevates them at the same time.

Being represents a dialectic of truth and the true. There is a distinction between the correct and truth. The correct can be untrue from the perspective of truth. In this case, 0 represents truth rather than the false. In statistics, 0, as a margin of significance, means that there is a low probability that a proposition or a thesis is true. Zero is false and 1 is true. However, 0 also points to truth lying outside correct statements instead of simply freeing us to look for the true in other statements. Truth represents something outside the statement that draws jouissance from the Real or the outside meaning.

The high probability that a hypothesis is true depends on the quality and magnitude of jouissance or the stillness of the statement rather than in a second statement devoid of jouissance that could ground, replace, or falsify the first. Zero is the point of equilibrium, or what grounds the truth of a number or letter rather than a false statement. The true follows from the false or is established on the basis of a prior false statement that can now be corrected with the aid of a margin of jouissance that has been drawn from the Real and embedded in a true act or statement. Zero *in* 1, or the One's own non-being, differs from the disjunction between 0 and 1(either is or is not). Only with 0 in 1 do we obtain or generate the correctness of representation, or truth within the true.

The metaphysics of presence refer to unconcealment in the adequacy or correspondence between truth and representation or the signifier. The metaphysics of presence does not refer to what is not fiction or true at the level of representation. Metaphysics here refers not to an idea that reveals the meaning of existence but to an experience of the jouissance of meaning that brings the 'soul' of jouissance into being (poiesis). Jouissance is the activity of blooming, or a threshold occasion within the blossom of the signifier. Not only is the signifier embedded in jouissance, but jouissance itself may not be pre-determined by any form of signification. Because jouissance may not be pre-determined by the signifier, or "ex-sists" in a moment outside the signifier, a true signifier may yet have to evolve that could process such undetermined form of jouissance (Truth). The word as jouissance is the truth outside meaning that structures meaning.

Jouissance withdraws or remains undisclosed in representation yet revealed in experience (something I experience but know nothing of with knowledge or *connaissance*). Savoir as *poiesis* draws something of the Real of jouissance. *Lethe* in *Aletheia*, or truth as forgetting, is not the shadow cast by the light but rather the darkness at the heart of the light. Hiddenness is the heart of unconcealment. The heart, or environment of light, is darkness. Dark matter or the void kindles the light. Frictions within dark energy or between dark matter, or dark frictions, give rise to light particles.

A-letheia is not truth but rather the true that makes it possible to speak of truth in the first place. The true is not truth but what allows us to speak of truth and half say it. Truth as jouissance or significance versus true signification within words and representation. Without hiddenness or jouissance, truth becomes dogma in the bad sense of what limits the Real of jouissance or emptiness to language or thinking. Thinking without non-thinking is dogma in the bad sense of the word. Thinking grounded in groundlessness or non-thinking is a different sense of dogma. Dogma instead refers to the meaning of words rooted in the experience of jouissance or the jouissance of meaning. It is Truth as jouissance (of meaning) that inspires Nous to bring forth first principles that are self evident and await confirmation by the secondary principles of science and other forms of reason. Convenience, or the correspondence between jouissance and speech, refers to an accord between the Real and the Symbolic (*accord du corps*, or an accord between the body and speech).

References

Heidegger, M. (1927). Being and Time. In: *Basic Writings*. Translated by D. F. Krell (Revised and Expanded Edition). London: Harperperennial/Modern Thought, 2008.

Heidegger, M. (1943). On the Essence of Truth. In: *Basic Writings*. Translated by D. F. Krell (Revised and Expanded Edition). London: Harperperennial/Modern Thought, 2008.

Heidegger, M. (1947). Letter on Humanism. In: *Basic Writings*. Translated by D. F. Krell (Revised and Expanded Edition). London: Harperperennial/Modern Thought, 2008.

Heidegger, M. (1969). The End of Philosophy and the Task of Thinking. In: *Basic Writings*. Translated by D. F. Krell (Revised and Expanded Edition). London: Harperperennial/Modern Thought, 2008.

Lacan, J. (1953–1954). *The Seminar of Jacques Lacan*. Book I. New York: Norton, 1988.

Lacan, J. (1966). Science and Truth. In: *Ecrits*. Translated by B. Fink. New York and London: Norton, 2006.

Lacan, J. (1971–1972). *The Seminar of Jacques Lacan. Book XIX*. Edited by J.-A. Miller. Cambridge: Polity Press, 2018.

Miller, J. A. (1974). An Introduction to the Reading of Television. In: J. Lacan. *Television*. Edited by J. Copjec. New York: London, 1990.

Index

Note: Page numbers in *italics* indicate a figure and page numbers in **bold** indicate a table.

For Product Safety Concerns and Information please contact our EU representative GPSR@taylorandfrancis.com
Taylor & Francis Verlag GmbH, Kaufingerstraße 24, 80331 München, Germany

www.ingramcontent.com/pod-product-compliance
Lightning Source LLC
LaVergne TN
LVHW020642300926
849161LV00004B/783
* 9 7 8 0 3 6 7 5 6 2 8 6 1 *